© 1996 Mac Keith Press
526/529 High Holborn House, 52–54 High Holborn, London WC1V 6RL

*Senior Editor:* Martin C.O. Bax
*Editor:* Pamela A. Davies
*Managing Editor:* Michael Pountney
*Sub Editor:* Pat Chappelle

Set in Times and Avant Garde on QuarkXPress

First published in this edition 1996

British Library Cataloguing-in-Publication data:
A catalogue record for this book is available from the British Library

ISSN: 0069 4835
ISBN: 1 898683 07 7

Printed by The Lavenham Press Ltd, Water Street, Lavenham, Suffolk
Mac Keith Press is supported by **Scope** (formerly The Spastics Society)

Clinics in Developmental Medicine No. 139

# Preschool Children with Inadequate Communication

## Developmental language disorder, autism, low IQ

Edited by

ISABELLE RAPIN
*Albert Einstein College of Medicine* New York

on behalf of the

AUTISM AND LANGUAGE DISORDERS NOSOLOGY PROJECT

*and including first publication of*
'Wing Autistic Disorders Interview Checklist (WADIC)'
*and*
'Wing Schedule of Handicaps, Behaviour and Skills (HBS)'
*by*
LORNA WING
*National Autistic Society Centre for Social and Communications Disorders*
Bromley, Kent, UK

1996
Mac Keith Press

*Distributed by* 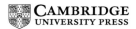 **CAMBRIDGE**
UNIVERSITY PRESS

# ACKNOWLEDGEMENTS

This study grew out of a request of the Child Neurology Society in 1978 to develop a better validated classification of the disorders of higher cerebral function in children than those which were then available. In 1985, with the encouragement of the Child Neurology Society and the International Neuropsychology Society, the investigators were able to obtain the support of Program Project grant #20489 from the National Institute of Neurologic and Communicative Diseases and Stroke of the United States Public Health Service (now the National Institute of Neurologic Disorders and Stroke— NINDS). The investigators thank the NINDS managers of the grant, Drs Martha Bridge Denckla, Sarah H. Broman and Giovanna M. Spinella for their unflagging encouragement, flexibility and enthusiastic support of the project. The Learning Disabilities Society of America invited the investigators to present preliminary findings from the study at their annual convention on March 4, 1992 in Atlanta, GA. The additional support of NINDS Conference Grant NS #30513 enabled the investigators to invite a panel of experts from relevant disciplines to a round table on March 5, 1992 to discuss issues raised by the previous day's presentations; the experts provided to the study many useful suggestions and criticisms. NINDS expressed its confidence in the value of the project by providing extra support for data analysis beyond the expiration of the grant. The investigators sincerely hope that the product of their efforts fulfils at least some of NINDS's expectations and will prove useful to clinicians, educators, and investigators concerned with the developmental disorders of preschool children.

The study was carried out through the collaborative effort of investigators at the following institutions. Atlanta, GA: Georgia State University; Boston, MA: Boston University School of Medicine; the Bronx, NY: Albert Einstein College of Medicine; Cleveland, OH: Case Western Reserve School of Medicine; Manhasset, Long Island, NY: North Shore University Hospital, then an affiliate of Cornell University Medical College; Providence, RI: Bradley Hospital, an affiliate of Brown University School of Medicine; Richmond, VA: St Mary's Hospital; Trenton, NJ: Trenton State College Child Development Project. In addition, investigators from the University of Arizona College of Medicine in Tucson, AZ, and from the University of Houston, TX, participated as consultants. The senior investigators designed the study collaboratively from its inception and participated in all its phases. Dr Robin Morris was responsible for management of the data base and provided the statistical analyses described in Chapters 4–9 and several of those in Chapter 10.

The project benefited from the advice of consultants from other institutions who served on the External Review Panels that met with the investigators at yearly intervals. The investigators acknowledge here the valuable contributions made by these outside consultants. The investigators are especially grateful to the parents and the children for their patience and their participation. They thank the children's teachers and therapists for their insightful answers to their many questions about the children's behavior and skills.

Finally, the investigators thank Dr Lorna Wing for preparing her questionnaires for the Appendix; and Dr Martin Bax and the anonymous reviewer, both of whom made valuable suggestions for improving the clarity and clinical implications of the text.

# CONTENTS

# STUDY PERSONNEL

**Principal Investigators**
Ronald B. David, St Mary's Hospital, Richmond, VA (1985–1988)
Isabelle Rapin, Albert Einstein College of Medicine, Bronx, NY (1988–1996)

**Methodologist**
Robin Morris, Georgia State University, Atlanta, GA

**Co-investigators**
Doris A. Allen, Albert Einstein College of Medicine
Dorothy M. Aram, Case Western Reserve School of Medicine, Cleveland, OH *and* Emerson
    College, Boston, MA
Michelle A. Dunn, Albert Einstein College of Medicine
Deborah Fein, Boston University School of Medicine, Boston, MA *and* University of Connecticut,
    Storrs, CT
Carl Feinstein, Brown University School of Medicine, Providence, RI *and* Johns Hopkins
    University School of Medicine, Baltimore, MD
Lynn Waterhouse, Trenton State College, Trenton, NJ
Barbara C. Wilson, North Shore University Hospital, Manhasset, NY *and* Cornell University
    College of Medicine, New York, NY

**Methodology Panelists**
Roger K. Blashfield, University of Florida, Gainesville, FL
David J. Francis, University of Houston, Houston, TX
Jack M. Fletcher, University of Texas Medical School at Houston

**External Review Panelists**
Gabrielle Carlson, State University of New York School of Medicine at Stony Brook, NY
Judith Johnston, University of Indiana and University of British Columbia, Vancouver, Canada
Steven Mattis, Cornell University College of Medicine, New York, NY
Ruth Nass, Cornell University College of Medicine
Bruce Pennington, University of Denver, Denver, CO
N. Paul Rosman, Boston University School of Medicine
Sara Sparrow, Yale University, New Haven, CT
Frank Wood, Bowman Gray School of Medicine, Winston Salem, NC

**Neurologists**
Robert DeLong, Massachussetts General Hospital, Boston, MA
Pauline Filipek, Massachussetts General Hospital
Susan Klein, Albert Einstein College of Medicine *and* Case Western Reserve School of Medicine
Carol Leicher, University of Connecticut School of Medicine, Hartford, CT
David Mandelbaum, Robert Wood Johnson School of Medicine, New Brunswick, NJ
Isabelle Rapin, Albert Einstein College of Medicine
Max Wiznitzer, Case Western Reserve School of Medicine *and* Albert Einstein College of
    Medicine

**Neuropsychologists/Psychologists**
Michelle A. Dunn, Albert Einstein College of Medicine
Deborah Fein, Boston University School of Medicine

Robin Morris, Georgia State University
Laurel Wainwright, Boston Universisty School of Medicine
Anne Walters, Brown University School of Medicine
Barbara C. Wilson, North Shore University Hospital

**Psychiatrists**
Carl Feinstein, Brown University School of Medicine
Edward Mikkelsen, Harvard University *and* Massachusetts Mental Health Center
Sonia Miles, Robert Wood Johnson School of Medicine
Alice Siegel, Albert Einstein College of Medicine
Eva Sperling, Albert Einstein College of Medicine
Morris Stambler, Tufts New England Medical Center, Boston, MA

**Psycholinguists**
Doris A. Allen, Albert Einstein College of Medicine
Ina Wallace, Albert Einstein College of Medicine
Lynn Waterhouse, Trenton State College

**Speech/Language Pathologists**
Dorothy M. Aram, Case Western Reserve School of Medicine
Judith Flax, Albert Einstein College of Medicine
Nancy Hall, Case Western Reserve School of Medicine
Judith Pierpont, Albert Einstein College of Medicine
Beth Tortolani, North Shore University Hospital (deceased)

**Grant Administrators**
Patricia Donohue, Albert Einstein College of Medicine
Bethany Einstein, Albert Einstein College of Medicine
Tera Yoder, St Mary's Hospital, Richmond, VA

**Research Assistants**
Albert Einstein College of Medicine:  Judith Adamo, Laura Bernstein, Saradee Cohen, Loretta
    Garin, Hillary Gomes, Eric Hershman, Rebecca Schwartz, Mary Joan Sebastian, Anita Smith,
    Robert Staffin, Charlotte Trott, Karen Zelman
Boston University School of Medicine:  Ann Aldershof, Christine Brumbach, Theresa Coyle, Judy
    Dwyer, Harriet Levin, Dorothy Lucci, Lori Nicoletti
Brown University School of Medicine:  Lisa Roccio Giordano, Julie Trecartin
Case Western Reserve School of Medicine:  Ann Forman, Melissa Meehan, Coleen Visconti
Georgia State University:  Kevin Baldwin, David Barrett, Elena Bettoli-Vaughn, Kelly Burgin,
    Bonnie Carlson Green, Mel Eldridge, Gene Farber, Vera Gabliani, Rob Godsall, William
    Haxton, Patricia Jones, Holly Keahey Middleton, Joseph Langford, Suzanne Lawry, Lorna
    Lazarus Benbinisty, Marcella Maguire, Duncan McArthur, Hamid Mirsalimi, Linda Owens
    Folsom, Pamela Parkinson, Stephanie Perleberg, David Woodsfellow
North Shore University Hospital:  Lois Black-Van Santen, Diane Frangipane, Karen Webb,
    Florence Wheeler
Trenton State College: Barbara Maher, Janet McGehean, Emily Nguyen, Linda Wiesner

**Editorial/Neurologic Consultant**
Peggy (Ferry) Copple

**Administrative/Secretarial**
Helene Manigault, Anita Smith, Christine Toomey

# FOREWORD

Disorders of communication in the broadest sense, including not simply language disorders but also disorders of social communication, are among the commonest problems reaching disability teams in the developed world. They also form a large proportion of child psychiatric referrals, and, of course, speech pathologists and therapists receive many direct referrals of children with these disorders. For these professions they are a problem. First, we know too little about their origin; second, we have major problems with diagnosis and deciding what sorts of investigations we should be doing; and finally, treatment or management presents an enormous challenge to many clinicians. The conditions are often poorly defined clinically, with all their characteristics not fully delineated. In this monograph, Dr Rapin and her colleagues have provided us with a mass of research-based information about four groups of children: those with high-functioning autistic disorders; those who have autistic disorders but are of lower intelligence; and two groups with developmental language disorders, those with normal cognitive function and those with lower levels of cognitive function.

What is unique about the study is, first of all, the size of the sample that the authors have collected. They have assessed no fewer than 487 children, including 201 with developmental language disorders of normal IQ range and 110 with nonverbal IQs below 80. The autistic group of 176 was divided into high- (N=51) and low-functioning (N=125) groups, cognitively. All these groups had information collected from them in a standardized and systematic way. Great care has been taken in ascertainment, so what we are provided with is a wealth of information on four very carefully delineated groups.

The next feature of note is the enormous range of material which has been collected on all these children; one can readily identify this by a look at the chapter headings. Apart from the history collected, they all had a full neurological examination; a mass of neuropsychological, language and behavioural data was collected; and, most importantly, there was an interesting study on play. We have information also from the children's parents and teachers.

The third unique feature is the care which has been taken in analysing these data and the clarity with which they have been presented. The methodology, described in the opening chapters, is necessarily rigorously presented and requires careful reading. The findings are no less rigorously described, but they come to life with the range of the clinical information which is presented to the reader.

A wide range of instruments was used in the study, and one might draw particular attention to the Wing Autistic Disorder Interview Checklist (WADIC) which is given full publication in the Appendix, as is the Wing Schedule of Handicaps, Behaviour and Skills, both tools which many clinicians will welcome being available in a published form.

What are the main outcomes of the study? It is not the role of a foreword to steal the author's thunder, and indeed, nor are the findings easily or quickly summarized. There are however a number of outcomes which seem of great significance. The study will allow us to define what the authors describe as 'pure' cases—groups of prototypic children with disorders tightly defined at the behavioural level—which, as they say, will minimize the 'noise' that falsely diagnosed cases introduce into biological studies. Nevertheless, perhaps the other finding to emphasize is the variability among the children, so that there is overlap among the groups in virtually all areas, confirming one's clinical experience. Interestingly, the single most discriminating measure was the WADIC.

The authors stress that in order to make the 'optimal diagnostic decision', everyone has to be involved in the diagnostic and assessment process. Such a thorough approach will allow the clinician to make crucial decisions about the way a programme of help for the child should be developed. The clinician will find, reading the book, a wealth of information which will form a background to this sort of decision-making. The authors do not make any suggestions about management of these often difficult children but they provide a springboard from which ideas can be developed. They conclude with a call for future research, stressing our need for information about the natural history of these conditions. Faced with the fact that these disorders are almost certainly becoming more rather than less common, an extremely useful outcome of their work is that it enables us to move toward more effective aetiological studies—and hopefully prevention.

MARTIN BAX
Charing Cross and Westminster Medical School
London, UK

# GLOSSARY OF ABBREVIATIONS

**AD** = autistic disorder

**APDD** = atypical pervasive developmental disorder

**COPDD** = childhood-onset pervasive developmental disorder

**CPP** = Collaborative Perinatal Project

**DLD** = developmental language disorder

**EOWPVT** = Expressive One-Word Picture Vocabulary Test

**HAD** = high-functioning autistic disorder (NVIQ ≥80)

**HBS** = Wing Schedule of Handicaps, Behaviour and Skills

**IA** = infantile autism

**LAD** = low-functioning autistic disorder (NVIQ <80)

**LIQ** = low (nonverbal) intelligence quotient (<80)

**MLU** = mean length of utterances

**NALIQ** = non-autistic, low NVIQ (<80)

**NICU** = neonatal intensive care unit

**NVIQ** = nonverbal intelligence quotient

**PDD** = pervasive developmental disorder

**PDD-NOS** = pervasive developmental disorder, not otherwise specified

**SAS** = standard age scores

**S-B** = Stanford–Binet Intelligence Scales

**SD** = standard deviation

**SES** = socioeconomic status

**SICD-R** = Sequenced Inventory of Communication Development—Revised

**SOC** = schizophrenia occurring in childhood

**SLI** = specific language impairment

**TELD** = Test of Early Language Development

**WADIC** = Wing Autistic Disorder Interview Checklist

# PREFACE

Developmental disorders of higher cerebral function have a major impact on the lives of many children and their families. In school-age children they result in a variety of specific learning disabilities and attention disorders, whereas in preschool children they are most likely to present as inadequate development of language and communication skills. The diagnosis and classification of such disorders pose major challenges. There are no universally agreed upon criteria for the detection, differential diagnosis or classification of developmental disorders, especially in preschool children. Detailed testing of children with these disorders is likely to reveal a variety of cognitive, language, visuospatial, attentional and other deficits that point to considerable neuropsychological heterogeneity among children with similar presenting symptoms. The more complex the affected behavior, the more likely it is that the symptoms of its dysfunction will overlap with those of other related conditions, and the less likely that professionals from different disciplines, who use different measures and attend to different aspects of behavior, will agree on the definition and boundaries of the disorder. Furthermore, preschool children with these disorders are difficult to evaluate, and few standardized tests have been developed for this age group. It is only recently that well-trained, knowledgeable clinicians and researchers have attempted to study preschool children's behaviors quantitatively.

The etiologies of developmental disorders are not yet well understood. The current view is that inadequate social opportunity, poor teaching or parental inadequacy provide an inadequate explanation for the occurrence of these circumscribed cognitive disorders in many if not most children; rather, they are attributable to dysfunction or maldevelopment of the immature brain, more often on a genetic than an exogenous basis. Further discoveries about the brain abnormalities responsible for these disorders and the devising of effective interventions are predicated on clearer definition of the neuropsychological deficits responsible for the children's deficient skills and on more uniform classification criteria.

This monograph describes the first stage of a study attempting to develop a statistically valid, useful clinical–empirical classification of preschool children with inadequate communication skills in whom neither hearing loss nor a known brain lesion or defined disease explained this inadequacy. In order to accomplish this goal it was necessary to assemble a sufficiently large sample of these children, selected according to uniform criteria and studied with uniform instruments. The study integrates the viewpoints of the children's parents and of the many professionals concerned with developmentally deviant preschool children. It reflects the efforts of investigators from child neurology and psychiatry, neuropsychology, speech–language pathology, psycholinguistics, early childhood education and biostatistics.

A total of 556 children were investigated in five study groups: 201 with specific developmental language disorders (DLDs), 176 who fulfilled DSM III-R criteria for autistic disorder (AD), 110 with nonverbal IQs (NVIQs) below 80[1] but without autistic features (non-autistic, low IQ—NALIQ), 51 clinically defined as language impaired who did not meet inclusionary criteria for the study, and 18 whose autistic features did not meet DSM III-R criteria for AD. The 69 children in the latter two groups are included only in the taxometric analyses described in Chapter 10, because there the issue was overall classification, which requires broadly defined samples.

This monograph presents a description of the findings in 487 children aged 3–7 years: the 201 with DLD, 176 with AD, and 110 in the NALIQ group. Because of the wide range of cognitive abilities among autistic children, the autistic sample was arbitrarily divided into two subgroups, 51 children with an NVIQ ≥80 (high-functioning autistic disorder or HAD) and 125 children with an NVIQ <80 (low-functioning autistic disorder or LAD). The HAD group was compared to the 201 DLD children, all of whom had NVIQs ≥80, and the LAD group was compared to the 110 NALIQ children, all of whom had NVIQs <80. The monograph focuses on comparisons among these four groups.

Our goal was to determine how best to discriminate among the four groups (DLD *vs* HAD *vs* LAD *vs* NALIQ), and to delineate the most salient differences among these groups in medical/historical features, cognitive function, communication skills, sociability and play. A novel regression-mixture taxometric method, developed by R.R. Golden (see Golden and Mayer 1995)[2], was used to attempt to determine whether autism represented a latent taxon (*i.e.* a 'natural' grouping) distinct from its non-autistic complement, supporting the hypothesis that it may have a distinct biological basis, and whether we could identify subtaxa among children with DLD and AD. Finally we compared the probability of group membership within statistically defined taxa with membership in the four clinically defined groups described in the monograph.

Measures selected included background information about the child's birth, family history, medical history and development. Each child underwent a standard neurological examination. Parents and teachers were asked to respond to questionnaires concerning the child's behavior and skills at home and in school. If the questionnaires suggested autistic behaviors, a child psychiatrist evaluated the child to confirm or refute the diagnosis of pervasive developmental disorder (PDD) based on DSM III (American Psychiatric Association 1980) and DSM III-R (American Psychiatric Association 1987) criteria. Each child was tested with standardized psychometric test batteries of cognitive function and language. In addition, the child was videotaped while playing with his[3]

[1]Our method of NVIQ assessment is described in Chapter 4. The 'low NVIQ' (LIQ) cut-off of 80 (rather than the ICD-10 criterion for mental retardation of a Full Scale IQ <70) was chosen because an IQ of 80 is the lowest widely accepted level for a diagnosis of developmental language disorder. In order to have four groups matched pair-wise for NVIQ, we had to make an arbitrary NVIQ cut-off of 80 in the entire population. This dictated the arbitrary NVIQ cut-off at 80 in the autistic sample and the recruitment of non-autistic cognitively subnormal children with an NVIQ <80. There were 28 children in the NALIQ sample (25 per cent) with an NVIQ between 70 and 80, making 'mental retardation' an inappropriate label.
[2]Preparation of a full description of Dr Golden's regression-mixture taxometric analysis method for publication has been delayed due to ill-health.
[3]As the majority of children affected by the disorders addressed by this study are male, the male pronoun is used throughout this monograph to refer to individuals of either sex.

parent or teacher and with a stranger, using a standardized set of toys. Spontaneous speech during play was transcribed for formal analysis, and play behaviors were assessed using a time-sampling methodology.

For measures for which there are standardized instruments, findings in the four groups were compared to stardardized norms. For analysis of spontaneous language and play, we recruited an additional group of 47 normally developing preschool children. Logistic considerations precluded the collection of historical and neurological data in the normal children, which limits comparisons for those measures to the four clinical groups.

The monograph begins with a consideration of the benefits and requirements of classification. Chapter 2 discusses classification of DLD, and Chapter 3 classification of AD. Chapter 4 describes the the selection of subjects, their demographic characteristics, and the instruments used. Chapter 5 presents the family histories and data from the children's medical and developmental histories. Chapter 6 describes the findings from the medical and neurological examination. Chapter 7 details data from the neurocognitive and language domains, and Chapter 8 those from the behavioral–social domain. Chapter 9 analyzes the children's play skills. Chapter 10 discusses issues posed by classification based on discrepancy criteria and questionnaires for diagnosis, and shows clinicians' judgments may be more sensitive to some deficits than standardized instruments. It also discusses issues of base rate, sensitivity and specificity in diagnosis. It introduces preliminary results using regression–mixture taxometric classification and compares this classification with clinical group membership. The final chapter summarizes the most salient differences among the four groups of children and the most powerful measures for substantiating this differentiation. Each data chapter makes some recommendations for clinical evaluation and intervention based on the study findings.

A note about authorship is required. The original intent of the group was to list no individual authors of chapters or editors of the monograph because it is impossible to allocate proportion of effort fairly inasmuch as all the senior investigators participated in all the phases of the study. However, Dr Martin Bax, Senior Editor of the *Clinics in Developmental Medicine*, pointed out that this was unworkable for bibliographic retrieval reasons. We reluctantly acceded to his request and listed as authors of chapters those investigators who wrote drafts of the chapters or made other major contributions to that part of the study. All senior investigators worked on the chapters so that, in reality, the entire group, including the many able research assistants and other collaborators listed on pp. vii–viii, should be credited for the entire monograph.

The focus of the book is classification of the major disorders: AD, DLD and NALIQ. Further work needs to be done to compare the subtypes of autism and language disorders described briefly in Chapter 10 with subtypes of language disorders proposed by Aram and Nation (1975), Rapin and Allen (1983, 1988), Wilson and Risucci (1986), and Allen (1989) and with several clinical classifications for autism such as those of Wing and Gould (1979) and Allen (1988), using behavioral and cognitive instruments employed in the project. In order to be able to carry out these future analyses, we gave the children a number of additional measures of language and sociability that were not used for analysis of the data presented in the monograph.

An important part of the validation of any classification of preschool communication disordered children is to study the developmental history of the disorders. Of particular interest are (a) the extent to which homogeneous groups remain homogeneous or diverge as development proceeds, (b) the extent to which relative strengths and weaknesses in the cognition and behavior of children in different groups remain characteristic of those children, and (c) the identification of features of early development which are the best predictors of outcome in childhood and adolescence. Outcome studies of the cohort at ages 7 and 9 are in progress, and we hope to follow the AD and NALIQ cohorts into adolescence.

This nosology research project is one of the largest multidisciplinary projects concerned with developmentally disabled children since the Collaborative Perinatal Project (CPP) of the 1960s (also supported by NINDS). That project raised as many questions in need of further research as it answered. Data collected by the CPP are still yielding new answers today, encouraging the investigators who are carrying out the present project to hope that their efforts will also continue to be useful for many years, both to them and to other researchers attempting to help the affected children and their families.

Autism and Language Disorders Nosology Project
December 1995

# 1

# INTRODUCTION

*R. Morris and I. Rapin*

This monograph reports data from a research project concerned with developing a validated classification of developmental disorders of communication skills in preschool children. It focuses on the relationships among those children traditionally described as having a developmental language disorder (DLD) or an autistic disorder (AD), or who have a low nonverbal IQ (NVIQ) but are not autistic (NALIQ). There is still no widely accepted classification and identification process for these disorders; professionals disagree on whether they represent developmental lags or intrinsic neurological disorders and on how to remediate them most effectively; and there is inadequate knowledge of their causes (etiologies), neurological basis and prognosis. Confusion is heightened by the fact that children who share the common symptom of inadequate communication skills often differ substantially in cognitive ability, social skills, associated deficits and long-term outcome. The need for a common basis for classifying children with these disorders is clear.

The ultimate objectives of the overall project are:
(1) to provide an empirically validated nosology, acceptable to researchers and professionals from diverse disciplines, in order to promote uniformity in subject selection and foster replicability of results, retrievability of data, and collaborative research and communication; and
(2) to provide a neuropsychological and behavioral foundation on which (a) to investigate the neurobiological basis of these disorders, and (b) to provide a basis for rational intervention and for improving the training of those who educate and care for these children.

The results presented in this monograph are the foundation for this larger effort. This chapter will outline the scope of the monograph but will also consider the broader subject of classification research. Although the focus of the monograph is a comparison among preschool children divided into three clinical groups (DLD, AD and NALIQ) on the basis of generally accepted behavioral criteria, the overall goal of the study is to develop an empirical classification and to compare this classification with the three clinical groups.

## Overall plan of the project
The project was conducted in the following steps.

### Definition of the population
The first step was to define the overall population to be studied. A series of decisions led

to a population with chronological ages of 3:0 to 5:11 for DLD, and of 3:0 to 7:11 for AD and NALIQ, so as to increase the range of mental ages in these more seriously affected children. The children were clinically referred to the study for deficient development of communication, and had no known brain lesions, gross sensory or motor impairments, or uncontrolled seizures, and were not on high doses of psychotropic or anticonvulsant medication. (Details of subject recruitment procedures, inclusionary and exclusionary criteria, and the rationale for these decisions are given in Chapter 4.)

*Selection of clinical criteria to define major groups*
The second step was the selection of clinical criteria for the definition of study groups. There are two fundamental approaches to defining groups within a population. The first is to adopt pre-existing theoretical notions about the existence of these groups and attempt to find a set of defining criteria that are reliable and valid: this is the clinically derived approach. The second approach is to begin with a set of observations, and let an empirically driven algorithm attempt to find naturally occurring groups; this is the statistical approach. A goal of this nosological study is to compare both approaches.

There are multiple and competing clinically derived classification systems for DLD and AD in the literature (see Chapters 2 and 3 for reviews). Kendell (1982) suggested that, given this state of affairs, using several alternative definitions simultaneously and testing rival classificatory systems makes a strong methodological contribution toward rational selection of a best system. In order to be able to incorporate and compare existing clinical ideas, we codified the rules for using some of these systems in the form of checklists or algorithms, with manuals to ensure their consistent application. Several of these traditional systems were tried for defining autism and language disorder. We monitored the number of subjects changing groups with each of the approaches, together with each classification's level of homogeneity and coverage of the sample of interest. The comparison of these various systems for language disordered children and the children with autism, using these methods, is mentioned briefly in Chapters 2, 3 and 10 and discussed in greater detail in separate publications (Aram *et al.* 1993, Waterhouse *et al.* 1996). The historically based, clinically derived classifications that were found generally to be most successful for each of the major disorders are the ones we chose to use for the present study; operationalized clinical criteria are described in Chapter 4. The results presented here serve as an anchor against which other classification systems can be compared and evaluated.

*Selection of a classification model*
The third step was the choice of a classification system, whereby some groups might be defined polythetically (*i.e.* on the basis of attributes which together define membership even though they do not do so individually) and others monothetically (*i.e.* on the basis of necessary and sufficient attributes), and with a two-level hierarchical structure. We defined Level I as differentiation of major disorders (autism, language disorder, low NVIQ). We then identified Level II behavioral subgroups or subtypes within each major Level I group. This monograph describes the Level I classification model (and lays the

2

foundation for investigations of alternative classification models); some Level II findings are also outlined in Chapter 10.

*Selection of measures*
The fourth step was the selection of behavioral and cognitive assessment instruments to compare children in the clinically defined groups and to develop the empirical classification. Both categorical and dimensional assessment measures were used in the study. Many were derived from standardized assessment instruments for preschool children; applying these instruments to disabled children brought to light major psychometric and measurement problems with many available standardized tests. These are discussed in Chapter 4. In addition, many of the important theoretical constructs relevant to the functioning of the children in this study, *e.g.* pragmatics, symbolic play and sociability, required that we develop new checklists and ratings scales for the scoring of behavior. These are also described in Chapter 4.

*Statistical recreation of groups*
The fifth step was to use empirical classification techniques to recreate groups. The data were analyzed with a regression-mixture taxometric method developed by R.R. Golden (see p. xii). Probability of membership in these empirically detected groups was then compared to membership in the clinically defined clinical groups. The result of these analyses is reviewed briefly in Chapter 10.

*External validation of clinically defined groups*
One way to validate clinically defined groups is to compare them using variables not used to define them. The four groups of developmentally disabled children described in this monograph were formed on the basis of behavioral and cognitive criteria; we compared these groups on external variates such as other behavioral and cognitive variables, medical and developmental histories of the children, family variables, and neurological examination findings. Chapters 5 and 6 give detailed results on these comparisons for the clinical classification system used. Additional means of external validation such as replication, using the original variables in new samples, and testing for external biological validity (*e.g.* genetic markers or other specific etiological correlates, or evidence that the groups differ neuroanatomically, electrophysiologically or biochemically), will be needed in the future but transcend the present project.

*Exploration of subtypes of major disorders*
As stated earlier, the classification model selected is a two-level hierarchical model, with AD, DLD and NALIQ at Level I, and behavioral subtypes of these disorders at Level II. Existing literature about hypothesized subtypes of language disorder and autism is reviewed in Chapters 2 and 3, and preliminary descriptions of taxometrically detected subgroups of AD and DLD are included in Chapter 10. The results of these taxometric analyses are described in greater detail by Waterhouse *et al.* (1996); further reports from the Nosology Project are currently in preparation.

**Research questions**

The study compares 176 preschool and young school-age children with Autistic Disorder as defined in DSM III-R (American Psychiatric Association 1987)—divided arbitrarily into 51 high-functioning children (HAD: NVIQ ≥80) and 125 low-functioning children (LAD: NVIQ <80)—with 201 children with DLDs (NVIQ ≥80) and 110 with low NVIQ (LIQ, <80) without autistic features, on a broad range of historical, neurological, neuro-psychological, linguistic, behavioral/social and play variables. The LIQ cut-off of 80 was selected so as to be able to match the groups because 80 is commonly accepted as the lower limit for a diagnosis of specific DLD. These groups of children were selected for study because they comprise the bulk of children with communication disorders of early life that are not accounted for by hearing loss or frank structural and neuromuscular abnormalities of the mouth and upper respiratory tract, or by identifiable lesions or diseases of the brain, and because overlaps in the children's communication disorders foster diagnostic disagreements among clinicians and investigators.

We began the study with four essential predictions to be tested:

(1) Because we did not enroll children with known brain lesions, identifiable diseases (except for a small group of children with Down syndrome selected for the NALIQ group), overt sensorimotor neurological abnormalities or severe epilepsy, and because genetics is now known to play an important etiological role in all the developmental disorders of brain function, we predicted that there would be no major differences in the prevalence of prenatal and perinatal abnormalities among the four groups. We did expect that the two LIQ groups (LAD and NALIQ) would have a higher prevalence of seizures and mild motor deficits and would show greater developmental impairment than the other groups in sociability and play skills, as well as in cognitive and language skills. We also expected to find family members with developmental disorders but did not know specifically how similar these would be to those of the children in the study.

(2) Inasmuch as impaired sociability is such a salient characteristic of AD children, we predicted that it would be reported by many observers, including parents, teachers, psychiatrists and neurologists, and that free play with a parent and a stranger would provide a sensitive way to bring it out. We predicted further that the symbolic play of all the clinically impaired children would be impoverished compared to that of normal children, and that the play of the autistic groups would be more severely affected than that of their comparison groups (*i.e.* normal>all groups; DLD>HAD; NALIQ>LAD).

(3) We theorized that the majority of children in the two AD groups would be more delayed in language acquisition than the majority of the DLD and NALIQ children, and that deficient pragmatic skills would be a strong predictor of membership in the AD group.

(4) We hypothesized that there would be empirically definable subtypes of AD and DLD.

The present monograph provides a broad and detailed description of young children with inadequate communication skills divided into three groups (AD, DLD, NALIQ) on the basis of widely accepted behavioral and cognitive criteria. As stated earlier, the ultimate goal of the project is to create an empirically defined nosology or classification

4

of these children based on both clinical/observational and test data. We are therefore providing, in the next two sections of this chapter, a discussion of classification theory research for interested readers. Those whose interest is primarily clinical may choose to skip over these sections.

## Classification research in disorders of higher cerebral function

Classification research is a bottom-up endeavor; it starts with a range of empirical observations in subjects selected as broadly as possible and attempts to detect common attributes that will enable the rational creation of homogeneous groups. Classification research of behaviorally defined conditions—in the present study, developmental disorders of communication and sociability—is particularly difficult because there are no dichotomous biological 'gold standards' to define class membership. Group membership depends on dimensional measures such as NVIQ. There will be some overlap between classes, with a variable—hopefully small—number of individuals whose classification remains indeterminate.

Typically, classification issues have not been the focus of either neurobehavioral or developmental research (Morris and Fletcher 1988). Most behavioral studies first identify a set of independent variables—*e.g.* age, gender, location of lesions—then formulate hypotheses about the relations of these to a set of dependent variables—*e.g.* expressive language, sociability, motor skill. If the study supports the hypotheses, it has established that the dependent variables were appropriately measured and were explicitly related to the independent variables; in addition, the study has provided implicit validation of the independent variables by confirming expected contrasts among them and their ability to classify observations appropriately. Conversely, if the hypotheses are not supported, then the study has highlighted theoretical problems with the hypotheses, or problems with the measurement of the dependent variables, or lack of validity of the implicit classification hypotheses that led to the selection of the independent variables (Fletcher *et al.* 1988, Morris and Fletcher 1988). Classification research thus addresses directly the reliability and validity of the independent variables that underlie the grouping of observations (Goodall 1966, Skinner 1981), whereas traditional research tends to focus on the adequacy of the dependent variables.

Most research on children with developmental disorders of higher cerebral function, such as autism and language disorders, assumes that these diagnostic groups and the criteria used to form them are reliable and valid, and that the groups represent true 'entities' or disorders with some biological reality. The focal point of this traditional research has been the differentiation among these clinically defined groups of children on the basis of such dependent variables as cognitive, language, social, and biological measures. This approach has yielded a mass of conflicting and inconsistent results that have hampered the adequate characterization of these developmental disabilities. One possible cause of these problems is inadequate study of the definition and formulation of the groups.

The literature on specific problems affecting classification of language disorders and autism is reviewed in Chapters 2 and 3. General problems that hamper attempts to classify all disorders of behavioral development include: (a) mixing different levels of classification; (b) changes in behavioral attributes with development; (c) difficulty measuring complex psychological constructs in disordered populations; and (d) the multidimensional nature of many of these behaviors.

*Mixing different levels of classification*
Classification of disorders can be carried out at many levels, from the descriptive classifications usually found early in the development of an area of knowledge, to pathological, pathophysiological and etiological classifications. Suspected disorders of the central nervous system have an added level—the anatomic. Neurological syndromes tend to be produced by dysfunction in particular (localized or distributed) brain systems, regardless of the etiology (*e.g.* stroke, malformation, epilepsy) or even the pathophysiology of their dysfunction.

These levels of classification, therefore, are far from overlapping exactly. Recent progress shows that a single etiology, *e.g.* inactivity of a particular enzyme, can cause vastly different diseases, and that a previously single, well-defined disease, like Tay–Sachs disease or poliomyelitis, may result from several distinct genetic mutations or viral types (*e.g.* see Johnson 1982). It is a rule that complex, behaviorally defined syndromes, like autism, tend to arise from a variety of entirely different genetic and acquired etiologies, although they may share some common pathophysiological mechanisms (Rapin 1987, Gillberg 1992).

Any of these multiple levels of classification may be valid and useful, but they must be kept distinct for initial research purposes. Hybrid classifications that mix classification domains (*e.g.* etiology—fragile X, and behavior—autism) are likely to create confusion (Gillberg 1992, Rapin 1992, Waterhouse *et al.* 1992). Discovery of the etiology of a disease is almost always insufficient to explain its symptoms. Understanding of symptomatology requires the unravelling of the pathophysiological and cellular consequences of the biochemical or anatomic alterations arising from a particular genetic mutation, infection, congenital anomaly or other etiology, and of their interactions with environmental influences. Thus, despite our assumption that the primary basis of the communication disorders under study is atypical or disordered brain function(s), classification research concerned with types of communication disorder is focused at the level of observable behaviors and skills; other types of data that might suggest the etiology, anatomy or pathophysiology of these behaviorally defined disorders are reserved for the external validation of any resulting classification schema (Skinner 1981).

*Changes in behavioral attributes during development*
The fact that the disorders under study affect developing organisms adds another set of difficulties. Classification of the disorders of higher cerebral function began with the study of adults with stable focal or diffuse brain lesions. As many investigators have pointed out (Fletcher and Taylor 1984, Segalowitz and Hiscock 1992), not only are brain–behavior inferences much less well understood for children than adults, but the changes in behavioral attributes, sometimes dramatic, over development make even strictly descriptive systems derived for one age group difficult to apply to another age

group. Therefore we have chosen to start with a classification for preschool and young school-age children. Tracing the natural history of the syndromes defined in early childhood will constitute an important later part of the project: longitudinal follow-up of these children will make it possible to investigate the stability of the classification across development and whether classifications at later ages have additional advantages.

*Difficulty in measuring complex concepts in disordered populations*
Developmental disorders that have a major impact on communication may be associated with deficits in 'simple' sensorimotor abilities, but have their major effect on so-called 'higher' cerebral functions such as memory, intelligence and affect. Higher cerebral functions are inferred psychological constructs serving to account for observed abilities to perform such complex cognitive tasks as reading, abstract reasoning and empathy. It is much more hazardous to make inferences about the precise localization of neurological dysfunction on the basis of abnormalities of such complex behavior(s) than on the basis of well-defined sensorimotor deficits. Complex human abilities call for the coordinated activity of often widely distributed networks in the brain; therefore they are vulnerable to a variety of focal lesions and diffuse pathologies which, in turn, are apt to be unselective and to affect multiple abilities. The variable timetable of brain maturation, the role of varying environmental influences on brain maturation, and the variant developmental trajectories of these abilities add another level of complexity.

In addition, measurement of complex cognitive and behavioral functions is problematic. Each function is multifactorial and may require sampling of many behaviors over time and across many situations in order to measure it accurately and reliably and to place it against the background of normal development. Researchers find some constructs, such as sociability, relatively easy to define but extremely difficult to rate reliably in the context of everyday spontaneous behavior.

*Multidimensional nature of behaviors measured*
Traditionally, classification of medical diseases has used categorical models that have been validated by external, biological criteria: a person does or does not have a brain tumor, a diagnosis validated by neuroimaging, surgical findings and pathology. Classification of the behavioral disorders of higher cerebral function is much less amenable to such a categorical framework. Their detection is based on departure from average performance on continuous variable(s) such as verbal or nonverbal cognition. Decisions about the presence or absence of a deficit thus rests on somewhat arbitrary cut-offs and statistical models, and consequently there may be no sharp, natural margin between normality and abnormality, or even between the boundaries of various groups with deficits. Mental retardation may be defined statistically as a score greater than two standard deviations below the mean on a test of intelligence. The use of such psychometric cut-offs, although it has the advantage of being operationalized, guarantees arbitrariness in the separation of normality and pathology; the difference between an IQ of 69 and an IQ of 71 is statistically, behaviorally and clinically meaningless; yet, according to commonly accepted classification, an IQ of 69, along with concordant adaptive behavior scores,

7

defines a mentally retarded individual, and an IQ of 71 defines one who is borderline normal, two labels that have very different implications for education and that imply different developmental outcomes.

In light of these general issues, the present investigators decided from the start: (i) to restrict the classification under development to a descriptive one, reserving etiological, pathophysiological and anatomic data for external validation; (ii) to restrict the age range for which the classification was intended; (iii) to measure as many behavioral and cognitive domains as we could, using standardized measures when possible and, rarely, devising new instruments when necessary; and (iv) to preserve as far as possible the dimensional nature of the classifying and dependent variables, and when reduction to categories was necessary, to explore the consequences of using different cut-off points between normality and pathology.

In the following section we describe the theoretical classification framework chosen, and the application of this framework in the overall plan of the current project.

**Classification framework**
Our research is based on the conceptual classification framework proposed by Skinner (1981). His construct validation approach to classification research integrates three basic components: theory formulation, and internal and external validation. Important elements of theory formulation include the following:
(1) decisions regarding the content domain, *i.e.* the variables to be employed for classification purposes—these are derived from an extant theory about the nature of the hypothesized disorder;
(2) specification of 'ideal type' constructs, *i.e.* a description of the expected (hypothesized) characteristics of subsets of subjects (groups and subgroups) in the population;
(3) selection of a classification model, *i.e.* the relation of subjects and subtypes to each other. There are many possible models for grouping children. Monothetic models propose that subjects be identified on the basis of a set of necessary and sufficient attributes. Polythetic models define attributes that are not necessary but which, when combined into sets to form types, are sufficient for membership. In this kind of model, membership is determined by the number of attributes possessed by a proposed constituent. Prototype models define an ideal type and its core set of attributes; membership is determined by the degree to which a subject resembles the ideal type. Hierarchical models specify types by partitioning subjects into the lowest possible number of groups, then systematically looking for relations among groups, with smaller subgroups possible within larger groups; and
(4) *a priori* specification of expected group interrelations and of the relations of hypothesized groups to external constructs and variables.

The internal validity component addresses the reliability of the classification. This component includes studies of replicability on another sample, homogeneity within groups, and coverage (the proportion of the relevant population classified by the system).

The external validity component involves the evaluation of hypotheses about differences among groups, employing variables other than those used to form the classification. Examples of external validity include the demonstration of different inheritance patterns of groups identified on the basis of behavioral measures, or of differential response to treatment between groups.

Relatively few published classification studies include an external validation component or attempt to evaluate *a priori* hypotheses explicitly. The goal of many classification studies has been, simply, to search for groups or subtypes; if these emerge, the research progresses no further. If validity is studied at all, the variables used for validation often either come from the same measurement domain or are the very ones used to form the classification, or else are selected *post hoc*. In future studies of our sample we will attempt to evaluate external validity by using measures from domains not used in forming the classification, and by evaluating the stability of the classification over time.

Kendell (1982) suggested further that comparing different classification systems on external variables such as family history, long-term outcome and response to treatment is necessary, but that it is not sufficient to guarantee validity. He concluded that 'The essential problem is that we can never be certain where the boundary between one syndrome and the next lies until we understand the underlying mechanisms, and we will have difficulty identifying these mechanisms unless we can draw the clinical boundaries in the right places first.'

External validation is therefore an ongoing bootstrap process that entails evaluation of a classification's generalizability, prognostic accuracy, descriptive validity, clinical utility and ability to predict response to treatment. Explicit in Skinner's (1981) framework is the concept that a classification scheme is an hypothesis arising from previous theory and research findings, an hypothesis subject to empirical test, refutation and revision. It is upon this explicit hypothesis-testing approach to classification framework that we built this longitudinal project.

**Conclusion**

This chapter has outlined the goal of the larger project: to develop a more quantitatively and clinically sophisticated classification system for preschool and young school-age children with developmental neurobehavioral disabilities, especially those affecting communication. We believe that the sample of children included in the study, with the particular range of developmental disorders, is the largest systematically investigated group of its kind assembled to date, and as such, the study provides a unique database for addressing a variety of issues about the similarities and differences in the development of such children, and the implications of the findings for clinical diagnosis and intervention.

# 2
# CLASSIFICATION OF DEVELOPMENTAL LANGUAGE DISORDERS (DLDs)

*N. Hall and D.M. Aram*

## History of the classification of DLDs

This chapter traces the history of the classification and terminology of DLDs, neither of which has yet achieved universal acceptance. What emerges is a patchwork of practices arising from diverse sources. We will then describe more recent attempts at a definition and systematic classification and the problems encountered. This will provide a background for the presentation of the classification criteria adopted in the Nosology Study which concludes this chapter.

We start with a preliminary note regarding the use of the label 'developmental language disorder' (or occasionally dysphasia) in this project. DLD is a term which has been used to reflect the developmental, as opposed to acquired, nature of the children's language disorders. While some investigators have suggested that 'specific language impairment' (SLI) may be a more appropriate label for these children (Johnston 1988; see also Aram 1991, Leonard 1991), many use DLD and SLI interchangeably (*e.g.* Leonard 1983, 1986; Johnston *et al.* 1985; Johnston 1988; Tallal 1988). Further, controversy persists relative to the 'specificity' of children's language disorders, and the usefulness of SLI as a construct (Leonard 1987, Clinical Forum 1991). We chose the term DLD for use in our study as it seemed to be more inclusive and to reflect the heterogeneous nature of language impairment in children better than SLI. We also felt that the term DLD, as opposed to SLI, implies that, potentially, the disorder can transcend the language domain. Readers may want to keep in mind that recently some in the field have begun to use the term DLD more broadly to refer to children who may exhibit other handicapping conditions in addition to impaired language, and to use the term SLI more narrowly to refer to children whose language deficits are not accompanied by concomitant conditions such as chronic middle ear effusion, mental retardation, learning disability, autistic behaviors, or identified neurological deficits or structural malformations.

The field of DLDs is relatively new, and it is difficult to determine when interest in this topic evolved into an identified area of study. Although reports of children with aberrant language appeared at least by the early 1800s (see Weiner 1974), the meeting of the Institute of Childhood Aphasia held at Stanford University in 1960 is generally accepted as the landmark for the coalescence of research and clinical interest in this group of children (see Miller *et al.* 1981, Johnston 1988). Major universities began offering courses in language disorders in children in the 1960s, and the American Speech–Language–Hearing Association (ASHA) added the 'Language' to its name in 1977, further evidence of the relatively recent advent of language disorders in children as a field of study and specialization.

Investigators of language and its development in the late 19th and early 20th centuries knew that language impairment can occur in the face of otherwise normal cognitive function and became aware that there are a number of different ways in which language can break down. Early attempts at classifying DLDs focused on their medical etiologies or causes and were carried out by neurologists and psychiatrists, as well as by educators of the deaf and developmentally disabled (Ewing 1930; Orton 1937; Chess 1944; Myklebust 1954; Strauss 1954; Ingram and Reid 1956; McGinnis *et al.* 1956; Morley 1957, 1965, 1972; Benton 1959, 1964; Hardy 1965).

*Contributions from neurology*
Adult aphasiology had a significant impact on the early work on DLD as investigators attempted to draw parallels between these two fields. Researchers modified classifications of acquired language disorders of adults and attempted to apply them to children with DLD. For example, Orton (1937) identified genetic and neurological causes of several DLD syndromes. His classification, directly transposed from adult aphasia, included developmental alexia (reading disorder), developmental agraphia (writing disorder), developmental word deafness, developmental motor aphasia, developmental apraxia, childhood stuttering, and a number of mixed syndromes. Myklebust (1954) divided children with DLD into four groups: children with predominantly expressive, predominantly receptive, mixed receptive–expressive, and central developmental aphasias. More recently, Rapin and Allen (1988) attempted to draw parallels between the various aphasic syndromes of adults with focal brain lesions and clinically defined developmental dysphasic syndromes in children.

*Contributions from psychiatry, psychology and pediatrics*
In addition to these neurologically based classification models for DLD, professionals in other fields published detailed case reports and clinical population studies (Worster-Drought and Allen 1930; Strauss 1954; Benton 1959, 1964). Strauss was among the first to include other aspects of child development in his descriptions of DLD; he used the term 'oligophasia', as 'signifying a deficit of language, or lack of language development' to distinguish childhood aphasia from adult aphasia. Using Piagetian principles, Strauss attempted to relate deficits in language development to sensorimotor aspects of cognition.

In 1956 Ingram and Reid described 78 children (aged 6–15 years) whom they identified as 'developmentally aphasic'. They characterized the speech and language deficits of these children in terms of their neurological status, and also considered their sociological, psychological and educational backgrounds. Each child received audiological, physical, neurological and ophthalmological examinations, electroencephalographic (EEG) testing, and assessments of handedness, speech, psychiatric and psychological functions, and reading and writing skills. They analyzed their data with respect to etiology of the DLD, its symptomatology, and other related developmental disorders such as dyslexia and dysgraphia. They reported a high percentage of ambidexterity among the subjects and their family members and severe reading and/or writing difficulties among individuals with receptive or expressive aphasia. Finally, they classified learning diffi-culties on the basis of three types of deficit: (1) inability to perceive the relationship of shapes and letters in space and reproduce them correctly; (2) failure to relate phonic and written symbols correctly to each other; (3) failure to perceive the meaning or signific-ance of the written or spoken word. It was this third factor which was most closely associated with the more severe learning disabilities.

*Contributions from deaf education*
Investigators working in schools for the deaf identified among their students children who had little or no hearing loss but significantly impaired language. They stressed the importance of the differential diagnosis between congenital hearing loss and DLD (*e.g.* Myklebust 1954). These investigators contributed significantly to the field of DLD by comparing the language of children with hearing impairment to that of children with defi-cits in receptive and/or expressive language (Ewing 1930, Myklebust 1954, McGinnis *et al.* 1956, Hardy 1965). They described specific remedial techniques based on principles from the oralist approaches to deaf education that were applicable to the education of dysphasic children, such as the use of written language in teaching phoneme production and sequencing.

*Contributions from case reports*
As the differential diagnosis and classification of DLD became recognized as worthy of study, detailed case reports led to the identification of specific subtypes of DLD (Town 1911, Worster-Drought and Allen 1930, Karlin 1951, deAjuriaguerra *et al.* 1976). For example, Worster-Drought and Allen described a 12-year-old boy with 'congenital auditory imperception' (also referred to as congenital word-deafness or verbal auditory agnosia) who, in the absence of hearing loss, mental retardation or significant emotional disturbance, was unable to understand the meaning of words. McGinnis (1963) illu-strated the similarities between adult aphasia and DLD in children through the case study of a brother and sister enrolled in the Central Institute for the Deaf who had significant deficits in language comprehension and expression despite having better hearing than the other children at the Institute. Likewise, Karlin (1951) used the case study of a 6-year-old girl with congenital verbal auditory agnosia to compare it with auditory agnosia or acquired word deafness in adults.

*Historical terminology*
Given the various disciplines involved in the study of DLD, it is not surprising that they introduced multiple terminologies. The terms developmental or congenital aphasia or dysphasia, borrowed from the medical terminology of acquired aphasia in adults, came into use. Such medically based terms, which imply a medical basis for DLD, have prompted considerable debate. The controversy revolves around the legitimacy of making a parallel between acquired aphasia seen in adults, *i.e.* disruption of a previously

intact language structure, and the developmental disorders observed in children. Further, the suitability of the term aphasia, which implies total loss of language, in contrast to dysphasia, referring to dysfunction, is questioned. Other terminology, such as congenital auditory imperception (an early precursor of verbal auditory agnosia and today's central auditory processing problems), presumes breakdowns in processing. Recent trends have led investigators away from pathogenic considerations and toward the use of categorically descriptive terms, such as developmental language disorder, specific language disability or specific language impairment. Yet this shift has not served to better define the population, rather it highlights researcher biases. As pointed out by Johnston (1988) in her review of the literature on child language disorders, 'differences in labels usually reflect theoretical emphasis rather than differences in population'.

## Differential diagnosis
### Application of exclusionary criteria
The early accounts, with their focus on differential diagnosis, led to the practice of diagnosing DLD by exclusion rather than on the basis of the characteristics of the child's language (see Tallal 1988). The use of exclusionary criteria for diagnosis grew out of attempts to identify causative factors for DLD. Myklebust (1954) introduced his discussion by stating that 'early life aphasia is readily confused with other conditions which affect language growth and development'. He initiated the practice of using exclusionary criteria in order to sharpen the identification of children with DLD. Following the publication of Myklebust's landmark text and those of Morley (1957, 1965, 1972), the use of exclusionary criteria for diagnosing DLD was popularized by Benton (1959, 1964), Adler (1964) and Wood (1964). By the 1960s this practice was well entrenched and it is still used today, although the debate on how best to standardize such an approach continues (Stark and Tallal 1981, Leonard 1987, Lahey 1990).

### Currently used exclusionary criteria
Children diagnosed as having DLD are assumed to exhibit language deficits which cannot be attributed to any of the following exclusionary criteria.
(a) *Mental retardation.* Children with documented mental retardation typically are excluded from studies of DLD, although some investigators have suggested that some retarded children demonstrate specific language deficits and that only a discrepancy between language functioning and nonverbal functioning is necessary for a diagnosis of DLD (Benton 1959, Miller *et al.* 1981; see discussion on discrepancy criteria below).
(b) *Hearing loss.* Documentation of normal hearing typically involves passing a standard pure tone audiometric screening of each ear at 20 dB for 1000, 2000 and 4000 Hz (American National Standards Institute 1970).
(c) *Frank neurological and neuromuscular deficits.* More recently, studies of specific language disorders have specified that children with frank neurological and neuromuscular deficits be excluded. 'Frank neurological deficits' usually refer to those that produce motor deficits (cerebral palsy), those with a known etiology, such as an intrauterine infection or metabolic brain disease, or those associated with brain malformations or

lesions detectable on neuroimaging by computed tomography (CT) scanning or magnetic resonance imaging (MRI). The intention is to exclude the possibility that dysarthria or motor involvement of the speech musculature is a primary limiting factor for the expression of language and to limit the term DLD to children without a specific etiology or anatomically definable brain lesion.

(d) *Severe emotional disorders*. Children with signs of severe emotional disorders and/or autism are typically excluded from studies of DLD.

(e) *Environmental differences and deprivation*. Recognition of the contribution of the environment to language development gained momentum in the 1960s, leading to the identification of social deprivation as an exclusionary criterion for DLD (Wood 1964). Language problems attributable to an impoverished environmental input are not considered DLD. Nonstandard dialectal variations, such as Black English, are not a disorder, and these variations must be taken into consideration in the differential diagnosis of DLD (American Speech–Hearing–Language Association 1983).

*Issues in the use of exclusionary criteria*

The most crucial of the many problems associated with the practice of establishing the diagnosis of DLD through exclusionary criteria is that the essential nature and causal bases for most forms of DLD remain unknown. Although it is widely assumed that neurological dysfunction underlies many forms of DLD, not all agree with this viewpoint, nor has it been unequivocally established. Some investigators (Inhelder 1966, 1976; Morehead and Ingram 1973; Cromer 1981, 1983), arguing from a psychologically oriented perspective, speculate that DLD represents a cognitive dysfunction which, while not specific to language, manifests itself in language. It is just as likely that the neurological deficit underlying DLD may result from one or a combination of factors, for example, a genetic predisposition that is exacerbated or pushed to expression by the occurrence of a fluctuating hearing loss (Ingram 1959, Ludlow and Cooper 1983). Those who advance such theories, however, generally do not address the neurological dysfunction that underlies the cognitive impairment or genetic predisposition.

In some respects, the field is limited by arbitrary definitions of the exclusionary criteria listed earlier. Although investigators have reached agreement on some specifications, such as the range of normal intelligence and what constitutes normal hearing, the appropriate boundaries for defining many of the factors critical to a diagnosis of DLD remain uncertain. Specific concerns regarding the use of each of the exclusionary criteria outlined above need to be addressed.

MENTAL RETARDATION

Studies of DLD have acknowledged that a particular range of IQ scores represents normal intelligence, yet no lower level for nonverbal abilities is universally accepted. Most investigators require an NVIQ of at least 80 or 85 as a means of ensuring that a child's language deficits do not merely reflect overall mental retardation. However, other investigators maintain that mentally retarded populations are not immune to specific language disorders; for these investigators, it is only necessary that a discrepancy between intelligence and language level be present, not a particular level of nonverbal intelligence (Benton 1959, Miller *et al*. 1981).

Basic to the issue of defining a suitable intelligence criterion for DLD is the manner and skill with which intelligence is measured in developing children. Several researchers have pointed out the critical dependence of cognitive scores on the choice of measures and have stressed the unevenness of the cognitive skills of children with DLD (Kamhi 1981; Johnston 1982, 1988; Johnston and Ramstad 1983; Nelson *et al*. 1986).

HEARING LOSS

No-one has resolved the question of how middle ear pathology and fluctuating hearing loss should be factored into the documentation of normal hearing. Whether or not fluctuating hearing loss due to middle ear pathology contributes to the occurrence of language disorders or later learning problems in children is disputed (for reviews of this literature, see Kavanaugh 1986, Klein and Rapin 1988, US Department of Health and Human Services 1994). The wide variation in language learning and reading abilities among children with hearing losses may not be entirely attributable to the severity of the hearing loss, age at diagnosis, native intelligence and effectiveness of habilitation, but may in some children be due to an associated language disorder.

NEUROLOGICAL AND NEUROMUSCULAR DEFICITS

The exclusion of children with 'frank neurological' impairments from studies of DLD have posed particular problems of definition and diagnosis of 'frank neurological' deficits. Clinical detection of these deficits can be difficult in young children and may, in some cases, depend upon whether the child has seen a neurologist or undergone neuro-imaging of the brain. This exclusionary criterion also presents a problem for those who view DLD as a manifestation of neurological dysfunction, rather than delayed brain maturation, which may or may not be expressed in other neurological or cognitive domains (Ingram 1959, Benton 1964, Eisenson 1968). These investigators point out that excluding neurological and neuromuscular deficits eliminates a portion of the population of interest.

BEHAVIORAL/EMOTIONAL DISORDERS

Procedures for screening out emotional disorders are even more imprecise than those for excluding potentially causal neurological conditions; in preschool children objective criteria for defining emotional, social, autistic, psychotic or 'atypical' behaviors are essentially lacking. Studies of language disordered children have often used imprecise and variable criteria to define these behaviors, decreasing the generalizability of their findings (Baker and Cantwell 1987, Howlin and Rutter 1987). The question of whether behavioral/emotional problems in children with DLD are primary or reactive to a severe communication disorder is often raised but is difficult to answer, at least in some cases.

In addition to factors specific to each exclusionary criterion, little is known about the developmental course and longitudinal manifestations of many of these variables over

time in both normal and DLD populations. As well, questions remain on how a definition of DLD based on exclusionary factors affects the measurement of outcome. For
example, while there is information about the stability of IQ over time in normally
developing children, little work has examined this aspect of development in DLD
children. A critical question is the predictive value of early nonverbal measures for later
outcome in DLD children, as evidenced by the variable findings of follow-up studies
(*e.g.* Aram *et al.* 1984, Bishop and Edmundson 1987, Bishop and Adams 1990, Haynes
and Naidoo 1991). Additionally, long-term studies of the effect of fluctuating hearing
loss on later auditory and language abilities are currently underway (Wallace *et al.* 1988,
US Department of Health and Human Services). These investigations are beginning to
shed light on the interaction between hearing sensitivity, language development and
time. Information on this interaction is critical for understanding the factors that contribute to DLD, as well as for identifying individuals at risk for language and/or learning
problems.

Finally, valid measures to define these exclusionary criteria reliably, measures that
are at the same time sensitive and practical for both clinical and research use in young
DLD children, have yet to come into general use. Assessments of motor, cognitive,
emotional and social functioning in young disabled children often depend on unreliable
measures or clinical judgments of undetermined reliability. Therefore one needs to be
aware of the arbitrary and often subjective nature of the exclusionary criteria upon which
the diagnosis of DLD rests. The issue of defining exclusionary factors in studies of DLD
remains a hotly debated subject, in need of careful exploration both for research purposes and for its clinical implications (Nye and Weems 1991).

*Application of discrepancy criteria*
Besides using exclusionary criteria to identify children with language disorders of
unknown etiology, investigators began using discrepancy criteria to document the degree
of language impairment. They argued that the diagnosis of specific language disorder
requires that there be a discrepancy between language skills and nonverbal aspects of
cognition, and that this discrepancy differentiates specific language disorder from more
generalized cognitive impairment, *i.e.* mental retardation.

Although current practice is to define DLD on the basis of a discrepancy between
nonverbal and verbal abilities, the reference points used in practice vary (Nye and
Montgomery 1989, Nye and Weems 1991).
• *Clinical reference.* The use of a clinical reference implies that an individual familiar
with normal development and with the particular child's development, *e.g.* a parent,
clinician, pediatrician or teacher, identifies the child's language skills as impaired, compared to other aspects of development. The use of a clinical referent constitutes the
expert diagnosis approach used in many studies (*e.g.* Strauss 1954, de Ajuriaguerra *et al.*
1976, Allen and Rapin 1980, Rapin and Allen 1983).
• *Quantitative discrepancy scores.* The other current practice for identifying DLD is to
use quantitative discrepancy scores. This approach includes the following alternatives.
(a) *Age reference.* The use of age reference points identifies a child as DLD when his

16

age score on a particular test of language falls below a specified age range. After exploring various approaches to establishing criteria for severity of language disorder, Stark and Tallal (1981) defined children with DLD as those with a combined receptive and expressive language age 12 months or more below their chronological age. They used different age reference points for receptive and expressive language.

(b) *Language test norms.* This approach identifies children as DLD if, on tests of language functioning, they perform one or two standard deviations below the norms for their age. For example, a child's performance on a particular test, such as the Peabody Picture Vocabulary Test—Revised (Dunn and Dunn 1981) might be compared to the age norms for that particular test to determine if a large enough discrepancy exists between the child's score and the norm.

(c) *Performance IQ.* A discrepancy of one or two standard deviations between NVIQ and a measure of language performance is also widely used in the identification of DLD children. This approach is based on the assumption that a child with a significantly lower language score than NVIQ is exhibiting a deficit that is specific to language as opposed to overall cognitive function, and is often referred to as 'cognitive referencing' (Cole *et al.* 1990).

*Issues in the use of clinical reference and discrepancy criteria*
Determining the presence of a language disorder on the basis of clinical reference may have considerable validity, especially in the hands of experienced clinicians sensitive to both delayed and deviant aspects of a child's language skills. Nation and Aram (1990), in discussing concepts of speech and language variation, suggested that, rather than depending on inclusionary or exclusionary criteria, a diagnosis of DLD should rest on the judgment of the clinician assessing the child who exhibits the problem or of others in a position to evaluate the child's ability. For example, the parents of a child who may be unaware of his language disorder may judge him to have a language problem; by the same token, a child who does consider himself to have a problem may not be so judged by his peers. From this perspective, a highly intelligent child who is verbally reticent may, in his parents' estimate, present a language problem. For that specific child, this apparent deficiency may represent almost as much of a perceived liability as the language inadequacies of the vast majority of criterion-determined DLD children, even though objective tests do not demonstrate subnormal verbal skills.

Perhaps parents and clinicians are better judges than any objective test data, given the complexity of language and the significant heterogeneity among children's levels of function. Tomblin (1983) uses a 'normative' perspective to define language disorders in children. This normative approach suggests that a language disorder is a function of the relationship between a level of language performance and some socially based evaluation of that performance.

However, the use of clinical reference for identifying language disorders in children is not without problems. The fact that parents and clinicians bring their own sets of expectations, bases of knowledge, and levels of expertise and training, suggests that relying on parental or clinical judgment would be too subjective to provide replicable findings. Recently, however, Records and Tomblin (1994) have demonstrated that clinical decision making can be objectified and that clinicians can have significant agreement in determining whether or not a child is language impaired.

The problems most often encountered in the application of discrepancy criteria involve the measurement of nonverbal intelligence and language abilities, and how best to define the scope of discrepancy (Casby 1992, Aram *et al* 1993). The use of IQ measures presents numerous difficulties, not only with regard to their validity, but also with respect to the appropriate choice of measures and how one uses them (Cole *et al.* 1990, 1994). One of the concerns with using IQ measurements to identify discrepancies is determining which aspect or aspects of nonverbal cognition should be compared to language skills. Investigators have speculated that some young DLD children demonstrate subtle deficits in symbolic representation which may be reflected in certain measures of nonverbal functioning (Snyder 1978, Kamhi 1981, Johnston and Ellis Weismer 1983, Johnston and Ramstad 1983, Masterson 1993). This issue raises concern about the interpretation of summary IQ scores when applied to an impaired population, such as children with DLD. Summary IQ scores may not be valid indicators of a child's abilities, but rather reflections of the child's impairments (Wilson 1986). Finally, several of the available nonverbal measures with normative information have psychometric weaknesses (*e.g.* Arthur Adaptation of the Leiter International Performance Scale—Arthur 1952; Merrill–Palmer Scale of Mental Tests—Stutsman 1931; see Johnston 1982), whereas others do not adequately assess the full range of abilities (*e.g.* Stanford–Binet Intelligence Scale, Revised—Thorndike *et al.* 1986).

These same issues, and others, are relevant when addressing the measurement of language abilities of children with DLD, and the application of discrepancy criteria. One of the main limitations in using a language discrepancy score is that psychometric language test scores in young children may or may not reflect language functions in a naturalistic setting. While it is assumed that scores are representative of a particular child's functioning, there are few means for quantifying actual language functioning in daily life settings. Recent studies have criticized the psychometric properties (*e.g.* reliability, validity, normative characteristics) of standardized language measures as well as their suitability for clinical practice (*e.g.* naturalistic, pragmatic characteristics) (Berk 1984, McCauley and Swisher 1984, Lieberman and Michael 1986).

The multiple aspects of language, and the question of how to test and quantify these aspects also present major problems for using discrepancy scores. Taking into consideration the multiple levels of language (*i.e.* phonology, syntax, semantics and pragmatics), as well as both comprehension and production, requires that a discrepancy score reflect any and all deficits at each of these levels. The issue then becomes one of arriving at a composite discrepancy score which represents the child's functioning adequately and accurately. As before, the discrepancy score assumes psychometric validity of the measures of all these levels, and implies an inherent understanding of the weight of each level and aspect of language, *e.g.* an understanding of whether a syntactic deficit should carry as much weight as a phonological deficit in determining a discrepancy. It is not clear whether difficulties with each and every one of the multiple aspects of language need to be consolidated when calculating discrepancy scores. Is impairment in one area sufficient, or must a certain overall threshold be exceeded for it to constitute a language disorder? Johnston (1988) has warned against the use of a single index as descriptive of a child's linguistic level, as asynchronies in the development of different aspects of language have been documented in children with DLD (Weiner 1974, Johnston and Schery 1976, Bloom and Lahey 1978, Leonard 1979, Steckol and Leonard 1979). It is likely that linguistic profiles, which take into account a number of language domains, ultimately will be most useful for characterizing children with DLD (Bishop and Edmundson 1987, Johnston 1988).

The final issue to be addressed here involves determining how large a discrepancy is required to diagnose a child as DLD. Typically, a discrepancy of one standard deviation or more is used to identify DLD. Questions remain as to how this number was selected and whether it represents a sufficient difference. Further, the field of developmental language disorders has not yet agreed upon any particular standard. For example, in their national survey of US state agencies, Nye and Montgomery (1989) found that several states did not require the use of standardized discrepancy formulas, and that for those states employing discrepancy criteria, the size of the discrepancy required varied considerably.

Furthermore, the issue of interpreting high NVIQs with respect to language functioning has not been addressed adequately. Whether the child with an NVIQ of 130 and a language score of 115 is really language disordered depends in part on the inter-test variability of the measures. Using a discrepancy implies that the inter-test variability of the measures is comparable, *i.e.* that norms for both tests were established on the same groups. Another problem involves regression to the mean; that is, the more extreme the scores the more variability is observed among scores. It may be that greater discrepancies between verbal and nonverbal scores are observed at the extremes of the distribution, thus raising the question of whether skill areas are comparable in this range. Regression to the mean also suggests that individuals with NVIQ scores at the extreme ends of the continuum will obtain scores in other skill areas, such as language, that are closer to the mean. Therefore, children with low NVIQ scores may not be identified as DLD because their language scores are likely to regress to the mean, and by the same token, children with high NVIQ scores may be over-identified.

We have little understanding of how discrepancies between language and other aspects of cognition change over time. The question is two-fold: is it appropriate to require the same discrepancy across all age levels, and do similar discrepancies at different ages have the same significance? A one-year or two standard deviation discrepancy is likely to signify a greater impairment at age 2 than at age 6. These issues have not yet been explored systematically.

**Classification criteria for the Nosology Study**

In consideration of the many pitfalls in defining and identifying children with DLD, the following set of criteria, based on the preceding review of practices, was chosen for the Nosology Study (see Chapter 4 for details).

- *Hearing.* No significant hearing loss in either ear.
- *Monolingual.* A predominantly English speaking family.
- *Neurological and craniofacial status.* No gross motor deficit or malformation, no uncontrolled seizures, no multiple or high doses of anticonvulsant or psychotropic drugs.
- *IQ.* An IQ of at least 80 on the Abstract and Visual Reasoning subtests of the Stanford–Binet (Thorndike *et al.* 1986).
- *Social behavior.* Lack of positive scores on the Wing Autistic Disorders Interview Checklist (see Appendix 1) or, when there were positive scores, evaluation by a psychiatrist for absence of a psychiatric diagnosis.
- *Language deficit.* Presence of a clinically significant language disorder. This was operationalized as a deficient score on the Test of Early Language Development (TELD) (Hresko *et al.* 1981), defined as less than 80 or greater than one standard deviation below NVIQ. Children who did not achieve basal scores on the TELD were identified using the Sequenced Inventory of Communication Development (Revised Edition) (Hedrick *et al.* 1984). Additionally, a one standard deviation discrepancy between chronological age and a mean length of utterances (MLU) age score (based on Miller's norms, 1981) was used to identify children with clinically defined language deficits not identified by TELD/Stanford–Binet criteria.
- *Age.* All of the DLD children were between the ages of 3 years and 5 years 11 months at the start of testing.

**Summary**
Review of both the historical and current uses of exclusionary and discrepancy criteria revealed a number of shortcomings in the application of these procedures for defining DLDs. There are difficulties in defining the scope of exclusionary factors adequately, and stringent application of these criteria may lead to the exclusion of a variable portion of the children with DLDs. Problems in using discrepancy criteria include the choices of references to be used in determining the discrepancy (*e.g.* clinical or psychometric), and the size of discrepancy required. We have summarized the variables we used to determine eligibility for the DLD group of the Nosology Study in light of the historical background on exclusionary and discrepancy criteria in the classification of DLD.

# 3
# CLASSIFICATION OF AUTISTIC DISORDER (AD)

*L. Waterhouse*

**History of diagnostic criteria for autism**

In 1943 Kanner identified a disorder he labelled 'early infantile autism'. In that paper he argued that the defining features of early infantile autism were aloofness and indifference to others, absorption in meaningless and repetitive activities, and good rote memory, accompanied by an attractive physical appearance. Fifty years have elapsed since Kanner defined the syndrome of autism, and during this period there has been a great deal of research and theoretical formulation, much of it directed at discovering the underlying basis for the cluster of features in the syndrome that he described.

Kanner's clinical vision of the syndrome of autism was followed by a series of redefinitions. At present most research workers and clinicians use one of two formal clinical diagnostic systems to identify cases of autism. The first of these comprises the variant definitions formulated by the American Psychiatric Association (APA) and published in three editions of their *Diagnostic and Statistical Manual of Mental Disorders*, *viz*. DSM III: Infantile Autism (APA 1980); DSM III-R: Autistic Disorder (APA 1987); and DSM IV: Autistic Disorder (APA 1994). The second formal clinical system is the World Health Organization (WHO) *International Classification of Diseases* (ICD-10, WHO 1993). As we began our project in 1985, we employed both the 1980 DSM III criteria for Infantile Autism and the 1987 DSM III-R criteria for Autistic Disorder (which were available in draft form) in a psychiatric clinical evaluation. We later constructed algorithms of symptoms to generate ICD-10 and DSM IV diagnoses. Research grouping in the present study is based on DSM III-R criteria because these were the standard criteria for classification at the inception of our project and because they offered the greatest sample coverage, as maximal coverage was crucial for our goals of exploring nosological boundaries and investigating possible subtypes (Waterhouse *et al*. 1993).

For most diagnostic formulations developed following Kanner's initial description of a cluster of features, there has been an awareness that autism is part of a larger spectrum of syndromes. The spectrum is now generally identified as 'pervasive developmental disorders' (PDDs) and is characterized by impairment in the development of reciprocal social interaction and communication skills, along with a markedly restricted repertoire of activities. Table 3.1 puts the criteria for subgroups within diagnostic systems for PDDs in historical perspective. The Group for the Advancement of Psychiatry (1966) classified Early Infantile Autism among the five 'psychoses' of childhood it identified. In contrast, DSM II (APA 1968) included only a single category for child-

**TABLE 3.1**
**Diagnostic classifications of severe childhood psychopathology**

**GAP** (1966)
*Psychotic Disorders*
a. Psychoses of infancy and early childhood
    1. Early Infantile Autism
    2. Interactional Psychotic Disorder (symbiotic)
    3. Other Psychosis of Infancy and Early Childhood
b. Psychoses of later childhood
    1. Schizophreniform Psychotic Disorder
    2. Other Psychosis of Later Childhood
c. Psychoses of adolescence
    1. Acute Confusional State
    2. Schizophrenic Disorder, adult type
    3. Other Psychosis of Adolescence

**DSM II** (1968)
295.8 Schizophrenia, childhood type

**DSM III** (1980)
*Pervasive Developmental Disorders*
299.0X Infantile Autism (full syndrome or residual)
299.9X Childhood Onset Pervasive Developmental Disorder (full syndrome or residual)
299.8X Atypical Pervasive Developmental Disorder
(NB: Adult-type schizophrenia with onset in childhood is identified but excluded from the pervasive developmental disorders)

**DSM III-R** (1987)
*Pervasive Developmental Disorders*
299.0 Autistic Disorder
299.80 Pervasive Developmental Disorder Not Otherwise Specified

**DSM IV** (1994)
*Pervasive Developmental Disorders*
299.00 Autistic Disorder
299.80 Rett's Disorder
299.10 Childhood Disintegrative Disorder
299.80 Asperger's Disorder
299.80 Pervasive Developmental Disorder Not Otherwise Specified (including Atypical Autism)

**ICD-9** (1978)
299    *Psychoses with origin specific to childhood*
299.0 Infantile Autism (=childhood autism, infantile psychosis, Kanner's syndrome)
299.1 Disintegrative Psychosis (=Heller's syndrome)
299.8 Other (=atypical childhood psychosis)
299.9 Unspecified (=child psychosis NOS, childhood schizophrenia NOS) (excludes schizophrenia of adult type occurring in childhood)

**ICD-10** (1993)
F84    *Pervasive developmental disorders*
F84.0 Childhood Autism
F84.1 Atypical Autism
F84.2 Rett Syndrome
F84.3 Other Childhood Disintegrative Disorder
F84.4 Overactive Disorder Associated with Mental Retardation and Stereotyped Movements
F84.5 Asperger Syndrome
F84.8 Other
F84.9 Unspecified

hood psychopathology, called 'Schizophrenia, childhood type'. The term 'psychosis' was retained up to the four-item classification proposed by the WHO's ICD-9 in 1978; DSM III (APA 1980) subsequently discarded it, introducing the term 'PDD' for children with autistic-like conditions. It was the first classification system to differentiate Schizophrenia Occurring in Childhood unequivocally from autism (PDD) by including it among the schizophrenias. DSM III PDD comprised three main types, plus residual states for children with Infantile Autism or Childhood Onset PDD who had in the past but now no longer fulfilled criteria for these diagnoses. DSM III-R (APA 1987) collapsed the five DSM III types of PDD into just two, Autistic Disorder and PDD Not Otherwise Specified (PDD-NOS). DSM IV (APA 1994) retained these two DSM III-R categories but added three new ones: Rett's Disorder, Asperger's Disorder and Disintegrative Disorder. The ICD-10 (WHO 1993) expanded PDD to include eight diagnostic types which overlap, but only partially, with the five DSM IV categories.

This shifting array of diagnostic categories reflects the problematic establishment of discrete syndromes of severe childhood psychopathology over the past 50 years (Green *et al.* 1984; Tanguay 1984; Coleman and Gillberg 1985; Quay 1985; Asarnow *et al.* 1986; Cohen *et al.* 1986; Waterhouse *et al.* 1987; Rutter and Schopler 1988; Wing 1988, 1993; Gillberg 1992). There are many reasons for diagnostic complexity (Cohen *et al.* 1976, Waterhouse *et al.* 1989, Rapin 1992, Waterhouse 1994), including major developmental variability in behavioral expression of symptoms. Symptoms may take many forms at different developmental and chronological ages. Another major cause of diagnostic complexity in autistic spectrum disorders is the very wide range of abnormal and impaired behavior including variation in the core deficit of social dysfunction as well as variation in patterns of cognitive function, *e.g.* abnormalities of memory, perception, attention, and motor and vegetative function.

Kanner at first considered that the cluster of abnormal behaviors he called early infantile autism formed a unique syndrome, separate from all other conditions. Later he was influenced by the arguments of Louise Despert to suggest that autism might be the earliest manifestation of schizophrenia; a number of other workers agreed with this view (Bender 1947, Goldfarb 1964, Fish 1977). For a period of time the term 'childhood schizophrenia' was used by many authors to cover all forms of severe childhood psychiatric syndromes (Creak *et al.* 1961, Creak 1963). However, a series of studies reviewed by Kolvin (1971) demonstrated the major differences between, on the one hand, the disorders involving impaired development of social interaction and empathy, usually from birth or early childhood, and, on the other, disorders with onset in later childhood which, in typical form, are characterized by delusions, hallucinations, and abnormal thought and will. The former, which include autism, are now referred to as the pervasive developmental disorders and the latter as schizophrenia occurring in childhood (SOC).

*Diagnosis and heterogeneity*
Although individuals with marked autistic features are now generally grouped under a diagnosis of 'autistic disorder', a variety of studies (Wing and Gould 1979; Waterhouse and Fein 1982, 1984; Dahl *et al.* 1986; Gillberg 1992) have shown that it is difficult to

make empirical groupings which clearly delineate differences between autistic children and the larger group with PDD or autistic spectrum disorders. This difficulty persists in part because some investigators and clinicians take the term autism to refer to a general global classification, while others apply it to a small group of children with a particular form of severe social deficit. It persists also because the assemblage of impairments which define autism also serve to define (with less specificity) non-autistic PDDs.

In 1973 Kanner published a follow-up of his original 11 cases of early infantile autism. In this paper he reported that he was surprised to find that the outcome as far as social and cognitive functioning was extremely variable. This wide variation in prognosis continues to be the case for individuals diagnosed as autistic today. Heterogeneity in etiology, neuroanatomic findings, cognitive functioning, social behavior and prognosis among persons with a diagnosis of autism has been blamed on the inadequacies of the systems used for diagnosis (Parks 1983), or on the incorrect use of diagnostic systems in research or clinical settings (Meehl 1986). Such arguments notwithstanding, it is unlikely that incorrect use of diagnostic systems is a major factor in the capture of heterogeneous samples of individuals diagnosed as autistic. It is more likely that the heterogeneity is real and inherent in autism defined behaviorally. Autism as a syndrome—the autistic spectrum of disorders—includes many different sorts of children who have many different sorts of brain dysfunction that have in common particular behavioral, social and communicative impairments. That they share dysfunction in a common brain system(s), with or without dysfunction in other systems, is a widely held but unproven assumption (Fein *et al.* 1987; Rapin 1987, 1991; Waterhouse 1994).

Behavioral heterogeneity among children with autistic disorder and PDD-NOS may be related in part to their many known etiologies. Genetic syndromes suggesting X-linked patterns of inheritance, including fragile X and Rett syndromes, have been associated with autism and PDD (Folstein and Piven 1991, Gillberg and Coleman 1992). There are families in which autism appears to be inherited as a particular genetic syndrome with an autosomal recessive or dominant pattern of inheritance (Ritvo *et al.* 1985, Folstein and Piven 1991). There is some evidence that deleterious perinatal events may be reported somewhat more often than expected in autistic children, although a majority of studies have shown no association between perinatal events and the presence of autistic spectrum disorders (Nelson 1991). Studies of the biochemistry of autistic individuals have suggested that there may be anomalies in the serotoninergic and dopaminergic systems of a substantial subset of autistic individuals (Coleman and Gillberg 1985). Furthermore, certain viral diseases like congenital rubella and cytomegalovirus, and metabolic diseases like phenylketonuria, abnormalities of purine metabolism and lactic acidosis can produce autistic symptoms, as can such well known genetic disorders as tuberous sclerosis, incontinentia pigmenti and others (for a review, see Gillberg and Coleman 1992).

Most importantly, of course, it is likely that at the level of pathophysiology, nearly all individuals who are diagnosable as autistic or as having PDD-NOS have some as yet undefined neurological deficit (Rapin 1987). Routine imaging of the brain in autism of unknown etiology is almost always unrevealing, and the few available pathological studies have disclosed no unitary major malformation nor any sign of inflammation or degenerative disease (Bauman and Kemper 1994). On the basis of morphometric analyses of MRI images, Courchesne and colleagues argue that developmental abnormalities of the cerebellar vermis play a critical part in the pathophysiology of autism (Courchesne *et.al.* 1988, 1994; Courchesne 1991). A variety of other neurological explorations have documented ventricular enlargement in a significant number of autistic individuals, and a variety of EEG and evoked potential abnormalities (Fein *et al.* 1987, Reichler and Lee 1987, Minshew 1991, Dunn 1994). None of these abnormalities is specific to autism. Quantitative analyses of whole brain serial sections from a few autistic individuals (Bauman 1991, Bauman and Kemper 1994) have disclosed evidence suggesting cellular maldevelopment in the hippocampus, amygdala and mesial limbic structures, as well as in the cerebellar hemispheres and inferior olive. Because the limbic system is well known to control emotional and social behavior, its malfunction had been predicted in autism (Maurer and Damasio 1982). The cerebellar abnormalities bring up new ideas about the role of the cerebellum in learning, attention and cognition.

*Attempts to subtype within the autistic spectrum*
A variety of attempts have been made to subtype the PDD spectrum on behavioral grounds. Wing and Gould (1979), for example, classified PDD children on the basis of their sociability (aloof, passive, active-but-odd), a classification validated by Volkmar *et al.* (1989), Castelloe and Dawson (1993) and Dawson *et al.* (1996). Allen (1988) classified children on the basis of communication and play as well as other specific behaviors. Other studies have attempted classification on the basis of cognitive or language abilities or disabilities (Simmons and Baltaxe 1975, Fein *et al.* 1985, Allen and Rapin 1992, Martineau *et al.* 1992), presence or absence of EEG abnormalities (Tsai *et al.* 1985), age of onset, or developmental course (Prior *et al.* 1975, Gillberg and Schaumann 1981, Burd *et al.* 1989, Percy *et al.* 1990, Kurita *et al.* 1992, Volkmar 1992), although no consistent findings have yet emerged relating onset to course or to outcome.

Degree of mental retardation has been found to be significantly correlated with degree of symptomatology in all three domains of autistic impairment (Volkmar *et al.* 1992). Some researchers, consequently, have suggested the use of IQ in defining subtypes (Rutter and Garmezy 1983). Cohen *et al.* (1987) and Tsai (1992) argue for a primary division between high- and low-functioning autism, pointing out important differences between them, in patterns of communication, educational needs, outcome, and likelihood of neurological signs. Level of intellectual functioning has also been found to be related to the Wing and Gould subtypes (Volkmar *et al.* 1989, Castelloe and Dawson 1993), to family history (DeLong and Dwyer 1988, Gillberg 1989, Piven *et al.* 1990), to pharmacological response (August *et al.* 1987, duVerglas *et al.* 1988), to co-morbidity with Tourette syndrome (Burd *et al.* 1987a) and with schizophrenia (Petty *et al.* 1985), to minor physical anomalies (Links 1980), to handedness (Fein *et al.* 1985, Soper *et al.* 1986), to developmental regressions and unevenness (Kurita *et al.* 1992), to the development of seizures (Bartak and Rutter 1976), and to seasonal birth differences (Konstantareas *et al.* 1986).

Some investigators have used a variety of empirical and statistical methods to define PDD subgroups (Prior *et al.* 1975, Bartak *et al.* 1977, Siegel *et al.* 1986, Overall and Campbell 1988, Bagley and McGeein 1989); although tantalizing findings emerge from each of these studies, there is little consistency in method or results among them. Beginnings have also been made in investigating etiologies that may correspond to certain behavioral or cognitive profiles (Deutsch *et al.* 1986, Reichelt *et al.* 1986, Ritvo *et al.* 1986, Ho *et al.* 1988, Coleman 1990, Gillberg 1992).

*Diagnosis of autism as a unitary disorder*

Although heterogeneity is a hallmark of the syndrome of autism and leads us to understand it as a spectrum disorder, there is a continuing impression of clinical unity for the disorder. Therefore, there continues to be research in which the syndrome is understood as a single entity. Despite this, researchers to date have found no single shared etiology, no uniquely pathognomonic neural deficit, no shared specific set of cognitive dysfunctions, and no shared specific life course or unity in response to drug treatment. A literature review suggested that only a subgroup of autistic individuals in a given sample will exhibit the particular validating biological marker under study (Waterhouse *et al.* 1989).

In the past 45 years trends in research have highlighted a series of features suggesting a unifying basis for disorders on the autistic spectrum. First, explanations centered on parents as causal agents in the generation of autistic behavior. Next, research focused on language deficits and then on cognitive functioning (Gillberg 1990). There has also been a clear focus on the possible neurological dysfunctions which are hypothesized to underlie both language and cognitive deficits in autism (Rutter 1974, Rapin 1987).

Current research addresses two sorts of questions. The first is 'What is the underlying neurological source for the wide range of behavioral deficit found in autism?' In this line of research efforts are being made through a variety of invasive and noninvasive methods to explore specific anatomic loci for autistic behavior. The second line of current research is direct exploration of the nature of the social impairment. Some researchers have argued that the direct basis for social impairment is a neurological deficit (Fein *et al.* 1986). Others have argued that mechanisms of impaired attention lead to dysfunction in the ability to attend to complex social events (Maurer and Damasio 1982, Dawson and Lew 1989, Ornitz 1994). Still others have argued that impaired social imagination (Wing 1981), or impaired social cognition, or impaired conceptualization of other people's inner thoughts or feelings (Baron-Cohen 1991, Rogers and Pennington 1991) define the core social impairment of autism.

While much of contemporary research focuses on a direct exploration of the social and other behavioral impairments in autism, a great deal of investigation and much speculation are taking place regarding the underlying locus or nature of a brain deficit that might give rise to such a behavioral syndrome. Controversy among investigators continues unabated. Could autism be defined as a specific brain disorder with a specific set of etiologies and a specific locus of cerebral pathology (Rutter and Schopler 1988)? Or is autism better understood as a consequence of multiple continua generating a behavioral syndrome of social and behavioral impairment (Waterhouse *et al.* 1989)?

**Differential diagnosis**

Even though autism is presently defined as Autistic Disorder in DSM-IV and as Childhood Autism in ICD-10, it has been repeatedly found in research sample selection and in clinical diagnosis that these formulations yield fuzzy boundaries, with a variety of disorders thought to lie outside the autistic spectrum. These boundary problems are similar to those found for autism within the spectrum of PDDs, although variation in social impairment is more complex within the PDD range of disorders.

*Autism and mental retardation*

Explorations of differential diagnosis have shown fuzzy diagnostic boundaries between autistic spectrum disorders and mental retardation. For example, Freeman *et al.* (1984) found that the behavioral expression of the syndrome of autism could exist in the behavior of mentally retarded individuals who had not been diagnosed as autistic by DSM III. In 1979, Wing and Gould reported in an epidemiological study that half of all the severely retarded children were also socially impaired in a variety of ways, some of which fitted diagnostic formulations for autism and some of which did not. Wing and Gould also reported that the lower the level of intelligence, the more likely it was that the social impairment would be aloofness and indifference.

In general, research findings have suggested that about one half of all individuals diagnosed as autistic have measured IQs <50 and that fewer than one third have IQs >70. It is important to note that the DSM definition of mental retardation includes some behaviors associated with the diagnosis of autism: stereotypies, self-injurious behavior and poor social relatedness. A diagnosis dependent on these behaviors may be indexing severe brain damage and thus indexing mental retardation.

Bartak and Rutter (1976) argued that high-functioning autistic individuals form a separate group from those who are mentally retarded. However, attempts to validate this have not supported a sharp behavioral distinction (Prior 1979, Wing 1988). Autistic children with higher IQs generally have a better prognosis than do those with lower IQs. This does not prove that there are two IQ subsyndromes within the autistic spectrum, it simply suggests that higher IQ is associated with better outcome. Burd *et al.* (1987*b*) argued that hyperlexia is also an index for future positive outcome in PDD. The presence of higher IQ or hyperlexia or both may signal that an individual autistic child's nervous system is initially less dysfunctional, or is capable of greater beneficent maturation during development. Clearly, higher versus lower IQ in autism cannot be seen as separating out mental retardation from the 'pure' disorder of autism.

In the present study, we have chosen to create two sample groups out of our larger group of children with AD. These two groups consist of children whose NVIQs are ≥80 and <80. We have chosen to do this not because we are committed to the notion that those children whose NVIQs are above 80 represent the 'pure' disorder of autism, but because it has allowed us to compare the social and communicative disorders of the autistic sample with contrast samples. Thus for children who receive a diagnosis of autism and whose NVIQs are below normal, the boundary problem between autism and mental retardation will exist. However, in Chapters 5 through 10 we report findings to suggest a variety of means for clinically differentiating individuals with autism from those with low NVIQ without autistic features (NALIQ).

*Autism and developmental language disorder*

For children who are diagnosed as autistic and who have low–normal or normal NVIQs, there is sometimes difficulty in defining the boundary between autism and receptive DLD (Bartak *et al.* 1975, Bishop and Adams 1989). One of the criterial features of autism common to all diagnostic systems is the presence of disorders in verbal communication. Paul and Cohen (1984*b*) studied a sample of adolescents who had been diagnosed as having DLD but had atypical features. They found that many of the behaviors of the DLD children in the sample would justify diagnoses of autism.

The language behaviors that exist at the fuzzy boundary of DLD and autism include a wide range of specific language disabilities, from total mutism to severe dysfluencies and impaired comprehension to language development characterized by normal syntax and phonology with impaired fluency or prosody (Allen and Rapin 1992). Some children with a primary diagnosis of DLD may have echolalia and prosodic impairment, both of which are characteristic of specific language impairments found in autism. When children have a variety of severe language disabilities and have near normal or normal NVIQs, the distinction between DLD and AD depends, in large part, on the individual child's expression of aberrant social relatedness (Allen 1988). Some DLD children do have impaired social relatedness, such as excessive shyness or even mutism, but most do not have the extreme aloofness or lack of social interest that characterizes children diagnosable as having AD.

A recent comparison of 40 DSM III-R autistic children, 40 PDD-NOS children and 40 children with DLD (Mayes *et al.* 1993) has suggested that impaired conversation was the only point of similarity between PDD-NOS and the language disorder groups, whereas indices of social deficit, such as withdrawal and the absence of friendships, clearly differentiated the socially impaired PDD-NOS children from children with language disorders. The method for determining the presence of a language disorder in the 40 children classified as having DLD is not outlined by the authors, thus limiting interpretation of these findings. Although subjects' IQs are not reported, it can be inferred from chronological age and mental age means that the average of study subjects' IQs must have been approximately 70. If so, then this study has compared mentally retarded children who have language disorders with retarded autistic and PDD-NOS children. Because the samples thus provide a sound basis for skill and symptom comparisons, these data suppose clear differentiation of language disordered children and PDD-NOS children.

In the present study we found 11 children among the 201 classified as having DLD (all with NVIQ ≥80) to have some behavioral autistic features. These features were largely limited to aspects of impaired social communication. The psychiatrist found that these 11 children did not meet diagnostic criteria for DSM III-R Autistic Disorder, nor did they express enough autistic-like features to classify them as PDD-NOS. In other words, their social deficits were not severe enough to place them on the autistic spectrum.

While essentially all verbal autistic subjects in the present study expressed some form of language disorder, the DLD children generally did not express the social impairments associated with autism and PDD-NOS. The issue of classification of individual children is addressed in Chapter 10.

*Autism and Asperger syndrome*

Still another boundary problem has been differentiating those children with AD who have higher NVIQs and generally good cognitive functioning from those with Asperger syndrome, another high-functioning group with developmental problems in social relatedness and social communication. Asperger syndrome refers to children with autistic features who are verbal or even verbose, whose language is often pedantic, who are obsessionally concerned with some narrow topic, and who are often clumsy (Frith 1991). The differential diagnosis between autism and Asperger syndrome currently included in ICD-10 and DSM IV proposes that autism and Asperger syndrome share two core diagnostic features, (1) impairments in reciprocal social interaction, and (2) restricted, repetitive and stereotyped interests and activities, but differ in that Asperger syndrome is not to be diagnosed if the child is significantly delayed in language or cognitive development. Wing (1991) has pointed out, however, that this diagnostic formulation contrast ignores a crucial feature of the four cases on which Asperger built his syndrome: aberrant language use. If the language features Asperger originally identified (topic fixation, persistent echolalia, empty speech, and pressured incessant speech) were incorporated in the current diagnostic formulations, Asperger syndrome would be indistinguishable from 'high-functioning' autism. In fact, one author (Happé 1991) has argued that she could find no difference between Asperger syndrome and able autistic persons if 'able autistic' means adequate language and normal intelligence.

Are less severe autism and Asperger syndrome separable disorders? Their paths of clinical discovery by Kanner and Asperger and current diagnostic formulations are nearly identical. What is really needed to identify Asperger syndrome as unique is empirical evidence (*e.g.* Szatmari *et al.* 1989*a,b*; Ozonoff *et al.* 1991). Research reported by Gillberg (1991) and Wing (1991) suggests that Asperger syndrome may have both a developmental and a genetic relationship to autism. Some individuals diagnosable as autistic in childhood meet criteria for Asperger syndrome in adulthood, and the investigation of the families of autistic individuals has revealed relatives with Asperger syndrome.

There are no comparative brain scan, brain physiology or neuroanatomical data with which to distinguish Asperger syndrome from autism, although two authors do invoke neurological models. Gillberg (1991) has proposed that Asperger syndrome may involve 'autism areas' in the brain plus other areas which regulate motor but not expressive language skills, whereas Wing (1991) has concluded that autism and Asperger syndrome are descriptors for overlapping parts of the same behavioral continuum. In our study sample of 176 (DSM III-R) AD children we found that no children were classified with Asperger syndrome. One child classified as part of our sample of 18 DSM III-R PDD-NOS children was diagnosed as having Asperger syndrome by both DSM IV and

ICD-10. Under the DSM III diagnostic system this same child was diagnosed as having COPDD. While it is likely that Asperger syndrome and autism in high-functioning individuals overlap, our uniform DSM III-R AD selection criteria at the young age of admission to the study meant that the majority of the children were seriously affected, virtually precluding referral of children with Asperger syndrome features.

**Classification criteria for the Nosology Study**

Selection of the study sample was accomplished in stages. Initially, children had to have been identified by a clinical professional as having marked impairment in social relatedness and communication. They were then screened for the presence of the claimed social impairment, using the Wing Autistic Disorder Interview Checklist (WADIC—Appendix 1). Children who met the initial screening requirements were seen by a child psychiatrist who conducted a structured psychiatric evaluation which included determination of DSM III and DSM III-R diagnoses. We chose to conduct data analysis on the sample defined by DSM III-R as AD because it provided the greatest coverage: 176 DSM III-R AD cases *vs* 98 DSM III Infantile Autism cases in the same sample of 194 children (Waterhouse *et al.* 1996). Selection methodology is discussed in more detail in Chapter 4.

In order to extend our knowledge of the behavioral repertoires of autistic children, we included in our study interviews of mothers and teachers, and behavioral observations by psychiatrists and neurologists (see Chapter 4 for details of the measures used). We have evaluated the children with standardized psychological tests and examined their language and play in some detail. The behavioral data we have collected has permitted us to generate DSM IV and ICD-10 diagnoses for the children in our sample. ICD-10 criteria yielded 125 positively diagnosed cases of Childhood Autism. DSM IV criteria yielded 115 positive diagnoses of Autistic Disorder. The rich diagnostic data we have collected will permit us to generate other diagnostic classifications in the future and have enabled us to develop a new empirical taxonomic approach for detecting autism and its subtypes (see Chapter 10) which we hope will be useful to clinicians as well as investigators of this complex developmental disorder.

**Summary**

Autism is part of a larger spectrum of disorders of sociability, social communication, and ritual or repetitive behaviors generally referred to as pervasive developmental disorder. There have been many variant clinical formulations of subgroups within this spectrum. For our study we used DSM III-R criteria for Autistic Disorder to form our sample because it provided the greatest coverage—crucial for our project because our goals were to explore the boundaries of the spectrum and to look for subtypes of autism.

# 4
# METHODOLOGY

*R. Morris, D.A. Allen, D.M. Aram, R. David, M. Dunn, D. Fein, I. Rapin, L. Wainwright, L. Waterhouse and B.C. Wilson\**

## Subjects

*Subject selection*

The major goal of recruitment and classification was to form reliable and meaningful clinical groups defined by operational criteria. Another goal was to achieve good coverage of the population under study: preschool and young school-age children with significant communication difficulties. These children were expected to fall into three major groups: developmental language disorder (DLD); autistic disorder (AD); and non-autistic, low IQ (NALIQ). The criteria for forming the four *a priori* groups contrasted in this monograph are described below. We divided the AD group arbitrarily into two subgroups on the basis of NVIQ in such a way that the DLD children would match the higher-functioning AD (HAD) children and the NALIQ group would match the lower-functioning AD (LAD) children, in nonverbal cognitive functioning. Normal controls were considered less crucial to the design of the classification project because they present less frequently for diagnosis of communication difficulties, and because the use of standardized test instruments provided normative data. A sample of normal children was included to collect normative data for non-standardized measures derived from videotaped play sessions.

A flow chart tracking the recruitment and classification of subjects is given as Figure 4.1, while the sample size at each stage of the process is shown in Table 4.1. Issues in classification and a comparison of the four *a priori* groups and similarly studied children excluded from the *a priori* groups with the empirically derived groups are discussed in Chapter 10.

RECRUITMENT

Children were recruited by (1) clinical referral for assessment or treatment of communication difficulties made to the clinician/researchers among the investigators, and (2) solicited participation of schools and programs for special needs children. Recruitment occurred at the six geographically separated sites where the investigators' institutions were located. The sites differed in the proportion of these two types of recruitment, in the type of children recruited, and in socioeconomic factors (see Tables 4.2–4.6).

---

\*R. Morris assumed major responsibility for this chapter; other participating investigators are listed alphabetically.

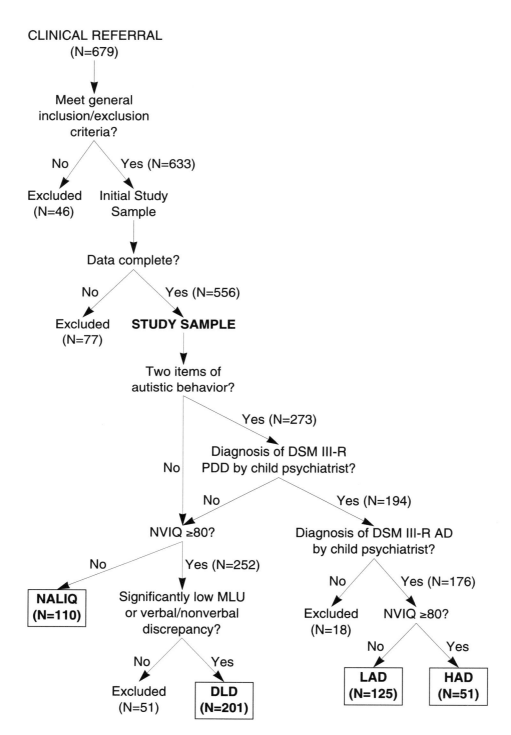

CLINICAL REFERRAL
(N=679)

Meet general
inclusion/exclusion
criteria?

No     Yes (N=633)

Excluded    Initial Study
(N=46)       Sample

Data complete?

No     Yes (N=556)

Excluded    **STUDY SAMPLE**
(N=77)

Two items of
autistic behavior?

Yes (N=273)

Diagnosis of DSM III-R
No    PDD by child psychiatrist?

No       Yes (N=194)

NVIQ ≥80?     Diagnosis of DSM III-R AD
by child psychiatrist?

No     Yes (N=252)     No     Yes (N=176)

**NALIQ**    Significantly low MLU    Excluded    NVIQ ≥80?
**(N=110)**    or verbal/nonverbal    (N=18)
       discrepancy?

No     Yes       No     Yes

Excluded    **DLD**     **LAD**    **HAD**
(N=51)     **(N=201)**    **(N=125)**    **(N=51)**

**TABLE 4.1**
**Sample sizes**

| | |
|---|---|
| **Total referred** | **679** |
| Normal | 46 |
| **Total sample** | **633** |
| Dropped out | 41 |
| Missing data | 36 |
| **Fully studied** | **556** |
| Referred as AD, failed inclusionary criteria | 18 |
| Referred as DLD, failed inclusionary criteria | 51 |
| **Final *a priori* sample** | **487** |
| DLD | 201 |
| HAD | 51 |
| LAD | 125 |
| NALIQ | 110 |

**TABLE 4.2**
**Distribution of clinical groups across sites*****

| Clinical group | Site | | | | | |
|---|---|---|---|---|---|---|
| | *Boston (N=65)* % | *Bronx (N=165)* % | *Cleveland (N=132)* % | *Manhasset (N=83)* % | *Trenton (N=42)* % | *All (N=487)* % |
| DLD | 4.6 | 23.6 | 75.0 | 71.1 | 2.4 | 41.3 |
| HAD | 10.8 | 21.2 | 2.3 | 0.0 | 14.3 | 10.5 |
| LAD | 46.2 | 37.0 | 3.0 | 0.0 | 71.4 | 25.7 |
| NALIQ | 38.5 | 18.2 | 19.7 | 28.9 | 11.9 | 22.6 |
| *Total* | 100 | 100 | 100 | 100 | 100 | 100 |

***$\chi^2$, p<0.001.

---

**Fig. 4.1.** *(Opposite)* Procedure for assignment of subjects to groups.

Children were referred clinically to the study. 633 met general exclusion/inclusion criteria. After 77 were excluded because of incomplete core data, 556 constituted the study sample. Based on whether they had at least two items in Area A or at least one each in Areas A, B and C of the Wing Autistic Disorder Interview Checklist (WADIC—see Appendix 1), children were referred to a psychiatrist who determined whether or not they fulfilled criteria for DSM III-R Autistic Disorder (AD). Of the 273 referred children, 194 met criteria for either AD (N=176) or for Pervasive Developmental Disorder Not Otherwise Specified (PDD-NOS) (N=18). The children in the AD group were later divided arbitrarily into two groups with nonverbal IQ (NVIQ) ≥80 (HAD group) or <80 (LAD group). The 79 children whom the psychiatrist diagnosed as not meeting criteria for AD or PDD-NOS were returned to the non-AD group. From this group of 362 children, those with an NVIQ <80 formed the NALIQ group (N=110). Of the remaining 252 children with an NVIQ ≥80, 201 fulfilled criteria (see text) for the DLD group, and 51 did not. The monograph is concerned with the children in the DLD, HAD, LAD, and NALIQ groups only (N=487). The 51 children who did not meet DLD criteria and the 18 who did not meet AD criteria were studied but are included only in analyses in Chapter 10 which is concerned with classification issues.

**TABLE 4.3**
**Children's gender across sites***

| Gender | Site | | | | | | |
|---|---|---|---|---|---|---|---|
| | Boston (N=65) % | Bronx (N=165) % | Cleveland (N=132) % | Manhasset (N=83) % | Trenton (N=42) % | All (N=487) % | Atlanta (N=46) % |
| Male | 84.6 | 78.2 | 68.2 | 68.7 | 83.3 | 75.2 | 62.5 |
| Female | 15.4 | 21.8 | 31.8 | 31.3 | 16.7 | 24.8 | 37.5 |
| Total | 100 | 100 | 100 | 100 | 100 | 100 | 100 |

*$\chi^2$, p<0.05.

**TABLE 4.4**
**Race of children across sites***

| Race | Site | | | | | | |
|---|---|---|---|---|---|---|---|
| | Boston (N=65) % | Bronx (N=165) % | Cleveland (N=132) % | Manhasset (N=83) % | Trenton (N=42) % | All (N=487) % | Atlanta (N=46) % |
| Caucasian | 80.0 | 64.2 | 65.2 | 89.2 | 78.6 | 72.1 | 83.3 |
| Black | 13.9 | 24.9 | 31.1 | 4.8 | 4.8 | 19.9 | 16.7 |
| Hispanic | 4.6 | 8.5 | 0.8 | 1.2 | 0.0 | 3.9 | 0.0 |
| Other | 1.5 | 2.4 | 3.0 | 4.8 | 16.7 | 4.1 | 0.0 |
| Total | 100 | 100 | 100 | 100 | 100 | 100 | 100 |

***$\chi^2$, p<0.001.

**TABLE 4.5**
**Socio-economic status (SES) across sites***

| SES level[1] | Site | | | | | | |
|---|---|---|---|---|---|---|---|
| | Boston (N=65) % | Bronx (N=165) % | Cleveland (N=132) % | Manhasset (N=83) % | Trenton (N=42) % | All (N=487) % | Atlanta (N=46) % |
| I (High) | 3.2 | 11.3 | 15.3 | 11.3 | 12.2 | 11.4 | 0.0 |
| II | 19.1 | 27.7 | 16.8 | 31.3 | 29.3 | 24.3 | 22.9 |
| III (Middle) | 34.9 | 36.5 | 31.3 | 30.0 | 43.9 | 34.4 | 54.2 |
| IV | 33.3 | 19.5 | 23.7 | 21.3 | 12.2 | 22.2 | 22.9 |
| V (Low) | 9.5 | 5.0 | 13.0 | 6.3 | 2.4 | 7.8 | 0.0 |
| Total | 100 | 100 | 100 | 100 | 100 | 100 | 100 |

*$\chi^2$, p<0.05.
[1]Hollingshead scale.

**TABLE 4.6**
**Mean nonverbal IQ[1] of children across sites**

| Boston (N=65) | | Bronx (N=165) | | Cleveland (N=132) | | Manhasset (N=83) | | Trenton (N=42) | |
|---|---|---|---|---|---|---|---|---|---|
| Mean | (SD) | Mean | (SD) | Mean | (SD) | Mean | (SD) | Mean | (SD) |
| 51.8 | (29.0) | 76.8 | (34.5) | 90.9 | (23.5) | 89.8 | (20.8) | 50.7 | (30.6) |

[1]NVIQ equivalent = ratio of nonverbal mental age to chronological age using scores from the Stanford–Binet or the Bayley (see text for details).

There was no significant difference between children from the Boston and Trenton sites, both of which recruited predominantly LAD children, or between children from the Cleveland and Manhasset sites, both of which recruited predominantly DLD children. Children from the Bronx site, which recruited children in all clinical groups, differed from all other sites (F=33.1, p<0.001).

All 46 normal children were recruited in Atlanta (Georgia). They served as controls for the analysis of spontaneous language, sociability and play measures. The normal children were attending a preschool for children of students and employees of Georgia State University, or a local private preschool program. Their demographics, described below, were reasonably, though not completely, similar to those of the children in the clinical groups. The other five sites were charged with recruiting different types of children: the Boston (Massachussetts), Trenton (New Jersey) and Bronx (New York) sites were to recruit AD children; the Cleveland (Ohio), Manhasset (New York) and Bronx sites were to recruit DLD children; each of the five sites was to recruit a share of the NALIQ cohort. Table 4.2 shows that small numbers of children with diagnoses other than those specifically sought were recruited at the Cleveland, Trenton and Boston sites. These were mainly children referred to the project as probably DLD who turned out to meet criteria for HAD or children referred as probably NALIQ who turned out to meet criteria for LAD. The absence of AD children recruited at the Manhasset site is explained by the transfer of these children to the Bronx site for testing.

Recruitment strategies also differed. In Boston and Trenton, investigators recruited AD and NALIQ children from specialized classes and schools for autistic children in the greater Boston–Rhode Island–Connecticut area and throughout the state of New Jersey. Most of these children were tested at their schools; occasional testing was done in the child's home. In the Bronx, children were recruited from two main sources: students and graduates of the Therapeutic Nursery in the Division of Child Psychiatry at the Albert Einstein College of Medicine, which treats 3- to 5-year-old non-retarded Bronx children with serious communication and behavior disorders, and children referred to the project from the medical center practice of one of the child neurologists. All children were tested at the Bronx site. The Cleveland site recruited children from two main sources: inner city children referred from the Cleveland Speech and Hearing Center, and children seen in consultation by one of the speech pathologists whose referral base encompasses the greater Cleveland area. These subjects were tested on-site. In Manhasset, all of the

TABLE 4.7
**TABLE 4.7**
**General inclusion and exclusion criteria**

| | |
|---|---|
| Age: | 36–59 mo (for DLD and normal children) |
| | 36–83 mo (for AD and NALIQ children) |
| Language of family: | English |
| Hearing: | 20 dB or better binaurally at 1000 and 2000 Hz |
| | 25 dB or better binaurally at 500 and 4000 Hz |
| Neurological status: | No gross sensorimotor deficit |
| | No known structural brain lesion |
| | No frequent seizures |
| | No high dose anticonvulsant drugs |
| | No high dose psychotropic medication |

DLD children were pupils at the specialized preschool affiliated with the North Shore University Hospital. The preschool enrolls children with communication disorders who are neither autistic nor mentally retarded. They were evaluated at the school. NALIQ children at all sites were recruited and tested in the same way as other children at the site.

The primary goal of recruitment efforts was to ensure an adequate number of children in low base-rate conditions (such as AD); thus no effort was made to sample randomly or consecutively from possible referral sources. Hence, the present project should not be regarded as epidemiological, and epidemiological conclusions cannot be drawn from it.

SELECTION CRITERIA

Before entry into the study sample, general inclusion and exclusion criteria were applied (Table 4.7). The age range was initially set at 3–5 years, when, typically, children with communication disorders present for initial assessment, and when differentiating language disorders, mental retardation and autism is most difficult. Because it was anticipated that there would be many children in the AD and NALIQ groups with very low mental ages who would be unable to complete many of the assessment tasks or who would score at the bottom of the distribution of scores on all tasks, and to ensure a wider range of functions for comparison purposes, the age of the NALIQ and AD children was allowed to go as high as 83 months.

All families had English as their only or primary language. Children's hearing was tested as part of the project (or else a hearing test, conducted by an audiologist within a year of the child's testing, was accepted); hearing had to be 20 dB or better binaurally at 1000 and 2000 Hz and 25 dB or better binaurally at 500 and 4000 Hz.

Because the goal of the project was to create a classification system for children with developmental disorders of higher cerebral function affecting communication, children were excluded if they had known and defined brain lesions, or diseases such as tuberous sclerosis or neurofibromatosis, or frequent, uncontrolled seizures.* Children were also excluded if they had significant motor or sensory disabilities that might create substantial assessment problems, or if they were on high doses of anticonvulsant or behavior altering medications.

For children who passed the general inclusionary and exclusionary criteria, completeness of their data was examined, and those lacking key measures (N=36), or who had dropped out of the study (N=41), were eliminated. These 77 children did not differ significantly in their demographic characteristics from other children recruited at the same site. Criteria for membership in clinical groups were applied to the remaining 556 children.

## Criteria for assignment to clinical groups

### AD GROUP

Selection criteria for the AD group were the most complex. Children were selected for the autistic sample by means of a three-step screening and diagnostic process (Fig. 4.1).
• *Step 1.* Children had to have been identified by a clinical professional as having significant impairment in social relatedness and communication. We then conducted a screening for each child to confirm the presence of the claimed social impairment, using the brief three-part Wing Autistic Disorder Interview Checklist (WADIC—Appendix 1), a questionnaire developed by Lorna Wing. The child's mother, or, in a few cases, his teacher or a psychologist, was interviewed with this instrument, and the child was excluded from the study if the mother (or teacher/psychologist) did not endorse either (1) at least one item from each of the three sections—(A) impairment in social relatedness, (B) impairment in social communication, (C) repetitive or restricted activities—or (2) at least two items from the A section of this 21 item interview. 273 children met the initial screening requirements for potential inclusion in the AD sample.
• *Step 2.* At each site, all children who met the initial screening requirement were seen by a child psychiatrist who conducted a structured comprehensive psychiatric evaluation. The three elements of this evaluation included: (1) determination of a DSM III diagnosis; (2) determination of a DSM III-R diagnosis; and (3) completion of a 21 item Social Abnormality Scale (Appendix 2). Data from the psychiatric interview, and from additional parent and teacher interviews and checklists (for the list of core measures, see Table 4.19, p. 47), permitted the determination of both an ICD-10 and a DSM IV diagnosis. 194 children were diagnosed as having PDD.

Comparative application of the four diagnostic systems for autism to these 194 children yielded samples of different sizes and slightly different compositions (for details, see Chapter 10 and Waterhouse *et al.* 1996). DSM III-R Autistic Disorder was most inclusive (176/194, 91 per cent); ICD-10 Childhood Autism (125/194, 64 per cent)

---

*Nine children in the NALIQ group were known to have Down syndrome. After enrollment, a pair of monozygotic twins in the LAD group were diagnosed as having Cornelia de Lange syndrome, and two LAD boys were found to have fragile X syndrome. One girl among the 18 excluded because they did not meet the criteria for AD was later diagnosed as having Rett syndrome.

and DSM IV Autistic Disorder (115/194, 59 per cent) gave intermediate results; and DSM III Infantile Autism was least inclusive (98/194, 51 per cent). Comparison of behaviors and cognitive and linguistic skills across these four overlapping samples of positively diagnosed 'autistic' individuals suggests to us that the continuum indexed is the same, regardless of the size of the sample netted by any one of the four systems. Therefore to maximize the study sample we chose to use the most inclusive diagnostic group: the 176 diagnosed with DSM III-R Autistic Disorder.

• *Step 3*. In order to evaluate the role of mental ages relative to behavioral deficits in the autistic and non-autistic children's communication difficulties, clinical groups were divided into normal and below-normal cognitive functioning groups on the basis of cognitive tests yielding an NVIQ equivalent (see description of measures) at or above 80, or below 80. Autistic children with NVIQs ≥80 were classified as HAD, and those with NVIQs <80 were classified as LAD. In this division of the diagnosed autistic sample, there were 2.5 times as many LAD (N=125) as HAD (N=51) subjects. Children who were not diagnosed by the child psychiatrist as autistic or as having PDD were placed back into the non-autistic subject pool as potential candidates for the DLD or NALIQ groups.

DLD AND NALIQ GROUPS

All the children referred to the project, whatever their referral diagnosis, were screened with the WADIC. The 283 children whose parent or teacher did not endorse at least two items from area A or one item from areas A, B and C were not seen by the psychiatrist and were considered candidates for the DLD or NALIQ groups. All non-autistic children with NVIQ equivalents <80 who fit the general selection criteria were placed in the NALIQ group, which therefore included both below average and truly mentally retarded non-autistic children. 25 per cent of the NALIQ children had an NVIQ between 70 and 80 and the remainder were <70. The 79 children from the DLD and NALIQ groups who fulfilled the WADIC criteria but whom the psychiatrist found not to fulfill criteria for AD or PDD-NOS were placed back in their respective groups.

Placement into the DLD group was based on having (1) a lack of autistic features on the WADIC or no PDD diagnosis by the psychiatrist, (2) an NVIQ equivalent ≥80, and (3) a significant relative deficiency in language measures. This deficiency was defined as a score on the Test of Early Language Development (TELD) (Hresko *et al*. 1981) that was 15 points (1 SD) below the mean NVIQ score or a mean length of utterance (MLU) score that was 1 SD below the mean for the child's chronological age (for details, see Chapter 10 and Aram *et al*. 1993). The application of these criteria resulted in a sample of 201 DLD children.

There were 69 children who were fully studied but did not meet criteria for any of these groups. Of these, 51 had been referred as having probable DLD and the other 18 are those mentioned earlier who had been referred as having probable AD and had the appropriate number of checks on the WADIC, but were not given a DSM III-R AD diagnosis by the psychiatrist. These 69 children were not included in the study but are discussed in Chapter 10 and in Dunn *et al*. (1996). They are being followed to school

**TABLE 4.8**
**Clinical groups**

| Group | Cognitive level | | Total |
|---|---|---|---|
| | Adequate (NVIQ ≥80) | Subaverage (NVIQ <80) | |
| Non-autistic | **DLD** (N=201) | **NALIQ** (N=110) | 311 |
| Autistic | **HAD** (N=51) | **LAD** (N=125) | 176 |
| Total | 252 | 235 | 487 |

age with the remainder of the cohort in order to determine whether they were normal, or did have the conditions for which they were referred to the study but were not captured by the inclusionary criteria, or had other conditions. Exclusion of these 69 children resulted in a total classified clinical sample of 487 children (Table 4.8).

*Subject characteristics and demographics*

No attempt was made to select subjects based on their gender. Boys outnumbered girls in all groups. Table 4.9 indicates that the gender imbalance was greater in the AD samples than in the other groups. Overrepresentation of boys among the normal controls reflected a deliberate effort to match the clinical groups.

The groups did not differ in racial distribution (Table 4.10), but there were significant differences across sites (see Table 4.4), with the highest proportion of Black children at the Cleveland site and of Hispanic children in the Bronx. The proportion of Hispanic children in the Bronx sample was lower than that of the local community because only children from English speaking homes were recruited to the study. The Manhasset site was overwhelmingly Caucasian, reflecting its community.

Significant age differences among groups (Table 4.11) resulted from setting the age range at 36–59 months for the DLD and normal children and at 36–83 months for the AD and NALIQ children. This was done to maximize the range of mental ages in the lower functioning groups. Table 4.11 shows the expected significant differences in NVIQ equivalents among groups, with the LAD group scoring the lowest; the notable exception was that the DLD and HAD groups had virtually equal mean NVIQs.

NVIQ equivalents differed among the children recruited at the five sites (see Table 4.6) depending on whether they were charged with recruiting DLD or AD subjects. There were differences among children from the three sites charged with recruiting AD children. Over 80 per cent of AD children recruited at the Trenton and Boston sites were mentally retarded, while this was true of only 60 per cent of those at the Bronx site. The Bronx site contributed 69 per cent of the HAD children because it had access to the pupils and graduates of the Einstein Therapeutic Nursery which only enrolls DLD and HAD children (Table 4.12). However, even at that site, LAD children outnumbered HAD children (see Table 4.2).

**TABLE 4.9**
**Children's gender across groups****

| Gender | Group | | | | | |
|--------|-------|-------|-------|-------|-------|-------|
| | DLD (N=201) % | HAD (N=51) % | LAD (N=125) % | NALIQ (N=110) % | All (N=487) % | Normal (N=46) % |
| Male | 73.6 | 82.4 | 84.0 | 64.6 | 75.2 | 62.5 |
| Female | 26.4 | 17.7 | 16.0 | 35.5 | 24.7 | 37.5 |
| Total | 100 | 100 | 100 | 100 | 100 | 100 |

$**\chi^2$, p<0.01.

**TABLE 4.10**
**Children's race across groups[1]**

| Race | Group | | | | | |
|------|-------|-------|-------|-------|-------|-------|
| | DLD (N=201) % | HAD (N=51) % | LAD (N=125) % | NALIQ (N=110) % | All (N=487) % | Normal (N=46) % |
| Caucasian | 74.6 | 58.8 | 73.6 | 71.8 | 72.1 | 83.3 |
| Black | 19.4 | 21.6 | 19.2 | 20.9 | 19.9 | 16.7 |
| Hispanic | 2.0 | 13.7 | 2.4 | 4.6 | 3.9 | 0.0 |
| Other | 4.0 | 5.9 | 4.8 | 2.7 | 4.1 | 0.0 |
| Total | 100 | 100 | 100 | 100 | 100 | 100 |

[1]No significant differences.

**TABLE 4.11**
**Mean age and nonverbal IQ (NVIQ) across groups**

| Characteristic | Group | | | | |
|----------------|-------|-------|-------|-------|-------|
| | DLD (N=201) Mean (SD) | HAD (N=51) Mean (SD) | LAD (N=125) Mean (SD) | NALIQ (N=110) Mean (SD) | Normal (N=46) Mean (SD) |
| Age (mo)[1] | 49.0 (10.9) | 57.8 (15.3) | 59.6 (16.6) | 55.9 (13.2) | 51.2 (13.0) |
| NVIQ[2] | 102.3 (17.1) | 102.9 (23.1) | 45.6 (19.4) | 55.5 (19.9) | — |

[1]LAD=HAD; LAD>NALIQ; HAD=NALIQ>DLD>Normal. F=18.29, p<0.001 (ANOVA).
[2]NVIQ equivalent = ratio of nonverbal mental age/chronological age based on Stanford–Binet or Bayley scores (see text for details). DLD=HAD>NALIQ>LAD. F=323.07, p<0.001 (ANOVA).

*Family characteristics and demographics*

A criterion for recruitment was that children come from families where English was the primary language. Only 3 per cent of the parents reported that another language was spoken by some family member; all stated that this second language was used infrequently or not at all in day-to-day family interactions. The groups did not differ in this respect.

40

**TABLE 4.12**
Sites' contribution of children to groups***

| Site | Group | | | | | |
|---|---|---|---|---|---|---|
| | DLD (N=201) % | HAD (N=51) % | LAD (N=125) % | NALIQ (N=110) % | All (N=487) % | Normal (N=46) % |
| Boston | 1.5 | 13.7 | 24.0 | 22.7 | 13.3 | 0.0 |
| Bronx | 19.4 | 68.6 | 48.8 | 27.3 | 33.9 | 0.0 |
| Cleveland | 49.3 | 5.9 | 3.2 | 23.6 | 27.1 | 0.0 |
| Manhasset | 29.4 | 0.0 | 0.0 | 21.8 | 17.0 | 0.0 |
| Trenton | 0.5 | 11.8 | 24.0 | 4.6 | 8.6 | 0.0 |
| Atlanta | 0.0 | 0.0 | 0.0 | 0.0 | 0.0 | 100 |
| Total | 100 | 100 | 100 | 100 | 100 | 100 |

***$\chi^2$, p<0.001.

The composition of families of children in the four clinical groups differed significantly (Table 4.13). 75–80 per cent of children lived in two-parent families. 19 children (4 per cent) were adopted, none in the HAD group.

The number of siblings and the order of the child in the family were examined because of the possibility that having a significantly disabled child would influence parents' decisions about family size. 21 percent of the children were only children at the time of enrollment (Table 4.14), 43 per cent had a single sibling, and 34 per cent had two or more siblings. There were highly significant differences among clinical groups in the number of children in the family, with children in the two AD groups having only one sibling on average, as compared to the NALIQ group who had 1.4 and the DLD group who had 1.7. In about 60 per cent of families the proband was the youngest in the family. Although we did not ask parents directly whether having a child with a developmental disorder had affected their decision about family size, we speculate that some parents may have limited their family after the birth of a child viewed as having a serious disability (Jones and Szatmari 1988). A limitation to the interpretation of these data is that most parents were still of child-bearing age and may not have completed their families at the time of the study, making it difficult to evaluate the impact on family size of having a seriously disabled child.

Although the final sample is reasonably representative of the population of the USA in racial composition and socioeconomic status (SES), differences across sites reflect the demographics of their respective communities (see Table 4.4). On average, children from the Boston site came from families with a lower socioeconomic and educational status than those from the other sites. At the Bronx site, the preschool served some inner city children, whereas subjects from the neurology practice were mostly middle class children who were referred from a wide area around New York City and from out-of-state. The higher proportion of Hispanic children among the HAD group reflects both the demographic characteristics of the Bronx and the prevalence of HAD children in the preschool. The Cleveland site resembled the Bronx site as far as demographics are con-

41

**TABLE 4.13**
**Family characteristics across groups[1]**

| Characteristic | Group | | | | |
|---|---|---|---|---|---|
| | DLD (N=201) % | HAD (N=51) % | LAD (N=125) % | NALIQ (N=110) % | All (N=487) % |
| Parents married | 80.6 | 78.4 | 76.8 | 73.6 | 77.8 |
| Parents separated/divorced | 7.0 | 13.7 | 14.4 | 11.8 | 10.7 |
| Parents single | 12.4 | 7.8 | 8.8 | 14.6 | 11.5 |
| Child adopted | 4.5 | 0.0 | 4.0 | 4.6 | 3.9 |

[1]No significant differences.

**TABLE 4.14**
**Family size across groups**

| Characteristic | Group | | | | |
|---|---|---|---|---|---|
| | DLD (N=201) | HAD (N=51) | LAD (N=125) | NALIQ (N=110) | All (N=487) |
| Child is only child (%)*** | 10.4 | 39.2 | 27.2 | 25.5 | 21.2 |
| Child is youngest (%) | 56.7 | 64.7 | 61.6 | 66.4 | 61.0 |
| Number of sibs (mean)[1] | 1.7 | 0.9 | 1.1 | 1.4 | 1.4 |

***$\chi^2$, $p<0.001$.
[1]DLD>HAD=LAD=NALIQ (ANOVA, F=9.23, $p<0.0001$).

**TABLE 4.15**
**Socio-economic status (SES) and race\*\*\***

| SES level[1] | Racial group | | | |
|---|---|---|---|---|
| | White (N=345) % | Black (N=92) % | Hispanic (N=18) % | Other (N=10) % |
| I (High) | 14.8 | 3.3 | 0.0 | 0.0 |
| II | 28.4 | 12.0 | 11.1 | 21.1 |
| III (Middle) | 35.4 | 23.9 | 61.1 | 42.1 |
| IV | 18.6 | 31.5 | 27.8 | 36.8 |
| V (Low) | 2.9 | 29.4 | 0.0 | 0.0 |
| Total | 100 | 100 | 100 | 100 |

***$\chi^2$, $p<0.001$.
[1]Hollingshead levels.

cerned; the children came from two main sources: inner city children, more often Black than Hispanic, referred from the Cleveland Speech and Hearing Center, and children seen in consultation by one of the speech pathologists whose referral base is much wider and encompasses the greater Cleveland area. Although the children from the Manhasset and Trenton sites were predominantly Caucasian, their SES [measured according to the

TABLE 4.16
Socio-economic status (SES) across groups**

| SES level[1] | Group | | | | | |
|---|---|---|---|---|---|---|
| | DLD (N=197) % | HAD (N=49) % | LAD (N=123) % | NALIQ (N=105) % | All (N=474) % | Normal (N=46) % |
| I (High) | 14.7 | 12.2 | 9.8 | 6.7 | 11.4 | 0.0 |
| II | 23.4 | 22.5 | 31.7 | 18.1 | 24.3 | 22.9 |
| III (Middle) | 33.5 | 49.0 | 31.8 | 32.4 | 34.4 | 54.2 |
| IV | 18.3 | 14.3 | 23.6 | 31.4 | 22.2 | 22.9 |
| V (Low) | 10.2 | 2.0 | 3.3 | 11.4 | 7.8 | 0.0 |
| Total | 100 | 100 | 100 | 100 | 100 | 100 |

**$\chi^2$, p<0.01.
[1]Hollingshead levels.

TABLE 4.17
Parents' education across groups[1]

| | DLD % | HAD % | LAD % | NALIQ % | All % |
|---|---|---|---|---|---|
| Fathers' education | (N=197) | (N=50) | (N=123) | (N=103) | (N=473) |
| College graduate or + | 42.6 | 50.0 | 48.8 | 35.9 | 43.6 |
| High school grad. | 47.7 | 48.0 | 40.7 | 51.5 | 46.7 |
| Not high school grad. | 9.6 | 2.0 | 10.6 | 12.6 | 9.7 |
| Total | 100 | 100 | 100 | 100 | 100 |
| Mothers' education | (N=200) | (N=50) | (N=123) | (N=109) | (N=482) |
| College graduate or +* | 38.5 | 54.0 | 41.5 | 26.6 | 38.1 |
| High school grad. | 55.0 | 42.0 | 52.0 | 62.4 | 54.6 |
| Not high school grad. | 6.5 | 4.0 | 6.5 | 11.0 | 7.3 |
| Total | 100 | 100 | 100 | 100 | 100 |

[1]Parents are those with whom the child is living.
[2]No significant difference.
*$\chi^2$, p<0.05; all other comparisons non-significant.

Hollingshead (1975) index] was quite similar to that of children at the other sites. The SES of the families of the normal children from Atlanta was more homogeneous than that of the clinical groups inasmuch as there were no children at the highest and lowest Hollingshead levels. There was a strong interaction of SES with race (Table 4.15): Black and Hispanic families were overrepresented in the lower SES levels, while almost half of the white families came from the highest two levels.

There were SES differences among clinical groups (Table 4.16), with the NALIQ significantly lower than the other groups in both SES and level of parental education (Table 4.17). It is not known whether endogenous or environmental factors related to unfavorable life circumstances, or more likely both, account for this finding. The finding is consistent with results from the Collaborative Perinatal Project which found that im-poverished social circumstances was one of the strongest contributors to mild to moder-ate mental retardation (Broman *et al.* 1987). An equally striking finding in our data is that the LAD group differed from the NALIQ group with respect to SES and level of parental education. This finding suggests that different pathogenetic mechanisms may be responsible for low IQ in autistic and non-autistic children, in the sense that, whereas low SES may contribute to the cognitive deficits of non-autistic children with low IQ, it makes much less of a contribution to the severe cognitive deficits of low-functioning autistic children. This difference fits with the hypothesis that AD is the result of a genetic or acquired abnormality in the development of the immature brain that is largely unrelated to the consequences of an unfavorable environment.

**Measures**
All children in the DLD, AD and NALIQ groups were given a common core battery of tests and measures (Table 4.18). In addition, children in the DLD and AD groups also underwent additional area-specific tests in order to assess functions of special interest. The selection of most of the measures was driven by considerations important to the success of a classification in that they were (i) well-known, (ii) widely used in standard clinical practice, and (iii) backed by research supporting their content and psychometric and other properties. Our choice of standardized instruments was guided by the need to reduce redundancy among measures, to assess a wide range of constructs and possible classification uses, to select tests with established reliability and validity, and to consider time constraints for testing. The development of 'better' psychometric measures fell outside the scope of this study, although we did devise standard assessment protocols in some areas such as history taking, neurological examination, and video play session, lin-guistic and pragmatic analysis. Our goal was to cover the major historical, neurological, cognitive, language and behavioral/social areas considered important for describing the range of children in the study. A full list of measures used, and the groups to which they were given, is provided in Table 4.19.

*Core assessment measures*
We discuss seven core assessments in this chapter: (1) family/medical/developmental history; (2) neurological/medical examination; (3) psychiatric inventory and evaluation; (4) adaptive developmental functioning; (5) cognitive functioning; (6) language develop-ment; and (7) play development (Table 4.18). Additional measures specific to the DLD and AD groups (listed in Appendix 4.1, pp. 55–57) are presented in the chapters report-ing findings from these measures.

FAMILY/MEDICAL/DEVELOPMENTAL HISTORY
A specially designed questionnaire regarding the child's developmental, medical and family history (Appendix 3) was mailed to each family so that it could be completed before the neurological examination, at which time we went over all the answers with a parent. This questionnaire was divided into sections providing information on: basic

**TABLE 4.18**
**Core measures**

1. Family/Medical/Developmental history (*informant:* parent)
2. Neurological/Medical examination
3. Behavioral inventory and evaluation
    —Wing Autistic Disorder Interview Checklist (*informant:* parent)
    —Psychiatric interview for DSM III and DSM III-R AD diagnoses
    —Social Abnormality Scales I and II (*informant:* parent)
4. Adaptive developmental functioning
    —Vineland Adaptive Behavior Scales (*informant:* parent)
    —Wing Schedule of Handicaps, Behaviour, and Skills (*informant:* teacher)
5. Cognitive functioning
    —Stanford–Binet Intelligence Scale, Revised/Bayley Scales of Infant
      Development—Mental Scale
6. Language functioning
    —Test of Early Language Development/Sequenced Inventory of Language
      Development
    —Spontaneous language sample (from videotaped play session)
7. Play development
    —Videotaped play session

demographics; parents; siblings; the mother's pregnancy; the child's birth and neonatal period; the child's history of medical conditions and past and current treatment with medications; the child's developmental history, including age at achievement of major behavioral milestones; the parent's report of atypical behaviors, including the child's age at their onset and disappearance, if applicable; and the (immediate and extended) family history of handedness, stuttering, speech/language disorders, motor difficulties, learning/behavioral disabilities, psychiatric disorders, neurological disorders, autoimmune and other medical diseases, and deaths.

NEUROLOGICAL/MEDICAL EXAMINATION
We developed a standardized neurological examination (Appendix 4) that emphasized those aspects of the neurological evaluation that were particularly relevant to the assessment of disorders of higher cerebral function, notably the mental status, language and play. The examination also encompassed the following classes of functions: gross motor, fine motor and oromotor skills; abnormalities of tone or posture; presence of abnormal involuntary movements; somatosensory function; cranial nerves; language and communication skills; behavior; and affect. There was also a short section that evaluated the child's general physical condition, including the presence of dysmorphic features, a screen for visual acuity, and an examination of the tympanic membranes.

PSYCHIATRIC INVENTORY AND EVALUATION
Following screening by the WADIC, as described above, each child at each site was evaluated by a board certified child psychiatrist. Each child psychiatrist, who was blind to all other questionnaire and test data, was asked to provide a DSM III and DSM III-R PDD diagnosis, if appropriate for the child. In addition, the psychiatrist rated each child

**TABLE 4.19**
**Core and specific measures used in Nosology Study***

| Domain/measure | Data used | Groups to which given |
|---|---|---|
| *Demographic/history/family history* | | |
| • Demographic–history interview (reviewed with parent) | Individual items | All |
| *Neurological examination* | | |
| • Standardized neurological examination (performed by child neurologist) | Individual items and composite scores | All |
| *Behavioral/social functioning* | | |
| • Wing Autistic Disorders Interview Checklist (completed by parent, rarely by teacher) | Individual items and area sum scores | All |
| • Wing Schedule of Handicaps, Behaviour and Skills (completed by teacher) | Individual items | All |
| • Vineland Adaptive Behavior Scales (interview with parent, rarely with teacher) Communication domain Daily Living Skills domain Socialization domain Motor Skills domain Adaptive Behavior Composite | Raw scores and domain standard age scores (SAS) | All |
| • Videotaped play session rating (parent/teacher and examiner are involved) | Frequency counts of types of play | All |
| *Psychiatric examinations/ratings* (completed by child psychiatrist) | | |
| • Psychiatric diagnosis | DSM III DSM III-R | AD[1] AD |
| • Wing Classification of Social Relatedness | Individual items | AD |
| • Social Abnormalities Scales I & II | Individual items | AD |
| *Cognitive functioning* | | |
| • Stanford–Binet Intelligence Scale, Revised Vocabulary subtest Comprehension subtest Absurdities subtest Pattern Analysis subtest[2] Copying subtest[2] Quantitative subtest Memory for Sentences subtest Memory for Digits subtest[3] Bead Memory subtest[4] Verbal Reasoning area score Abstract/Visual Reasoning area score[2] Quantitative area score Short-term Memory area score Test Composite score | Subtest raw and SAS; area SAS; and composite score | All |

| | | |
|---|---|---|
| • Bayley Scales of Infant Development—Mental Scale (only for children who could not do Stanford–Binet) | Raw score MDI; Kent factor scores | All[1] |
| • Hiskey–Nebraska Test of Learning Aptitude Visual Attention Span subtest Picture Identification subtest | Raw score; standard score | All |
| • McCarthy Scale of Children's Ability Verbal Fluency subtest Verbal Memory II subtest | Raw score | DLD All |

*Cognitive/verbal/language functioning*

| | | |
|---|---|---|
| • Test of Early Language Development (TELD) | Raw score; standard score | All |
| • Sequenced Inventory of Communication Development—Revised (given only to children who could not do the TELD) | Age equivalent | All[1] |
| • Peabody Picture Vocabulary Test—Revised | Raw score; standard score; age equivalent | All |
| • Expressive One-Word Picture Vocabulary Test | Raw score; standard score | All |
| • Illinois Test of Psycholinguistic Abilities Manual Expression subtest[4] | Raw score; standard score | DLD |
| • Photo Articulation Test Tongue, Lip, Vowel scores Total score | Raw score; standard score | DLD |
| • Analysis of Spontaneous Language Transcripts from play session analyzed using automated system and ratings of semantics and pragmatics | MLU; type/token ratios | All |

*Motor functioning/handedness*

| | | |
|---|---|---|
| • Seguin Formboard | Time # placed | All |
| • Annett Pegboard | Time with each hand | All |
| • UCLA Handedness Tasks | Handedness ratio | All |

*See Appendix 4.1 for description of measures.
[1]Used only if the child could not perform the primary measure.
[2]Used as best estimate of nonverbal IQ.
[3]There are no standard scores on this subtest for the youngest children in the study.
[4]Not used in scoring the Stanford–Binet.

on the Social Abnormalities Scales I and II (Appendix 2), which is a listing of typical social abnormalities found in individuals manifesting autistic spectrum symptomatology.

ADAPTIVE DEVELOPMENTAL FUNCTIONING

We used the Vineland Adaptive Behavior Scale (Sparrow *et al.* 1984) to assess the general adaptive functioning of all children. It is an inventory completed by a trained examiner during an interview with the child's mother or someone who knows the child well. The scale provides standard scores in four primary domains, each of which are composed of subdomains: (1) Communication domain (Receptive, Expressive, Written); (2) Daily Living Skills domain (Personal, Domestic, Community); (3) Socialization domain (Interpersonal Relationships, Play and Leisure Time, Coping Skills); (4) Motor Skills domain (Fine and Gross). The Scale also provides overall Maladaptive Behavior composite scores (Scale I—Dysfunctional Behaviors; Scale II—Disordered Thinking).

In addition, the child's teacher was asked to complete the Wing Schedule of Handicaps, Behaviours and Skills (HBS). This multi-item instrument is reproduced as Appendix 5.

COGNITIVE FUNCTIONING

The tests used were the Stanford–Binet Intelligence Scale, Revised (S-B) (Thorndike *et al.* 1986) or the Bayley Scales of Infant Development—Mental Scale (Bayley 1969). The S-B is standardized from age 2 years to 32 years 6 months and encompasses four content areas with various subsets of its 15 subtests. Eight subtests have norms for children under 6 years of age: within the Verbal Reasoning area, there are three subtests (Vocabulary, Comprehension and Absurdities), within the Abstract/Visual Reasoning area there are two subtests (Pattern Analysis, Copying), within the Quantitative Reasoning area there is one subtest (Quantitative), and within the Short-term Memory area there are two subtests (Bead Memory, Memory for Sentences).

Because of the wide range of cognitive abilities of the children in this study, the S-B was not entirely adequate psychometrically, and we had to make a number of decisions regarding its use, scoring and analysis in order to ensure the usefulness of the measures obtained. Our main reason for using this test was to provide a measure of nonverbal cognitive functioning and to use an instrument that would be appropriate for longitudinal follow-up of the children. Our original plan was to use either the Abstract/Visual Reasoning or Quantitative Reasoning standard age scores (SASs) as our proxy index of nonverbal intellectual abilities. After publication of the S-B Technical Manual in 1986, and after we gained experience in evaluating preschool children with a wide range of abilities, we decided that the Abstract/Visual Reasoning SAS, which is made up of the Pattern Analysis and Copying subtests, would be the better measure of nonverbal abilities for the children. The Abstract/Visual Reasoning composite has slightly better reliability than Quantitative Reasoning for the age groups being evaluated, a slightly lower correlation with the Verbal Reasoning SAS (although it was still surprisingly high, at 0.69), greater independence and specificity in confirmatory factor analytic models for this age group, and more children in the study were able to complete the required subtests.

Although the majority of children could perform some items in the Abstract/Visual area, there were a number who functioned at such low levels that they failed every item on both subtests. As the S-B Guide for Administering and Scoring clearly indicates, zero scores on various subtests occur frequently and restrict the 'lowest composite score that can be obtained on a scale' both at ages below 4 years and in children with disabilities. This problem also occurs because the S-B currently provides no standard score norms for raw scores of 0. Because of both this psychometric limitation and the need to assess the nonverbal functioning of children with mental ages in the vicinity of 2 years or below, we decided also to evaluate such low-functioning children with the Bayley Scales of Infant Development—Mental Scale (Bayley 1969), a test designed to assess infant development between the ages of 2 and 30 months. This scale provides a composite Mental Development Index with a normalized standard score of 100 (SD = 16), and combines items with verbal/language, visual/spatial, and motor and other behaviors. In order to generate a measure of nonverbal abilities, the Kent scoring (Reuter *et al.* 1981) of the Bayley was used. This measure provides separate composite scores for a child's verbal, nonverbal and motor functioning in age equivalents.

In order to be included in the study, children had to be assessed adequately either by Pattern Analysis and Copying of the S-B or, if they obtained 0 scores on these measures, by the Bayley. All children testable with the S-B were given as many of the eight subtests as they could perform. In addition, although there are no normative data for this age group on the Memory for Digits subtest, it was given to those children who could complete it so as to obtain digit recall/sequencing information. A large majority of the children in the study, especially children in the AD group, found the Bead Memory subtest very difficult (score = 0), and it was dropped as a required subtest after the first year.

Because the S-B has a somewhat complex scoring system, it was important to use systematic rules for developing composite and area scores. Children received scores in a particular area based only on those subtests on which they could perform. Consequently, children's Verbal Reasoning SAS was typically based on their Vocabulary, Comprehension and Absurdities subtest scores; their Abstract/Visual SAS on their Pattern Analysis and Copying subtest scores; their Quantitative Reasoning SAS only on their Quantitative subtest score; and their Short-term Memory SAS only on their Memory for Sentences subtest score. The overall test composite score was based on all four area SASs when available. Given the significant disabilities of some of these children, we were unable to obtain scores for all four areas in all children.

The scoring system described in the S-B manual presents some difficulties for the interpretation of area and composite scores. For example, a nonverbal child who could not perform the tasks required in the Verbal Reasoning and Short-term Memory areas might have a test composite score of 100 based solely on the Abstract/Visual Reasoning and Quantitative Reasoning areas. A verbal child able to complete all areas, who obtained identical scores as the first child in the Abstract/Visual and Quantitative Reasoning areas, might nevertheless receive a test composite score of only 88 because he performed at lower levels in the other two areas. The lack of 0 score normative SASs within subtests and composite areas puts a significant limitation on the interpretation of the test composite on the S-B. This same problem can occur within areas comprising multiple subtests. Therefore we recommend caution in interpreting the composite scores presented in this monograph.

We also developed a common metric to express a child's ranking on the two measures of nonverbal ability used. This task was not straightforward, given the normative data and unique characteristics of the S-B and Bayley Scales. The underlying assumption that the Bayley visual/spatial items measure similar constructs to those in the Abstract/Visual Reasoning area of the S-B may be unfounded. There were also technical problems. First, only children who could not do the S-B were given the Bayley; therefore, all such children's scores should have fallen below the lowest score on the S-B. Secondly, the Bayley does not provide normative standard scores for children over 30 months of age, which was the case for all the children in our study tested with the Bayley.

Therefore, in order to obtain an estimated index of children's relative ranking on nonverbal abilities, (1) we transformed the S-B Abstract/Visual Reasoning subtest raw scores into age equivalents and took the average of these age equivalents to yield a nonverbal mental age; (2) we used the Kent cognitive (nonverbal) mental age (Reuter *et al.* 1981) from the Bayley items; and (3) we compared the lowest possible S-B nonverbal mental age level (24 months) with the highest possible Bayley nonverbal mental age (30 months). Because of the overlap in the range of 24–30 months mental age, and because of our assumption that all children who received the Bayley items had to be lower functioning than the children who were testable with the S-B, we decided to adjust the Bayley nonverbal mental age scores by subtracting a constant of 6 months (the amount of overlap) from all children. This resulted in a nonverbal mental age range between 6 and 24 months on the Bayley. These different nonverbal mental age scores were then combined and, in order to develop an age adjusted composite which would be comparable to other age adjusted/normed scores, we derived a ratio by dividing the nonverbal mental age (MA) by the child's chronological age (CA). This nonverbal 'intelligence' ratio score was compared in children tested with both instruments to the original S-B Abstract/Visual Reasoning SASs and to the Bayley MDI scores; we found the scores to be highly correlated and similar in magnitude.

The limitations of using age equivalent scores, MA/CA ratios, and of combining scores from different instruments are well known. Age equivalent and ratio scores are not necessarily comparable between children at different ages as standard scores are. The growth in abilities represented by a one year difference in age equivalence may vary widely for different developmental periods. Ratio scores are less and less meaningful as the rate of development slows with age. Different instruments, even those that purport to measure the same skill, may call for different cognitive abilities; combining such scores may mask within- or between-subject variability in cognitive functions that might be measuring somewhat different constructs using different approaches to assessment. Nevertheless, because we were evaluating such a diverse sample of subjects with such a wide range of abilities and deficits, we had no choice but to devise a composite score, given the lack of a single standardized test to assess all children adequately at all ages. We consider the resulting composite nonverbal score an acceptable estimate of each child's relative ranking within the sample.

Given that many of our analyses were carried out on two distinct groups of children, as defined by their nonverbal abilities (NVIQ <80 *vs* NVIQ ≥80), this composite nonverbal ratio score was used only for analyses which included both the higher and lower functioning groups (all the children who obtained an NVIQ of at least 80 were able to complete the Abstract/Visual Reasoning area of the S-B and only the lower functioning children in the LAD and NALIQ groups required the Bayley). The nonverbal composite score, despite its limitations, was one of the few indices that could be used as a covariate for the entire population, or used in multiple regression models.

LANGUAGE FUNCTIONING

The tests chosen were the Test of Early Language Development (TELD) (Hresko *et al.* 1981) or the Sequenced Inventory of Communication Development—Revised (SICD-R) (Hedrick *et al.* 1984). The TELD provides a standardized measure of language function and was given to all the children in the study. Again, some children with limited language abilities were unable to complete the TELD and were given the SICD-R, a measure that evaluates both receptive and expressive language skills.

Because the SICD-R was used as a lower-extension for children who could not perform the TELD, we used a similar approach to the one used with the S-B for developing a combined score. The TELD provides both a standard score and an age equivalent score. The lowest age equivalent score on the TELD is 24 months. The SICD-R yields age equivalent scores for both the receptive and expressive areas, which were averaged and ranged between 3 and 48 months, but does not provide standard scores. Using a similar method to the one used in combining the S-B and Bayley age equivalent scores, children with SICD-R scores were considered to be functioning below the lowest level of the TELD (<24 months). Because a number of children had SICD-R age equivalent scores above 24 months, yet were untestable with the TELD, their age equivalent scores were transformed so as to range between 0 and 24 months. This method maintained the child's individual rank within the sample and provided a lower extension of age equivalents for children who could not do the TELD. These language age equivalent scores were then divided by a child's chronological age to provide a ratio-based language score comparable to the ratio-based NVIQ score. Again, a comparison of these ratio-based language scores to the original TELD or SICD-R scores indicated a high concordance.

In addition, the spontaneous language of those children who were verbal, intelligible and produced at least 25 utterances during the play session discussed below was transcribed and analyzed for mean length of utterances (MLU), conversational pragmatics and errors in meaning, structure and verbal pragmatics.

LEVEL OF PLAY

Each child's play and spontaneous language were evaluated on the basis of a 25 minute structured play session. The session was carried out either in available space in laboratory facilities or at the child's school or home. The session was video and audio recorded for later analysis. A specific set of toys, which covered a broad range of developmental levels, was used and included sensorimotor toys, functional/constructional toys and symbolic toys. The session was divided into three parts. During the first five minutes each child was introduced to the play area, offered a simple snack and invited to play with whatever toys he liked. The examiner and a familiar adult (a parent or teacher) sat to the side of the play area and talked. This provided an opportunity to record the child's choice of toys and style of solitary play. Next, the examiner played with the child for a further 15 minutes and attempted to elicit his highest level of play and language, using the available toys. Lastly, the familiar adult then returned and played with the child for another five minutes. This final period provided a means for comparing the child's play, language and sociability when engaged with familiar *vs* unfamiliar persons.

## Data analysis

### Group comparisons

We decided to divide the children into conventionally accepted diagnostic groups—DLD, AD and NALIQ—and to compare these groups using as broad a range as possible of developmental, neurological, cognitive, language and behavioral function. As already stated, we divided the AD group arbitrarily into HAD and LAD subgroups so as to have a four group 2×2 matrix (see Table 4.8), with NVIQ along one dimension (a group was defined as either ≥80 or <80), and autistic behavior along the other dimension (a group was defined as either autistic or non-autistic). In this model, the DLD and HAD groups occupied the two higher NVIQ cells, while the NALIQ and LAD groups occupied the two lower NVIQ cells, with stratification on NVIQ controlling some of its effects. The entire sample thus could be collapsed into a two group design along either dimension (*i.e.* autistic *vs* non-autistic or higher functioning *vs* lower functioning children).

Another approach for addressing the issue of developmental or functional level was to assess the effect of NVIQ on various measures directly, using regression modeling. We used multiple regression to investigate the effects of developmental level and two other potentially important confounding variables, *viz.* age of the children at time of testing, and family socioeconomic status (SES), on the measures taken of these children. These analyses yielded information regarding the amount of independent or combined variance in scores from each test or measure that could be attributed to NVIQ, age or SES, and was not necessarily related to group membership.

Because many researchers prefer analysis of covariance (ANCOVA) designs for interpreting the effects of these possibly confounding variates, we also performed between-group ANCOVA analyses using NVIQ, age and SES as the covariates, with *post hoc* least-means square group comparisons, in order to provide additional information regarding the effects of each of these variables on our results. Traditional non-covaried ANOVAs were also performed for comparison purposes.

### Missing and specially coded data

There were two kinds of missing data in this study; they were coded and treated differently. The first type was data which were never collected, either because the child was not given the test, due to the project's design or by error, or because the child did not return for a final evaluation session. Data missing for these reasons explains the unequal numbers of subjects for some analyses.

Missing data also occurred in situations where the child was given the test or task but either refused to do it, or could not do it because of severe language, cognitive, behavioral or motor disabilities. It was not always possible to discern whether a child could not, or would not, perform. Regardless of the underlying reason for lack of performance, including these subjects in the analysis posed problems. Some children did not obtain a score because the measures did not have a 0 score (*e.g.* speed on the pegboard test), while on S-B subtests, a 0 score had no SAS equivalent. We also had to consider whether a child who produced no behavior in a particular domain (*e.g.* expressive vocabulary for a nonverbal child) should be given a score along a measurement dimension of that domain. If we did not find a way to include these children in the analyses, then only those who could perform the test would be included. Such an approach would yield biased group means, especially for the two lower functioning groups of children.

Because of this problem we compared several approaches to data interpolation and, for group comparisons, decided to assign the lowest possible value that the measure allowed to children who could not or would not do a specific test or subtest. Thus, for example, children who were untestable with the One-Word Expressive Picture Vocabulary Test (Gardner 1979) because they were nonverbal were assigned the lowest possible raw score (0) and standard score (55) for their age. Data from groups in which this situation was frequent tended to be significantly skewed, which made the mean an inadequate estimate of the group's central tendency. In most such cases we also determined group medians, which provided more accurate estimates of the children's performances on the given measure.

*Classification using regression-mixture taxometrics*
AD and its subtypes and DLD and its subtypes are behavioral syndromes for which we lack an accepted diagnostic gold standard. We started with the hypothesis that the diagnostic criteria used to identify autistic children in this study would yield reasonable AD *vs* non-AD groups, but set out to determine whether the cut-off between them could be 'fine tuned' empirically, using a regression-mixture method developed by R.R. Golden (see footnote, p. xii). We also expected that the widely accepted receptive(/expressive) *vs* expressive subtypes of DLD and those defined on clinical grounds by Rapin and Allen (1983) would be found by empirical analysis. We did not hypothesize any subtypes within AD beyond the widely conjectured high- and low-functioning subtypes described in the literature (*e.g.* Bartak and Rutter 1976, Freeman *et al.* 1981, Wing and Atwood 1987). The presumption is that subtypes reliably defined at the behavioral level may reflect some 'fundamental' underlying abnormality of brain function or structure. Not much is known about the conjectural brain abnormality or abnormalities that might determine each clinically defined syndrome, whereas previous research has identified many genetic and acquired etiological factors associated with the behavioral syndromes (for a discussion of classification issues, see Rapin 1992).

The following sequence of tests was performed (until failure) for each clinically conjectured autism and language disorder syndrome. (1) Logistic regression and regression classification trees were used to develop and identify those indicators (test scores or scales comprising items assessing related behaviors)—taken singly and in combination —which best predicted clinical diagnosis. (2) Next, these indicators were used to attempt taxometric detection of a latent 'taxon' or 'subtaxon' (conjectured 'natural' group or subgroup), employing consistency requirements across methods and indicators. (3) If a taxon was detected, then, for each individual child, the probability of being a member of the taxon was estimated and used for classification. (4) Estimates of taxon base rate, misclassification rates, indicator validities, and other latent parameters (and associations with diagnosis and other classification systems, measurements and ratings) were used to learn more about the nature of the detected taxon. The regression-mixture method, its rationale, its pitfalls and the ways in which it differs from other multivariate approaches to classification are discussed in the chapter by Golden and Mayer (1995) and other works quoted therein.

## Summary

Classification is a dynamic process that undergoes continuous revision and that will advance as our understanding of the complexities of children with neurobehavioral disorders improves. There are numerous options and limitations to the classification of these disorders. The methodology we used is a beginning step toward reaching a better understanding of the consequences of choosing particular classification systems on the resulting nosologies, and on theories regarding the nature of the neurobehavioral disorders of early childhood.

# APPENDIX 4.1
## MEASURES USED IN THE STUDY

**Neuropsychological/language measures**
• *Peabody Picture Vocabulary Test—Revised (PPVT-R)* (Dunn and Dunn 1981). The PPVT-R is one of the most widely used language tests. It has extensive norms and provides a lexical comprehension measure for children aged 2 and above. The children are presented with a four-choice picture array from which they are required to point to the picture representing the noun or verb spoken by the examiner. A raw score, standard score and age equivalent score were obtained for all children in the study on this measure.

• *Expressive One-Word Picture Vocabulary Test (EOWPVT)* (Gardner 1979). The EOWPVT, which has norms for children over 2 years of age, is a measure of the expressive lexicon. It requires confrontation naming of black and white line drawings. Raw, standard and age equivalent scores were obtained for all children.

• *Hiskey–Nebraska Test of Learning Aptitude (H-N)* (Hiskey 1966). Two H-N subtests, Picture Identification and Visual Attention Span, were administered to all children in the study. This test does not require verbal instructions or verbal responses. Raw and standard age scores were derived for the two subtests.

• *McCarthy Scales of Children's Abilities* (McCarthy 1972). Two subtests from the McCarthy—Verbal Fluency and Verbal Memory Part II—were given to all children. Raw and standard scores were derived for each subtest. The Verbal Memory Part II subtest was used to assess memory for sentences, whereas Verbal Fluency (referred to below) provided an index of categorical word retrieval.

**Tests of motor function and handedness**
• The 10-form *Seguin Formboard* (Stutsman 1931), which assesses visuospatial and motor abilities, was completed by all children under timed conditions. Both time to completion and total number of forms placed were recorded.

• The *Annett Pegboard* (Kilshaw and Annett 1983) requires children to place, with each hand, a set of ten pegs into a sequence of holes as quickly as possible. Each child received three trials with each hand, and the average for each hand was calculated.

• The *UCLA Handedness Measure* (Soper *et al.* 1986) requires each child to show how he would use a set of six objects (hammer, coin, etc.). The hand used was recorded. Each child completed this task twice in order to provide a set of 12 items for deriving a handedness ratio score [(R–L)/(R+L)].

• *Illinois Test of Psycholinguistic Abilities (ITPA)* (Kirk *et al.* 1968). The Manual Expression subtest of the ITPA provides a measure of the ability of the child to show how to use common tools and objects in response to a picture and is thus a measure of apraxia. It was given to approximately half the subjects in each diagnostic group during the videotaped play session.

**DLD-specific language measures**
A number of additional tests for assessing various components of speech or language function were given to all the DLD children. They were also given to some NALIQ and HAD children, depending on their overall level of functioning and on available testing time.

• *Photo Articulation Test (PAT)* (Pendergast *et al.* 1984). The PAT is a measure of the phonetic and phonemic characteristics of single word responses in a picture naming task. This task assesses single consonants and vowels, blends and diphthongs. Norms are available for children 3 years of age and older for tongue, lip and vowel sounds. The test also provides a total score that combines all three areas. Raw error scores were converted to standard age scores, using the age norms available in the manual. This test was used for the identification of the expressive DLD subtaxon (see Chapter 10).

• *McCarthy Scales of Children's Abilities* (McCarthy 1972). The Verbal Fluency subtest was given to DLD children. This subtest requires a child to generate a list of words within a specific category. Raw and standard scores were derived.

• *Curtiss–Yamada Comprehensive Language Evaluation—Receptive Measures (Cycle-R)* (see Curtiss *et al.* 1992). This instrument provides an in-depth assessment of comprehension within the semantic, syntactic, morphological and phonological domains. It has norms for children between the ages of 2 and 9 years and provides both global and specific domain age-equivalent scores. We devised a ratio score for this measure by dividing the age equivalent score by the chronological age used for DLD subtyping described in Chapter 10.

## Analysis of spontaneous language

Our analysis of the children's spontaneous language was informed by the psycholinguistic literature dealing with language acquisition in normal children. While a language sample collected within a given time frame may not be entirely representative of a child's total repertoire, it is at least partially so. Despite the labor-intensive time necessary to transcribe and analyze spontaneous language samples in a large population study, we felt that this kind of information was required in order to accomplish our goal of determining the similarities and differences in the population under study by comparing the linguistic performance of the four groups (DLD, HAD, LAD, NALIQ) with that of a group of normal preschool children.

### Method for data collection, transcription and scoring

Using both audio- and videotape recordings, all adult and child utterances were transcribed along with a description of the context within which each utterance occurred (following conventions described by Bloom 1970). Two different kinds of data treatment were used: (1) computer-assisted analysis, which provided quantitative data, and (2) manual analysis of elements which required clinical interpretation of the language samples. For the computer analysis, we used the Lingquest 1 software package (Mordecai *et al.* 1985). A split-half analysis of the first 50 tapes confirmed that the first 100 utterances of the child were representative of the entire transcript, and transcription was subsequently reduced to 100 utterances per child for the Lingquest analysis. The program contains a limited dictionary and a large set of linguistic rules that are used to identify, analyze and count grammatical structures and form classes (parts of speech) in the speech sample ('corpus').

Tapes transcribed for analysis included 128/201 (64%) of the DLD group, 32/51 (63%) of the HAD, 41/125 (33%) of the LAD, and 55/110 (50%) of the NALIQ, and 46/46 (100%) of the control group. The proportion of tapes that were not transcribed because of lack of intelligibility or for technical reasons (other than production of less than 25 utterances) ranged from 25% in the NALIQ group to 33% in the HAD.

*Mean length of utterances (MLU), different parts of speech classes and verb forms.* The Lingquest Program was used to compute MLUs for each language sample and counts of different parts of speech classes and verb forms. The spontaneous language sample analysis could be performed only if the child had at least partially intelligible expressive language. The Lingquest analysis required a minimum of 25 utterances. In order to preserve most of the population, we assigned an arbitrary MLU of 1.0 for children who spoke but produced fewer than 25 utterances, and an MLU of 0.1 for those who were totally nonverbal. A total of 110 children fell into these categories (8% of the DLD, 4% of the HAD, 53% of the LAD, and 24% of the NALIQ groups). Children who spoke but were totally unintelligible could not be assigned an MLU. Pragmatic and error analyses were performed if the subject produced five or more utterances, and the semantic analysis was performed on all subjects who spoke.

Although the use of computer-assisted analysis was useful for counting discrete forms and structures, there were a number of more abstract kinds of analysis that could only be carried out by a person who could take into account the context within which an utterance was produced in order to judge meaningfulness, appropriateness and errors. For this analysis, we devised coding systems: one for doing a multi-level pragmatic analysis of communicative use of language, and another for determining errors in meaning, structure and communicative use of language. The pragmatic and error analyses were performed by four pre-trained raters who held graduate degrees in speech–language pathology or psycholinguistics. The first 50 transcripts were scored by two raters, and their scores were compared. Discrepancies were resolved by a third rater. Throughout the analyses of the remaining transcripts, questionable judgments were likewise resolved by submitting the transcript to another rater. Periodic cross-checks of transcripts and of the semantic, pragmatic and error analyses were conducted throughout the study for quality assurance purposes.

*Analysis of conversational pragmatic skills.* Determining a child's knowledge of pragmatic rules for verbal communication involves a multi-level analysis. The analysis reported here is confined to the discourse level in which we determined the 'speaker role' played by the child in conversation with the adult during the play session. The child-as-speaker can assume one of four roles in the communicative interchange with a conversational partner: (1) child initiates conversation; (2) child responds to partner's initiation; (3) child continues the conversational topic; (4) child echoes or repeats what has just been said. Performing this analysis entails examining each of the child's utterances within the context of the surrounding utterances of his adult playmate. We computed the percentages of utterances in each child's corpus in which he performed each of these discourse functions by dividing the number of initiations, responses, continuations or echoes by the total number of utterances in the child's corpus. Using percentages was necessary because of the uneven numbers of utterances across and within groups.

*Error analysis.* Total transcripts were also subjected to error analysis, up to a maximum of 200 utterances. We tallied errors in (1) meaning, (2) structure, and (3) verbal pragmatics. *Meaning errors* included substitutions of lexical items or phrases that resulted in an inappropriate utterance given the context, as well as situations in which the child's meaning was unclear or ambiguous due to omission of obligatory content. *Structural errors* included incorrect use of morphological or syntactic elements, omission of obligatory function words (telegraphic speech) and incorrect word order. *Pragmatic errors* subsumed violations of the rules for conversational dialogue, including failure to take appropriate turns for speaking, failure to answer or acknowledge direct questions, failure to maintain topic, and failure to provide sufficient context for the listener's understanding. Other types of pragmatic errors included self-contradiction, addressing inanimate objects, talking to oneself and using memorized scripts. For each of the error analyses, we counted the number of utterances containing an error of a specific type and converted the numbers into percentages by dividing the number of occurrences of each error type (meaning, structural or pragmatic) by the total number of utterances in each child's corpus. An overall error score was also computed for each subject (*i.e.* number of utterances containing errors divided by total number of utterances).

## Assignment of children to clinically defined DLD subtypes
Investigators at the sites where DLD children were being tested were asked to classify the children's language disorders into the clinical subtypes proposed by Rapin and Allen (1983, 1988): (1) children with comprehension deficits at the level of phonology and, therefore, with severe expressive deficits as well, are classified as having either verbal auditory agnosia if comprehension (and expression) are very severely compromised, or mixed receptive (phonological–syntactic) deficit if their comprehension is superior to their expression; (2) children with vastly better comprehension than expression (or normal comprehension) are classified as having either verbal dyspraxia if expressive language is minimal, or speech programming deficit if they speak much more but do so unintelligibly; (3) children with adequate phonology and syntax but comprehension deficits at the level of the sentence and with word retrieval deficits are classified as having semantic–pragmatic deficit if they are verbose or lexical–syntactic deficit if expressive speech is sparse and phonology and syntax immature. For almost all the children, language was rated by more than one of the investigators. A diagnosis was accepted as reliable if all examiners rating the child agreed on their clinical classification. Children for whom there was disagreement were not included in these analyses. Clinical ratings were available for 313 children. The purpose of this analysis was to compare the empirically derived DLD subtaxa with these clinically defined subgroups. These analyses are summarized in Chapter 10.

## Behavior rating scales
• The *Social Abnormality Scales I and II* (Appendix 2) were developed in order to document a range of 21 socially abnormal behaviors characteristic of many autistic children. They were used by the child psychiatrists in their clinical assements of the children.

• The *Wing Schedule of Handicaps, Behaviour and Skills* (HBS—Appendix 5) is an interview protocol created as a modification to the Vineland Social Maturity Scale (Doll 1965). It contains all the original items from the Vineland, plus additional items focused on aberrant developmental behaviors. It provides a detailed assessment of language, play, educational achievement, abnormal sensory and motor behavior, daily living skills, behavior problems, attention and social skills. It was constructed specifically for use with children and young adults with (a) moderate, severe or profound mental retardation, (b) AD, and (c) DLD. (The original Vineland Social Maturity Scale was designed to document the development of mentally retarded individuals.) All items serve to discriminate very low levels of performance, hence it is appropriately focused for administration to the caretakers of preschool disabled children. Each child's teacher completed the interview for all groups of children. The data were used for the assessment of behavior described in Chapter 8 and for the taxometric analysis described in Chapter 10.

# 5
# HISTORICAL DATA

*I. Rapin*

Developmental disorders of higher cerebral function are thought to reflect dysfunctions of the brain arising as a consequence of a variety of genetic or acquired causes (etiologies). A problem in the clinical evaluation of children with these disorders is that in most cases there is no precisely definable brain lesion or specific finding on neurological examination to provide a clear-cut etiology or evidence on the localization and nature of the brain dysfunction.

The history form used for this project enabled us to collect systematic data on the families and on the medical and developmental histories of the children, in an attempt to evaluate possible causes and early signs of the children's disorders. We had to rely on parental reports because of logistic limitations to the type and amount of historical data we could gather. Examination of family members in such a large sample of children would have been prohibitively expensive and time consuming, as would have been documentation of all previous hospital and physician records. While these limitations restrict somewhat the validity of the evidence we are presenting, most parents are adequately reliable historians* (*e.g.* Pyles *et al.* 1935, Hefner and Mednick 1969, Knobloch *et al.* 1979, Majnemer and Rosenblatt 1994) and there is no reason to believe that there are systematic biases in their reports, which were collected uniformly across the entire sample.

We predicted that the prevalence of similarly affected family members would be higher in the AD and DLD groups than in the NALIQ group because of a stronger genetic contribution to the etiology of AD and DLD. We further predicted that sociocultural deprivation would not contribute as much variance to the AD sample as to the NALIQ sample since environmental factors are well known contributors to mild mental retardation, in contrast to acquired biological and genetic factors' strong contribution to severe mental retardation. We predicted that low socioeconomic status might also be prevalent in the families of children with DLD, because DLD, which may be inherited, often jeopardizes school performance and thus may have compromised the vocational opportunity of some of the affected parents. We did not expect a particularly high prevalence of perinatal factors in any group because we had excluded children with overt motor deficits

---

*In order to assess the reliability of parental reports, we reviewed the hospital birth records of 23 children. Correlation for number of previous pregnancies was 0.94, number of miscarriages 0.73, bleeding 0.58, length of pregnancy 0.75, birthweight 0.98, caesarian section 1.0, forceps delivery 0.76, induced labor 0.73, use of an isolette 0.45, sucking problems 0.55, need for phototherapy 0.82, remaining in hospital after mother's discharge 0.51. These correlations are based on small numbers and are provided only for information; in some cases correlations were lowered by parents responding that they did not know the answer to a question.

(cerebral palsy) and severe seizure disorders. We expected that parents would report delayed language development in all groups, that AD children would have ubiquitous comprehension deficits and impaired language use, and that nonverbal children would be most numerous in the LAD sample. Finally we anticipated that reports of deviant behaviors such as impaired sociability and play, a limited range of interests, and prevalent temper tantrums and lability of mood would be highest in the AD sample.

## Method

We developed a questionnaire that encompassed medical, developmental, behavioral, and cultural and socio-economic domains in the children and their families. We mailed questionnaires to the children's families in advance of their evaluation. In 51 per cent of cases a child neurologist, in 4 per cent a psychologist, and in 45 per cent a research assistant went over each question with the parent so as to make sure that all questions had been understood as intended and filled out as fully as possible. The mother was the informant in 92 per cent of cases. The data collected are therefore parental—mostly mothers'—reports.

Highlights of the data are presented here. The questionnaire (as used) is provided in Appendix 3. Mothers had little difficulty answering the majority of the questions. Questions which the interviewers found to be ambiguous or which the parents found difficult to answer reliably are not included in this review. Some of these omitted questions, such as those regarding use of medicines, alcohol and drugs in pregnancy, were insufficiently detailed to yield meaningful data; others could not be answered because parents had forgotten precise ages at attainment of milestones such as age at sitting, crawling or answering questions.

Data are expressed in the tables as percentage of subjects with data. Data are available on the entire sample of 487 children for most items. They are presented so as to contrast the four groups defined in the previous chapter: 201 children with DLD, 51 with AD with adequate nonverbal intelligence (NVIQ equivalent ≥80, HAD), 125 with AD with low NVIQ (<80, LAD), and 110 NALIQ. As mentioned in Chapter 4, another 69 children who completed the study were excluded because they did not meet one or more subject selection criteria for DLD or AD, and 36 children were dropped because of incomplete collection of core data. Chi-squared analysis was used to assess the significance of intergroup differences. Mean age at attainment of milestones was tested with analysis of variance with *post hoc* evaluation of intergroup differences.

## Findings

*Family histories*

We drew a pedigree of both the maternal and paternal biological families and asked a common set of questions about each of the parents, sibs, grandparents, uncles, aunts and first cousins of the probands. The questions encompassed handedness, a history of language delay or disorder, motor problems, scholastic difficulties, mental retardation, autism, attention deficit disorder, psychiatric problems, antisocial behavior, and a variety of medical and neurological conditions.

**TABLE 5.1**

**Reported conditions in immediate and extended maternal and paternal biological families (N=468)—percentage of families with at least one member with condition**

| | Immediate family | Extended family | |
| --- | --- | --- | --- |
| | | Mother's | Father's |
| *Medical condition* | | | |
| Cancer | 1.9[†] | 18.4 | 20.3 |
| Thyroid condition | 4.5 | 8.8 | 4.5 |
| Colitis, Crohn's disease | 1.5 | 3.4 | 1.7 |
| Asthma | 15.8 | 13.0 | 10.0 |
| Diabetes mellitus | 3.0[†] | 18.6 | 14.3 |
| Other | 19.2[†] | 26.7 | 26.5 |
| | | | |
| *Neurological conditions* | | | |
| Seizures | 5.8 | 4.0 | 4.1 |
| Migraine | 15.0 | 12.4 | 10.7 |
| Tics, Tourette syndrome | 1.5 | 1.1 | 0.9 |
| Stroke | 0.0[†] | 8.1 | 8.3 |
| Head injury/brain damage | 4.1 | 3.9 | 4.5 |
| Other | 4.3 | 3.4 | 4.3 |
| | | | |
| *Psychiatric conditions* | | | |
| Schizophrenia | 1.1 | 1.3 | 1.9 |
| Major depression | 5.8[†] | 10.0 | 8.6 |
| Manic–depression | 1.3 | 1.5 | 2.8 |
| Psychiatric hospitalization | 2.6[†] | 6.0 | 6.8 |
| Anxiety | 6.8 | 6.2 | 7.3 |
| Eating disorder | 3.4 | 3.4 | 3.4 |
| Antisocial behavior | 8.8 | 6.6 | 6.8 |
| Other (incl. substance abuse) | 4.9 | 7.3 | 9.6 |
| | | | |
| *Developmental conditions* | | | |
| Dysphasia or delayed speaking | 26.7 | 6.5 | 16.7 |
| Stuttering | 7.3 | 6.2 | 5.8 |
| Difficulty reading | 23.3 | 16.5 | 15.4 |
| Difficulty writing | 11.1 | 8.3 | 8.3 |
| Difficulty spelling | 15.4 | 10.9 | 10.7 |
| Difficulty with mathematics | 10.0 | 7.5 | 7.9 |
| Attention deficit | 9.6 | 8.3 | 3.8 |
| Hyperactivity | 7.5 | 7.1 | 3.4 |
| Motor deficit | 7.7 | 7.1 | 4.5 |
| Tics/Tourette syndrome | 1.5 | 1.1 | 0.9 |
| Mental deficiency | 2.4 | 1.9 | 3.0 |
| Autism | 2.6 | 1.7 | 0.6 |

No reliable difference between maternal and paternal extended families ($\chi^2$ test).

[†]Significant differences between immediate and extended families for such disorders as stroke, cancer, and diabetes mellitus are accounted for by increased prevalence in grandparents.

The data presented in this section were collected uniformly and are suitable for making comparisons among the four clinical groups and between immediate and extended families. They cannot be used to judge whether reported prevalences of particular conditions are higher in the families of the children in the study than in the general population because families were scored as having a condition whenever a family member was stated to have that particular condition, without adjustment for numbers of individuals in each family. Except for demographic variables, data concerning medical, neurological, psychiatric and developmental disorders are reported only for the biological families of 468 children, excluding adopted children.

FAMILY CHARACTERISTICS

Because mothers overwhelmingly were the providers of historical information, they might have known more about abnormalities in their own families than in the fathers' families. However, data in Table 5.1 show little difference in the reported prevalence of disorders of interest in the fathers' and mothers' extended families across the entire sample. Grandparents account for the excess of conditions of later life such as diabetes mellitus, cancer, cardiovascular diseases and depression in extended families compared to immediate families. Better information about immediate than about extended families may account for a trend toward the report of higher prevalences of some developmental disabilities in immediate families, a finding also commented upon by Lewis (1992) in pedigree analysis of families of children with phonological disabilities.

MEDICAL HISTORY

We collected data on the prevalence in the family of medical disorders, including cancer, thyroid problems, diabetes mellitus, asthma, Crohn's disease or colitis, migraine headaches and other medical conditions. We found no difference across the four groups in either immediate or extended families for any of these disorders (Table 5.2). The particular conditions about which we chose to ask specifically were influenced by the report by Geschwind and Galaburda (1984) that there is an excess of autoimmune disorders in the families of developmentally disordered children. Other investigators (*e.g.* Urion 1988, Hynd *et al.* 1990, Wood and Cooper 1992) have attempted to duplicate these findings in families of dyslexic children, with mixed results.

Among the neurological conditions in family members, we inquired particularly about disorders that may be familial and those reported to be associated with developmental disorders such as convulsive disorders, tics or Tourette syndrome, migraine, stroke and head injury. There was no difference across groups for any of these variables (Table 5.2). A 4–6 per cent familial prevalence of seizures seems somewhat high but is consonant with a 4 per cent cumulative life expectancy to age 80 for epilepsy (Engel 1989) and, probably, with the inclusion of some family members with provoked seizures, *e.g.* febrile seizures, rather than epilepsy.

PSYCHIATRIC HISTORY

A major concern was whether there were differences among the families of the four

TABLE 5.2
**Reported medical and neurological disorders in immediate and extended families—percentage of biological families with at least one member with condition[1]**

| | DLD (N=192) | HAD (N=51) | LAD (N=120) | NALIQ (N=105) | All (N=468) |
|---|---|---|---|---|---|
| **A: Immediate family** | | | | | |
| *Medical conditions* | | | | | |
| Cancer | 1.6 | 0.4 | 2.5 | 1.0 | 1.9 |
| Thyroid conditions | 3.1 | 7.8 | 5.8 | 3.8 | 4.5 |
| Colitis, Crohn's disease | 0.5 | 2.0 | 2.5 | 1.9 | 1.5 |
| Asthma | 16.7 | 13.7 | 18.3 | 12.4 | 15.8 |
| Diabetes mellitus | 3.1 | 3.9 | 1.7 | 3.8 | 3.0 |
| Other | 18.8 | 13.7 | 25.8 | 15.2 | 19.2 |
| *Neurological conditions* | | | | | |
| Seizures | 6.8 | 0.0 | 7.5 | 4.8 | 5.8 |
| Migraine | 15.1 | 21.6 | 13.3 | 13.3 | 15.0 |
| Tics, Tourette syndrome | 2.6 | 2.0 | 0.8 | 0.0 | 1.5 |
| Stroke | 0.0 | 0.0 | 0.0 | 0.0 | 0.0 |
| Brain injury/damage | 6.3 | 2.0 | 0.8 | 4.8 | 4.1 |
| Other | 4.2 | 4.0 | 1.7 | 7.6 | 4.3 |
| **B: Extended family** | | | | | |
| *Medical conditions* | | | | | |
| Cancer | 36.5 | 33.3 | 35.0 | 28.6 | 34.0 |
| Thyroid conditions | 12.5 | 11.8 | 8.3 | 16.2 | 12.2 |
| Colitis, Crohn's disease | 6.3 | 5.9 | 5.0 | 1.9 | 4.9 |
| Asthma | 21.4 | 25.5 | 21.7 | 18.1 | 21.2 |
| Diabetes mellitus | 31.3 | 35.3 | 24.2 | 28.6 | 29.3 |
| Other | 40.6 | 43.1 | 45.0 | 41.9 | 42.3 |
| *Neurological conditions* | | | | | |
| Seizures | 8.3 | 3.9 | 10.0 | 5.7 | 7.7 |
| Migraine | 19.3 | 15.7 | 22.5 | 21.0 | 20.1 |
| Tics, Tourette syndrome | 3.7 | 0.0 | 1.7 | 0.0 | 1.9 |
| Stroke | 15.6 | 13.7 | 16.7 | 12.4 | 15.0 |
| Brain injury/damage | 8.9 | 2.0 | 8.3 | 7.6 | 7.7 |
| Other | 7.3 | 3.9 | 6.7 | 10.5 | 7.5 |

[1]No significant difference among the four groups ($\chi^2$ test).

groups in the prevalence of depression or manic–depressive illness (reported to be linked to some high-functioning autistic children—DeLong and Dwyer 1988, DeLong 1994, DeLong and Nohria 1994), schizophrenia, and antisocial behaviors such as substance abuse, that might have had deleterious fetal effects. There was a trend for immediate but not extended families of LAD children to have a higher prevalence of psychiatric disorders than the other groups, but differences among the four groups failed to reach significance for any disorder (Table 5.3). The prevalence of major depression was highest in the immediate families of LAD children but was low in those of HAD children, and that of manic–depressive illness was equal in both AD groups. Again, our data are

**TABLE 5.3**
**Reported psychiatric conditions in immediate and extended families—**
**percentage of biological families with at least one member with condition**

| | DLD (N=192) | HAD (N=51) | LAD (N=120) | NALIQ (N=105) | All (N=468) |
|---|---|---|---|---|---|
| **A: Immediate family**[1] | | | | | |
| Schizophrenia | 1.0 | 0.0 | 1.7 | 1.0 | 1.1 |
| Major depression | 5.2 | 2.0 | 8.3 | 5.7 | 5.8 |
| Manic–depression | 1.0 | 2.0 | 1.7 | 1.0 | 1.3 |
| Psychiatric hospitalization | 2.1 | 2.0 | 5.0 | 1.0 | 2.6 |
| Anxiety | 6.8 | 3.9 | 7.5 | 7.6 | 6.8 |
| Eating disorder | 2.1 | 0.0 | 5.0 | 5.7 | 3.4 |
| Antisocial behavior | 8.3 | 5.9 | 14.2 | 4.8 | 8.8 |
| Other (incl. substance abuse) | 2.6 | 5.9 | 7.5 | 5.7 | 4.9 |
| **B: Extended family** | | | | | |
| Schizophrenia | 3.1 | 0.0 | 5.0 | 2.9 | 3.2 |
| Major depression | 13.0 | 23.5 | 20.0 | 15.2 | 16.5 |
| Manic–depression | 3.7 | 3.9 | 5.0 | 4.8 | 4.3 |
| Psychiatric hospitalization | 10.4 | 9.8 | 14.2 | 10.5 | 11.3 |
| Anxiety | 8.9 | 21.6 | 15.8 | 10.5 | 12.4 |
| Eating disorder | 5.7 | 5.9 | 8.3 | 6.7 | 6.6 |
| Antisocial behavior | 8.3 | 15.7 | 18.3 | 10.5 | 12.2 |
| Other (incl. substance abuse)* | 9.9 | 11.8 | 22.5 | 12.4 | 13.9 |

[1]No significant difference among the four groups ($\chi^2$ test).
*Significant difference among the four groups ($\chi^2$, p<0.05).

unsuitable to determine whether prevalences in these families are generally higher than expected in the non-impaired population.

DEVELOPMENTAL AND EDUCATIONAL PROBLEMS

We asked about late development of language or language disorder, stuttering, motor problems (unspecified on the form but clarified by the interviewers as clumsiness, as well as mild cerebral palsy or other motor deficits), scholastic difficulties, attention deficits, mental retardation and autism. Parents of DLD children reported a significantly higher prevalence of language disorders in their immediate families (33 per cent) than parents of NALIQ and autistic children (20–24 per cent) did in theirs (Table 5.4). Although other differences among groups were non-significant, there was a trend for parents of DLD and NALIQ children to have been late speakers and also for siblings of DLD and LAD children to have been late speaking in sentences (Table 5.5). Parents of DLD children reported about twice as high a prevalence of reading (29 per cent) and spelling (19 per cent) disorders in their immediate families as parents of AD children (19 per cent and 8 per cent). Parents of NALIQ children reported prevalences of reading and spelling disorders in their immediate families similar to those of parents of DLD children. Among extended families, the only discrimination was language disorders in DLD families. Prevalences of learning disabilities of less than 10 per cent in the general

## TABLE 5.4
### Reported developmental disorders in immediate and extended families— percentage of biological families with at least one member with disorder

| | DLD (N=192) | HAD (N=51) | LAD (N=120) | NALIQ (N=105) | All (N=468) |
|---|---|---|---|---|---|
| **A: Immediate family** | | | | | |
| Dysphasia/delayed speech* | 33.3 | 19.6 | 24.2 | 21.0 | 26.7 |
| Stuttering | 6.8 | 5.9 | 9.2 | 6.7 | 7.3 |
| Difficulty reading** | 29.2 | 15.7 | 14.2 | 26.7 | 23.3 |
| Difficulty writing | 15.1 | 5.9 | 6.7 | 11.4 | 11.1 |
| Difficulty spelling* | 18.8 | 7.8 | 9.2 | 20.0 | 15.4 |
| Difficulty with mathematics | 12.5 | 3.9 | 7.5 | 11.4 | 10.0 |
| Hyperactivity | 10.4 | 11.8 | 11.7 | 4.8 | 9.6 |
| Attention deficit | 6.3 | 11.8 | 9.2 | 5.7 | 7.5 |
| Motor deficit* | 12.0 | 7.8 | 4.2 | 3.8 | 7.7 |
| Tics/Tourette syndrome | 2.6 | 2.0 | 0.8 | 0.0 | 1.5 |
| Mental deficiency | 2.1 | 3.9 | 1.7 | 2.9 | 2.4 |
| Autism | 2.1 | 3.9 | 5.0 | 0.0 | 2.6 |
| **B: Extended family** | | | | | |
| Dysphasia/delayed speech** | 37.0 | 27.5 | 20.0 | 27.6 | 29.5 |
| Stuttering | 15.1 | 11.8 | 8.3 | 9.5 | 11.8 |
| Difficulty reading | 30.7 | 31.4 | 25.8 | 23.8 | 28.0 |
| Difficulty writing | 17.2 | 11.8 | 15.0 | 14.3 | 15.4 |
| Difficulty spelling | 20.8 | 21.6 | 18.3 | 18.1 | 19.7 |
| Difficulty with mathematics | 13.5 | 15.7 | 14.2 | 15.2 | 14.3 |
| Hyperactivity | 10.4 | 19.6 | 10.8 | 10.5 | 11.5 |
| Attention deficit | 13.0 | 13.7 | 6.7 | 6.7 | 10.0 |
| Motor deficit | 8.9 | 9.8 | 9.2 | 16.2 | 10.7 |
| Tics/Tourette syndrome | 3.7 | 0.0 | 1.7 | 0.0 | 1.9 |
| Mental deficiency | 5.7 | 0.0 | 5.8 | 3.8 | 4.7 |
| Autism | 1.6 | 3.9 | 3.3 | 1.9 | 2.4 |

*Significant difference among four groups ($\chi^2$, p<0.05).
**Significant difference among four groups ($\chi^2$, p<0.01).


## TABLE 5.5
### Parents and siblings[1] with developmental disorders—percentage of children with affected relative

| | DLD (N=192) | HAD (N=51) | LAD (N=120) | NALIQ (N=105) | All (N=468) |
|---|---|---|---|---|---|
| Parent with DLD | 19.4 | 7.8 | 10.4 | 15.5 | 15.0 |
| Sib with DLD | 22.8 | 19.4 | 22.0 | 11.0 | 19.8 |
| Sib 1st words >19 mo | 9.4 | 0.0 | 8.8 | 2.4 | 7.0 |
| Sib 1st sentence >25 mo | 15.6 | 6.5 | 12.1 | 8.5 | 12.5 |
| Parent with AD | 0.5 | 0.0 | 0.0 | 0.0 | 0.2 |
| Sib with AD* | 1.7 | 6.5 | 6.6 | 0.0 | 2.9 |

[1]Only 384 children have siblings, 103 are only children (see Chapter 4).
*Significant difference among groups ($\chi^2$, p<0.05).

TABLE 5.6
**Disorders in the immediate family by socioeconomic status (SES) level—percentage of 455 biological families with at least one affected member**

**A. Neurological and psychiatric disorders**

| SES level[1] | Mental deficiency | Autism | Manic– depression | Depressive illness | Schizo- phrenia | Tics |
|---|---|---|---|---|---|---|
| I (High) | 2.0 | 4.0 | 0.0 | 0.0 | 0.0 | 6.0 |
| II | 0.0 | 5.5 | 1.8 | 10.0 | 1.8 | 0.9 |
| III (Middle) | 1.3 | 0.6 | 2.5 | 7.6 | 1.3 | 0.6 |
| IV | 2.0 | 3.0 | 0.0 | 3.0 | 0.0 | 2.0 |
| V (Low) | 16.2 | 0.0 | 0.0 | 2.7 | 0.0 | 0.0 |
| All | 2.4 | 2.6 | 1.3 | 5.9 | 0.9 | 1.5 |
| p ($\chi^2$) | 0.001 | ns | ns | ns | ns | ns |

**B. Language/learning disabilities**

| SES level[1] | DLD | Stuttering | Reading | Spelling | Mathematics | ADD |
|---|---|---|---|---|---|---|
| I (High) | 24.0 | 16.0 | 14.0 | 12.0 | 2.0 | 10.0 |
| II | 20.9 | 6.4 | 19.1 | 9.1 | 8.2 | 11.8 |
| III (Middle) | 25.9 | 6.3 | 24.5 | 15.7 | 12.0 | 6.9 |
| IV | 33.3 | 7.1 | 24.2 | 18.2 | 10.1 | 11.1 |
| V (Low) | 46.0 | 5.4 | 37.8 | 29.7 | 18.9 | 13.5 |
| All | 27.3 | 7.5 | 23.1 | 15.4 | 10.1 | 9.9 |
| p ($\chi^2$) | 0.02 | ns | ns | 0.04 | ns | ns |

[1]Hollingshead score.

population are often quoted (*e.g.* Stevenson and Richman 1976), but higher figures are reported by Silva (1980) and Beitchman *et al.* (1986*b*) in population surveys of pre-school children with language disorders.

Parents of AD children reported an increased prevalence of autism in their immediate and extended families: although differences among the four groups did not reach statistical significance, there was a significantly higher prevalence of autism (6.6 per cent) among the siblings of both HAD and LAD children (Table 5.5). We enrolled four pairs of siblings in the study, three concordant for DLD and one for autism. In addition there were seven pairs of twins, three said to be dizygotic (two concordant for DLD, one with one DLD and one autistic twin) and four said to be monozygotic (three concordant for autism, one with one DLD and one autistic twin). (One pair of concordant autistic twins was diagnosed as having Cornelia de Lange syndrome after they were enrolled in the study.)

SOCIOECONOMIC CHARACTERISTICS

Socioeconomic and demographic data were collected because of reports indicating that variables such as poverty, lack of education, and low cognitive skills of mothers are correlated with suboptimal outcome in children with developmental deficits (*e.g.* Richardson 1981, Broman *et al.* 1987). With few exceptions (discussed in Chapter 4), differences among the four groups were negligible in regard to race, gender, parents' level of education and socioeconomic status (SES), and language spoken in the home. Therefore we examined the effects of these social variables across the entire sample (Table 5.6), hypothesizing that low NVIQ (LIQ), DLD and reading difficulty would be inversely correlated with SES. The data support this well-documented correlation. There was no relation between SES and AD or any of the psychiatric disorders.

DISCUSSION

None of the medical, neurological or psychiatric conditions we enquired about discriminated strongly among the families of the four groups of developmentally disabled children in the study. This lack of difference is consonant with probably heterogeneous genetic factors playing a substantial role in DLD and AD (for a review, see Rapin 1994). Lack of discrimination between groups in terms of prevalence of affected family members is not surprising if one considers that these disorders are likely to have a variety of genetic and non-genetic etiologies. It is in families with a dominant or X-linked mendelian genetic etiology that histories are apt to identify affected members in multiple generations, whereas siblings are likely to be selectively affected in autosomal recessive disorders. Same-sex twin studies or segregation analyses of specific neuropsychological traits in multiple large families are required to discern specific inheritance patterns in the developmental disabilities. Our study does not provide such data.

Because of the role of genetic factors in the developmental disabilities, we had hypothesized that the prevalence of family members with DLD would be higher in the families of DLD children than of AD children, and that there would be more family members with AD in the families of AD than of DLD children. We made no hypothesis about the NALIQ group which was viewed as an etiologically diverse control group. The fact that DLDs and reading and spelling difficulties were somewhat more prevalent in the families of the DLD than of the AD children supported our hypothesis, which was based on reports of dominantly inherited expressive DLD and dominant dyslexia (*e.g.* Lewis *et al.* 1989, 1992; Pennington 1991; Lewis 1992). Similarly, the high prevalence of AD was limited to the siblings of children with AD. These negative and positive findings in the families of DLD and AD children are consistent with the notion that DLD and AD are etiologically distinct rather than the nonspecific manifestation of one or more shared genetic or environmental causes for developmental disorders (August *et al.* 1981).

• *Autism.* Although it is not possible to rule out the effects of a shared environment, the high prevalence of AD in sibs supports a strong genetic contribution to its etiology (Folstein and Piven 1991, Gillberg and Coleman 1992). Folstein and Rutter (1977) found that 2 per cent of autistic children have an autistic sibling, while Smalley (1991) quotes a figure of 3–5 per cent; these figures are lower than the 6.5 per cent reported in the present study but dramatically higher than prevalence figures in the general population (see below). Our figure is closer to the overall recurrence risk of 8.7 per cent reported in the epidemiological study of autism in Utah (Ritvo *et al.* 1989*b*). This high prevalence of autism in the families of children with autism needs to be stressed. Asperger (1944) stated that the parents of high-functioning autistic children often have autistic traits, a finding confirmed by others (Gillberg 1989). Ritvo and colleagues (1988, 1989*b*) evaluated family members of children with autistic symptomatology in Utah and found an apparent genetic etiology in a substantial number of families, including 11 families with an affected parent (usually the father) and one or more affected children, suggesting dominant inheritance in those families. These two-generation families indicate that the social skills of some mildly affected autistic individuals with adequate intelligence are sufficient to enable them to marry. This seems to be a rare event, judging from the absence of autistic parents reported in the present study.

Probably the most reliable study on the prevalence of AD is a whole population survey carried out in a prefecture of Nagoya, Japan in which every infant born over a 10 year period was followed to age 3 years. This survey suggests a prevalence of around 1.6–2.0/1000 preschool children (Sugiyama and Abe 1989, Sugiyama *et al.* 1992), considerably higher than the figure of 3–5/10,000 that is often quoted for the condition (Van Bourgondien *et al.* 1987). Estimates from the surveys by Wing and Gould (1979) in London, Gillberg (1984) in Göteborg, Sweden, Ritvo *et al.* (1985, 1989*a*) in Utah, and Bryson *et al.* (1988) in Nova Scotia, are closer to these lower figures, although the more recent study of Gillberg *et al.* (1991) in Sweden quotes a prevalence of 8.4/10,000 for 'nuclear' autism.

Reviews of prevalence figures for autism by Gillberg and Coleman (1992) and Wing (1993) indicate that one reason for discrepancies among different series is lack of consensus on diagnostic criteria for 'autism' and 'autistic-like' conditions, despite the publication of descriptive criteria in the various editions of the DSM and ICD manuals. Another reason for the lower figures may be that, however careful, these regional surveys relied on referrals and on programs for the disabled to identify probands. As a result they no doubt missed some less severely affected children attending regular classes, some of whom would have fulfilled criteria for HAD, PDD-NOS or Asperger syndrome. It is not clear at this time whether such children represent separate disorders or the upper end of the distribution of children on an autistic spectrum (Wing 1988, 1991; Szatmari *et al.* 1989*b*; Frith 1991). These children tend to be more easily detectable in very early childhood than at school age, because they often appear much more classically autistic before they become verbal than in mid-childhood or adolescence when their social skills may have improved substantially. This may explain in part the higher prevalence figure from Nagoya and suggests that, when the entire PDD spectrum is considered, the usually quoted figure of only 20–30 per cent of AD subjects with IQs above 70 may have to be revised upward.

We asked specifically about tics and Tourette syndrome in the families of the children because of the recent speculation that autism may be the homozygous manifestation of the gene for Tourette syndrome (Comings and Comings 1991, Sverd 1991). Our data do not provide supporting evidence for a link between autism and Tourette syndrome or for linkage of autism with manic–depressive illness in family members (DeLong and Dwyer 1988, DeLong 1994, DeLong and Nohria 1994). This lack of evidence must be viewed tentatively since ours are not primary data based on personal assessment of all family members.

• *Developmental language disorders and reading disability.* We reiterate that the significantly high prevalence of DLD and learning disabilities in the families of children in the DLD group corroborates the significant role of genetics as a cause of both language disorders and learning disabilities, and that in a sizable number of cases, reading disability may be the later manifestation of DLD (*e.g.* Weiner 1985, Kamhi and Catts 1986, Bishop and Adams 1990, Rissman *et al.* 1990). Genetic contribution to the etiology of dyslexia has been known for a long time (*e.g.* Hallgren 1950, Finucci *et al.* 1976, Pennington and Smith 1983). This has been shown convincingly for dyslexia in a large Colorado family (Smith *et al.* 1983, Pennington 1991, Pennington *et al.* 1991) in which the trait appears to be autosomal dominant and linked to chromosome 6 (Cardon *et al.* 1994). DLD across three generations of a British family (Hurst *et al.* 1990, Vargha-Khadem and Passingham 1990, Gopnik and Crago 1991) also suggests dominant inheritance. A genetic contribution to attention deficit disorder with hyperactivity (Biederman *et al.* 1986, Goodman and Stevenson 1989) and to some cases of verbal dyspraxia, a severe developmental disorder of verbal expression with good comprehension, is suspected (Lewis *et al.* 1989, 1992; Lewis 1992). Tallal *et al.* (1991) reported an extremely high frequency (70 per cent) of positive histories of language/reading deficits in the parents of DLD children in San Diego, again suggesting dominant inheritance, but with the added twist that the 4:1 ratio of boys to girls was found only in children with positive family histories. Similarly, recent studies of developmental speech and language disorders among twins have shown monozygotic twins to have higher concordance than dizygotic twins (Lewis and Thompson 1992, Tomblin and Buckwalter 1994).

Interpretation of the increased prevalence of delayed or deficient language acquisition and learning disabilities in the families of children in the NALIQ group is difficult, owing to the fact that a significantly larger number (43 per cent) of these families came from the two lower SES groups than was the case in families with DLD (28 per cent) and AD (24 per cent). Without first-hand data on family members it would be hazardous to try to disentangle genetic (whether mental retardation or developmental disorder), environmental and social factors as causes of this high prevalence of language and learning disabilities.

In summary, the high prevalence of specific developmental disorders in the families of the four groups of children in this study is probably real. Although published prevalence figures for DLD in the general population range from less than 5 per cent to over 20 per cent (Levine 1980, Beitchman *et al.* 1986*b*) because of the lack of agreed-upon diagnostic criteria for DLD (Aram *et al.* 1993) and of variability of age at ascertainment (for a review, see Beitchman *et al.* 1986*b*), the rates in our four groups are higher than the highest estimates for the general population. Prevalence estimates for DLD are strongly linked to age and are highest in preschool children (Silva 1980, Tallal 1988), because most children with DLD learn to speak before school entry. This observation has led to the widely held but biologically unproven hypothesis that DLD may be but the reflection of a lag in brain maturation rather than a disorder, especially in the case of children with exclusively expressive disorders (Locke 1994, Whitehurst and Fischel 1994). The maturational delay hypothesis contradicts the persistence of spelling deficits for non-words in compensated ('recovered') dyslexics (Pennington *et al.* 1991) and of temporal processing deficits in former dysphasics (Tallal *et al.* 1993).

### TABLE 5.7
**Characteristics of the pregnancy**

|  | DLD (N=189) % | HAD (N=50) % | LAD (N=116) % | NALIQ (N=102) % | All (N=457) % |
|---|---|---|---|---|---|
| Length of pregnancy (N=439) |  |  |  |  |  |
| <33 weeks (N=19) | 5.1 | 0.0 | 2.6 | 7.1 | 4.3 |
| 33–37 weeks (N=84) | 19.7 | 27.1 | 14.9 | 19.2 | 19.1 |
| 38–42 weeks (N=316) | 73.0 | 66.7 | 76.3 | 67.7 | 72.0 |
| 43–44 weeks (N=20) | 2.3 | 6.2 | 6.1 | 6.1 | 4.6 |
| Bleeding (N=457) | 11.1 | 16.0 | 8.6 | 6.9 | 10.1 |
| Infection (N=455) | 3.7 | 4.0 | 7.0 | 4.9 | 4.8 |
| Diabetes mellitus (N=457) | 3.7 | 4.0 | 2.6 | 3.0 | 3.3 |
| Toxemia (N=457) | 9.5 | 10.0 | 11.2 | 7.8 | 9.6 |
| Other (N=449)* | 9.6 | 16.0 | 21.1 | 8.2 | 13.0 |

*Significant difference among the four groups ($\chi^2$, p<0.05).

### Medical histories

Despite the strong evidence for the significant role of genetics in the etiology of the developmental disorders of higher cerebral function, acquired disorders of brain development are frequently invoked in their causation. Non-genetic dysplastic disorders, gestational complications, preterm birth (Volpe 1991), perinatal insults resulting in hypoxia or intracranial bleeding (Volpe 1995), and serious postnatal illnesses or trauma that might damage the brain are often cited as risk factors for mental retardation, language and learning difficulties, and autism. The history form therefore inquired about these aspects of the child's history.

PRENATAL AND PERINATAL HISTORY

Questions put to mothers included the length of their pregnancy, any abnormalities of the pregnancy or delivery, the infant's birthweight, and any neonatal complications such as assisted ventilation and admission to the neonatal intensive care unit (NICU).

Table 5.7 summarizes the gestational variables in the four groups. There was no statistically reliable difference among the groups. Overall, 77 per cent of pregnancies lasted 37 or more weeks. None of the HAD children was born of a pregnancy lasting less than 33 weeks, in contrast to 7 per cent of the NALIQ and 5 per cent of the DLD children. Mean birthweights were within the normal range and similar in all groups (Table 5.8), with the exception of the NALIQ children who were somewhat more likely than other groups to have been born extremely preterm. The high prevalence of infants whom their mothers considered to have a low weight for their gestational age should be viewed with caution in the absence of corroborative evidence.

Complications of the pregnancy (Table 5.7) and delivery (Table 5.9) did not differentiate the groups. The large number of reports of neonatal cyanosis or depression may be exaggerated in view of the considerably smaller proportion of infants requiring assisted ventilation or admission to an NICU (Table 5.10). Infants with birthweights of

### TABLE 5.8
### Birthweight

|  | DLD (N=196) % | HAD (N=50) % | LAD (N=122) % | NALIQ (N=108) % | All (N=476) % |
|---|---|---|---|---|---|
| Birthweight |  |  |  |  |  |
| <1.5 kg (N=15) | 2.0 | 2.0 | 1.6 | 7.4 | 3.2 |
| 1.5 to <2.5 kg (N=53) | 8.7 | 12.0 | 15.6 | 10.2 | 11.1 |
| 2.5 to 4.0 kg (N=369) | 80.6 | 74.0 | 74.6 | 76.9 | 77.5 |
| >4.0 kg (N=39) | 8.7 | 12.0 | 8.2 | 5.6 | 8.2 |
| Small for gestational age (N=463) | 4.5 | 11.8 | 13.7 | 11.1 | 9.1 |
| (Mean birthweight, kg) | (3.33) | (3.33) | (3.29) | (3.17)* | (3.28) |

No significant differences among 4 groups ($\chi^2$ test).
*Significantly lower than DLD ($p < 0.05$, ANOVA).


### TABLE 5.9
### Characteristics of the delivery

|  | DLD (N=200) % | HAD (N=51) % | LAD (N=124) % | NALIQ (N=108) % | All (N=483) % |
|---|---|---|---|---|---|
| Labor induced (N=478) | 19.3 | 21.6 | 24.4 | 27.1 | 22.6 |
| Breech (N=351)[1] | 10.8 | 15.0 | 11.4 | 13.2 | 12.2 |
| Forceps (N=474) | 12.8 | 5.9 | 15.5 | 12.4 | 12.7 |
| Caesarian section (N=483) | 21.0 | 21.6 | 29.0 | 29.6 | 25.1 |
| Labor >24 hrs (N=475) | 8.7 | 11.8 | 11.4 | 14.2 | 11.0 |
| Asphyxia, neonatal depression[2] (N=468) | 30.2 | 31.4 | 37.5 | 39.1 | 34.2 |

No significant difference among groups ($\chi^2$ test).
[1]Percentage calculated after removal of 121 children born by caesarian section.
[2]At least one of six potential problems reported (*i.e.* nuchal cord, no immediate cry, cyanosis, oxygen administration, breathing problems, use of ventilator).


### TABLE 5.10
### Neonatal problems

|  | DLD (N=199) % | HAD (N=51) % | LAD (N=124) % | NALIQ (N=108) % | All (N=482) % |
|---|---|---|---|---|---|
| Intensive care (N=482) | 14.1 | 13.7 | 13.7 | 20.4 | 15.4 |
| Ventilator (N=480) | 3.5 | 0.0 | 2.4 | 6.5 | 3.5 |
| Neonatal seizures (N=482) | 0.5 | 0.0 | 2.4 | 4.6 | 1.9 |
| Other problem(s)[1] (N=468)* | 20.3 | 21.6 | 30.8 | 33.3 | 26.1 |
| Not discharged with mother (N=481) | 16.2 | 15.7 | 16.9 | 17.6 | 16.6 |

[1]At least one of eight potential problems reported (*i.e.* abnormal movements, seizures, problems with heart rate, difficulty sucking or swallowing, limpness, stiffness).
*Significant difference among groups ($\chi^2$, $p < 0.05$).

<1.5 kg and 1.5–2.5 kg respectively accounted for 15.7 per cent and 30 per cent of admissions to these units, and infants <2.5 kg for 43.4 per cent of those who were not discharged home with their mothers. There was no difference among the four groups in the percentage admitted to the NICU. Phototherapy for hyperbilirubinemia and, in some hospitals, routine admission to NICUs for 24 hours of infants born by caesarian section (N=121) and breech presentation (N=43) may have contributed to NICU admissions and prolonged hospital stays of infants who did not have low birthweights.

Somewhat more neonatal problems that were potential risk factors for brain damage (see Table 5.10) were reported in the two LIQ groups (LAD, NALIQ) than in the DLD and HAD groups. There were nine children with Down syndrome among the NALIQ children, but they accounted for only two of the children admitted to NICUs.

POSTNATAL HISTORY

A criterion for inclusion in the study was a hearing level of 20 dB or better binaurally at 1000 and 2000 Hz, and 25 Hz or better binaurally at 500 and 4000 Hz, documented by an audiologist. Chronic middle ear effusion has been implicated as a cause of delayed language acquisition (Zinkus and Gottlieb 1980, Brookhouser and Goldgar 1987), although its pathogenic importance is debated, at least for otherwise normal children (Klein and Rapin 1988, US Department of Health and Human Services 1994). We asked parents whether the child had had any episode of otitis media or middle ear effusion, and if so how many, and whether he had undergone tympanostomy for insertion of ventilating tubes. There was no significant difference among the groups for any of these variables (Table 5.11). A third of the parents reported that their child had been essentially otitis-free, and 50 per cent that the child had had no more than two episodes. Close to a third of parents (29 per cent) reported six or more episodes of otitis, with 10 per cent of the children undergoing tympanostomy. Figures on the prevalence of middle ear disease may be imprecise but do not suggest that middle ear effusion played a major role as a causative agent for language impairment in our cohort. Our data are almost identical with those in Haynes and Naidoo's (1991) study (a 45 per cent report of middle ear problems and 16 per cent of tympanostomy among 121 DLD children).

The questionnaire included a number of items about postnatal potentially encephalopathic events (Table 5.12). Only nine parents reported meningitis or encephalitis in their children, six of them in the LAD group. There was no difference among groups in the prevalence of head injury with loss of consciousness or of other illnesses, including hospitalizations and surgical interventions. Inasmuch as these latter illnesses were not associated with seizures, loss of consciousness or other evidence of an encephalopathy, their relevance is highly questionable.

What did differentiate the groups was a history of seizures, even though frequent seizures or the need for high dose anticonvulsants was an exclusionary criterion for the study. The prevalence of epilepsy (more than one unprovoked seizure, an episode of status epilepticus, or a history of infantile spasms) was 7 per cent overall, with generalized seizures reported in 6 per cent of the children. 6 per cent of the children were currently taking anticonvulsant drugs, which corroborates the reported prevalence figures.

## TABLE 5.11
### Middle ear problems

| | DLD (N=201) % | HAD (N=51) % | LAD (N=125) % | NALIQ (N=110) % | All (N=487) % |
|---|---|---|---|---|---|
| Ear infection | | | | | |
| Never | 29.3 | 27.5 | 34.4 | 41.8 | 33.3 |
| 1–2 times | 19.9 | 19.6 | 16.0 | 12.7 | 17.3 |
| 3–6 times | 24.9 | 16.6 | 18.4 | 17.3 | 20.9 |
| >6 times | 25.9 | 33.3 | 31.2 | 28.2 | 28.6 |
| Myringotomy + tubes | 10.5 | 2.0 | 8.0 | 9.1 | 8.6 |

No significant difference among the four groups ($\chi^2$ test).


## TABLE 5.12
### Child's medical history

| | DLD (N=201) % | HAD (N=51) % | LAD (N=125) % | NALIQ (N=110) % | All (N=487) % |
|---|---|---|---|---|---|
| *Events* | | | | | |
| Encephalitis/meningitis (N=487)* | 1.0 | 0.0 | 4.8 | 0.9 | 1.8 |
| Epilepsy (N=487)* | 4.5 | 0.0 | 11.2 | 9.1 | 6.8 |
| Infantile spasms (N=487)*** | 0.0 | 0.0 | 7.2 | 2.7 | 2.5 |
| Currently on anticonvulsant drug (N=438)* | 4.5 | 2.1 | 4.6 | 11.8 | 5.9 |
| Febrile seizures (N=487) | 6.5 | 2.0 | 4.0 | 8.2 | 5.8 |
| 'Staring' (N=487)*** | 5.5 | 15.7 | 34.4 | 17.3 | 16.6 |
| Concussion/coma (N=487) | 3.0 | 0.0 | 1.6 | 3.6 | 2.5 |
| Other illness (N=487) | 19.9 | 19.6 | 28.0 | 24.6 | 23.0 |
| *Tests performed* | | | | | |
| Imaging (CT, MRI) (N=487)*** | 11.0 | 5.9 | 32.8 | 32.7 | 20.9 |
| EEG (N=487)*** | 11.9 | 17.7 | 51.2 | 41.8 | 29.4 |

*Significant difference among the four groups ($\chi^2$, p<0.05).
***Significant difference among the four groups ($\chi^2$, p<0.001).


Seizures were more than twice as prevalent in the NALIQ and LAD groups as in the DLD group, and no seizures were reported in the HAD group. The LAD and NALIQ groups were the ones most likely to encompass children with diffuse brain pathology who are prone to seizures (Goulden *et al.* 1991, Tuchman *et al.* 1991*b*). Significantly, infantile spasms, a seizure type linked with mental retardation and autism (Taft and Cohen 1971), were reported in 12 children, all in either the LAD or NALIQ groups, with almost three times as many in the LAD group. Status epilepticus, which, in any case, generally has a benign prognosis in childhood (Maytal *et al.* 1989), had occurred too infrequently to enable any judgment to be made about its importance, being reported in only seven children, four in the DLD, two in the LAD, and one in the NALIQ group.

TABLE 5.13
**Sleep problems**

|  | DLD (N=201) % | HAD (N=51) % | LAD (N=125) % | NALIQ (N=110) % | All (N=487) % |
|---|---|---|---|---|---|
| *Type of problem* | | | | | |
| Falling asleep*** | 15.9 | 25.5 | 38.4 | 15.5 | 22.6 |
| Waking up early*** | 16.9 | 17.7 | 37.6 | 20.9 | 23.2 |
| Waking > 1 time during the night | 33.3 | 35.3 | 48.0 | 37.3 | 38.2 |
| *Number of problems*** | | | | | |
| None | 60.7 | 56.9 | 40.8 | 54.6 | 53.8 |
| Any one | 21.4 | 15.7 | 15.2 | 26.4 | 20.3 |
| Any two | 9.0 | 19.6 | 23.2 | 10.0 | 14.0 |
| All three | 9.0 | 7.8 | 20.8 | 9.1 | 11.9 |

*Significant difference among the four groups ($\chi^2$, p<0.05).
***Significant difference among the four groups ($\chi^2$, p<0.001).

In contrast to epilepsy, the prevalence of febrile seizures, which are most often the result of a genetic predisposition without other evidence of brain dysfunction (Frantzen *et al.* 1970), was not expected to differ across groups. Febrile seizures were reported in 6 per cent of the children overall, with no reliable difference among the four groups. This figure is somewhat higher than the prevalence of 2–4 per cent quoted for normal children (Annegers *et al.* 1990). Staring spells were reported in all groups but predominantly in the LAD group. While some of these staring spells may have been partial complex seizures, it is likely that most of them were not seizures but reflected inattention or autistic unresponsiveness to verbal stimuli.

One hundred and two children (21 per cent) had been subjected to a neuroimaging study, usually CT, less often MRI. These studies were unevenly distributed, with the LAD and NALIQ subjects being much more likely to have undergone testing than the other two groups. Virtually all tests were stated by the parents to be normal but we did not have the opportunity to review them. A third of the children had undergone an EEG scan; we did not request copies of EEG reports because the variability of administration and interpretation would render them non-comparable. About half of the LAD and NALIQ children had been tested, as opposed to 12–18 per cent of the other two groups, no doubt because of a higher prevalence of seizures and obvious or suspected neurological abnormality in children with LAD and NALIQ.

Finally, we inquired about the prevalence of sleep difficulties because sleep problems are common in the histories of children with severe attention disorder with hyperactivity and of children with autism (Segawa *et al.* 1992a,b). The prevalence of sleep problems differed significantly across groups (Table 5.13). Children in the autistic groups were more likely than those in the other groups to have difficulty falling asleep, and those in the LAD group were more likely to wake up early in the morning. Almost half of these children still awoke more than once during the night and they were more than twice as likely to have all three sleep problems than the other two groups. There was no correlation between number of sleep problems and age. The relation of these sleep problems to attention problems noted by the neurologists is discussed in Chapter 6.

DISCUSSION

The information collected in the present study is limited by the fact that it consists entirely of parental reports. It does not provide reliable overall prevalence data but does enable comparisons among the four clinical groups of interest. Our data will be considered against those of the Collaborative Perinatal Project (CPP) (Broman *et al*. 1975, 1987), even though differing presentation of the findings precludes exact comparisons.

The main findings in the present study are that most pre-, peri- and postnatal events did not differentiate among the four groups, with the exception of a marginally lower birthweight in the NALIQ group. A postnatal history of encephalitis or meningitis, although rare in all groups, was more common in the LAD group; epilepsy was more prevalent in the LAD and NALIQ groups; and sleep problems were more common in the two AD groups.

The sleep problems are a provocative finding for autism. Segawa *et al*. (1992*b*) report that abnormalities of the sleep/wake cycle in autism may be ameliorated through concerted efforts at diurnal stimulation and more normal entrainment of sleep time, and that this may have a favorable effect on other autistic behavioral symptoms. They argue that these abnormalities of the circadian sleep/wake cycle provide a window on the balance of serotonergic/noradrenergic/cholinergic neurotransmitter release in the brainstem. Future systematic study of the relationship of circadian patterns to neurotransmitter release, though difficult to carry out in such children, are clearly needed because they may shed some light on the pathophysiology of autism.

• *Pre- and perinatal events*. In the 1950s and up to the 1970s perinatal problems were widely accepted as a major contributor to the etiology of the developmental disorders of higher cerebral function without a clear etiology (*e.g.* Knobloch and Pasamanik 1959). Data from the CPP (Broman *et al*. 1975, 1987) which followed over 50,000 children and their mothers from early pregnancy to age 7 years, indicate that retrospective attribution of a child's developmental problem to perinatal events may be plausible but is entirely conjectural and statistically unsound. A major finding of the CPP was that suboptimal perinatal events, including preterm birth, were less detrimental to cognitive outcome than socioeconomic factors, especially in the case of mild mental retardation (Broman *et al*. 1987). Even in the case of severe mental retardation, its major causes were not perinatal factors, but prenatal factors such as anomalies of embryological or fetal development that often result in cerebral palsy and other frank neurological signs. It is now clear that most of the excess morbidity attributable to very low birthweight unassociated with major malformations is due to definable complications of preterm birth such as intraventricular hemorrhage, severe hypoxic/ischemic encephalopathy, malnutrition and infection (Volpe 1995).

In the CPP, children were divided at age 7 years into a severely retarded group (IQ <50), a mildly retarded group (IQ 50–69), and a non-retarded group with three subgroups: children with borderline IQ (70–89), average IQ (90–119), and above average IQ ($\geq$120). Abnormal behavior summary scores were recorded in about 75 per cent of the severely retarded group, and 'several' of the children in this group 'without major neurological disorders' were said to be autistic.

In our study, 70 (56 per cent) of children in the LAD sample, but only 34 (31 per cent) of those in the NALIQ group, which included nine children with Down syndrome, had NVIQ equivalents <50; thus two thirds of the NALIQ and slightly less than half of the LAD children in our study correspond to the mildly mentally retarded and borderline groups of the CPP. The low IQ groups in the present study differ from the majority of those in the CPP in that the children were selected not to have severe seizures, a frank motor deficit or a known brain lesion, whereas half of the severely mentally retarded children in the CPP walked late, about a quarter had cerebral palsy, and 15 per cent had epilepsy.

In the present study there were only 17 babies (4 per cent) said to be born at 32 weeks or earlier, a group too small to evaluate, especially as our exclusionary criteria selected against very low birthweight associated with overt brain damage. In the CPP, 6 per cent of pregnancies ended at less than 37 weeks among White families, *vs* 11–18 per cent among Black families, with the highest prevalence of preterm deliveries occuring in the lowest SES group. In our sample the reported figure for delivery before 37 weeks was higher, at 23 per cent, and the relation of SES to birthweight was non-significant. The 19 per cent of children born between 33 and 37 weeks were at low risk for significant neurological damage. In any case, neither gestational age nor birthweight differed significantly across the four groups (except for marginally lower mean birthweight in the NALIQ group).

A number of recent studies have examined the prevalence of deleterious perinatal factors in autism and mental retardation, comparing autistic or mentally retarded probands to their normal siblings or to normal controls. Although some studies (*e.g.* Gillberg and Gillberg 1983, Lord *et al.* 1991) found a small effect of perinatal suboptimality, studies in over 300 autistic children (Finegan and Quarrington 1979, Deykin and MacMahon 1980, Mason-Brothers *et al.* 1990) failed to uncover significant differences. In mentally retarded children, Gillberg *et al.* (1990) and Gillberg and Coleman (1992) reported that perinatal suboptimality played a smaller role than in children with autism or cerebral palsy. These data, those from the CPP, and those from our study provide strong evidence against perinatal events playing a strong causative role in the developmental disorders, thereby supporting our hypothesis.

Recent pathological studies have disclosed subtle prenatal dysplastic abnormalities in some of the brains of the few persons with DLD, AD and dyslexia who have come to necropsy (Galaburda *et al.* 1985, Cohen *et al.* 1989, Bauman 1992*b*, Kemper and Bauman 1992, Bauman and Kemper 1994). These microscopic abnormalities may be detectable only by detailed neuropathological study after death. Some of them may be directly or indirectly genetic. Their cause and relation to the developmental disorders remain

75

speculative (*e.g.* Galaburda 1993). Whether they have any correlates in gestational histories is not known.

• *Postnatal events.* There was no postnatal illness or potential brain insult that differentiated among the four groups, with the exception of encephalitis or meningitis which, though rare, was more prevalent in the LAD group (4.8 per cent). This finding is provocative in view of a few reports of autistic-like syndromes arising in the aftermath of herpes simplex encephalitis (DeLong *et al.* 1981). Unfortunately we have no further details about these children's illnesses.

Epilepsy was the other sign of neurological dysfunction that had a different prevalence in the four groups. In the CPP, the prevalence of seizures was less than 1 per cent in the three non-retarded groups of children, 2 per cent in the mildly retarded group and 15 per cent in the severely retarded group. In our study, which excluded children with uncontrolled or very frequent seizures, the prevalence of seizures approximated 10 per cent in the LAD and NALIQ groups, 4.5 per cent in the DLD and 0 per cent in the HAD group, consonant with the CPP data. This study confirms once again that infantile spasms are a significant risk factor not only for severe mental retardation but also for autism (Taft and Cohen 1971), although not exclusively so inasmuch as, in the Tuchman *et al.* (1991*b*) study, infantile spasms were reported with equal frequency in epileptic children with DLD and with autism. Several other studies have found a correlation of seizures with the severity of mental retardation and the presence of a motor disability in autistic and non-autistic children (Goulden *et al.* 1991). Tuchman *et al.* (1991*b*) found a somewhat higher prevalence of epilepsy (8 per cent in DLD children and 7 per cent in autistic children without severe mental retardation or motor disability) than in our study, but theirs was a clinically referred sample that excluded no children. In the Tuchman *et al.* study, seizures were correlated most strongly with verbal auditory agnosia or word deafness (Rapin 1985), the most severe receptive language disorder which presumably reflects temporal lobe pathology, in both autistic and non-autistic DLD children. The relationship of acquired epileptic aphasia (Landau–Kleffner syndrome—Landau and Kleffner 1957, Rapin *et al.* 1977) to verbal auditory agnosia and to autistic regression and disintegrative psychosis—which is autistic behavior acquired after the age of 3 years or after the ability to speak in full sentences (Kurita 1985, 1988; Kurita *et al.* 1992; Rapin 1995)—requires further investigation.

*Developmental and educational histories*

MOTOR MILESTONES AND TOILET TRAINING

The milestones we enquired about included age at smiling, reaching for objects, rolling over, sitting, crawling and walking, as well as age at attainment of toilet training. Previous studies showed that age at walking is a developmental milestone that mothers remember quite reliably (Pyles *et al.* 1935, Hefner and Mednick 1969, Knobloch *et al.* 1979, Majnemer and Rosenblatt 1994), and that, if they make errors, they tend toward reporting younger rather than older ages at achievement of milestones. Because many parents told the interviewers that they did not remember other motor milestones such as age at sitting and crawling reliably, these data are not presented. There were reliable differences among groups for these unreported milestones which were in the same direction as those for age at walking (Table 5.14). Age at walking was delayed in the LAD and NALIQ groups and was thus generally correlated with LIQ.

Mean ages at achieving other developmental milestones are summarized in Table 5.14; these means underestimate delay because they do not include the substantial number of children in some groups who had not yet attained particular skills. Table 5.15A lists the proportion of children in each group who had not yet achieved these milestones, and those who had been substantially delayed beyond expected norms. For toilet training we tabulated only the mean age at which children were trained for bladder and bowel during the day because of the great variability in the age at which even normal children achieve nocturnal continence. The average at day-time training for the DLD group was close to $2^1/_2$ years, compared to $3-3^1/_2$ years for those in all other groups who had reached this milestone. On average, only 12 per cent of the normal IQ children were not toilet trained at the time of the study, compared to 22 per cent in the NALIQ group, and 42 per cent in the LAD group (at a mean age of 5 years).

We examined how much of the developmental delay in the LAD and NALIQ groups was attributable to the severity of mental retardation by recalculating these milestones after removal of the 70 LAD and 34 NALIQ children with NVIQ equivalents of 50 or below (Table 5.15B). Removal of these severely mentally retarded children resulted in only a modest decrease in the proportion of children who had not achieved the milestones, suggesting that factors other than mental retardation contributed substantially to the delay.

PLAY SKILLS

We inquired about the age at which the child could engage in pretend play, engage another child in play, and follow the rules of a game. Parental reports summarized in Table 5.14 indicated that the DLD group was superior in all respects, a finding supportive of the observational data on play described in Chapters 6 and 9. Reported age at ability to engage in pretend play separated the autistic groups sharply from the non-autistic groups. This was particularly striking for the children in the HAD group; none of them had an NVIQ equivalent below 80, and their mean NVIQ equivalent of 100 was identical to that of the children in the DLD group, yet they were stated to have achieved the ability to pretend a year later than the DLD children, only four months earlier than the NALIQ children. Also, the HAD children were almost three times as likely as the DLD children not to have achieved that milestone by 36 months (Table 5.15A). Although children in the two autistic groups who achieved play skills did so at about the same age, they differed markedly in the proportion who had not yet achieved these skills at the time of testing, inasmuch as 46 per cent of the LAD group reportedly had no pretend play at a mean age of 5 years, compared to 16 per cent of the HAD and NALIQ groups. Mothers of children in both the HAD and LAD groups reported that they were severely impaired in their ability to engage another child in play. Children in the two autistic groups who achieved this milestone did so at essentially the same age and did so significantly later than those in the NALIQ group; children in the LAD group were more

**TABLE 5.14**

**Mean ages (months) at achievement of milestones by group[1]**

| Milestone | Group | | | | | | | | F | Significant contrasts |
|---|---|---|---|---|---|---|---|---|---|---|
| | DLD | | HAD | | LAD | | NALIQ | | | |
| | Mean | (SD) | Mean | (SD) | Mean | (SD) | Mean | (SD) | | |
| Walking alone | 13.0 (N=197) | (3.5) | 12.3 (N=50) | (2.2) | 15.7 (N=120) | (6.4) | 17.0 (N=105) | (6.6) | 19.6*** | DLD=HAD<LAD<NALIQ |
| Toilet training (day bladder) | 32.0 (N=174) | (7.6) | 36.5 (N=44) | (8.4) | 41.9 (N=70) | (11.9) | 37.1 (N=78) | (11.4) | 19.3*** | DLD<HAD=NALIQ<LAD |
| Toilet training (day bowel) | 32.3 (N=163) | (8.1) | 38.3 (N=44) | (8.5) | 43.7 (N=56) | (12.9) | 37.7 (N=76) | (11.6) | 20.3*** | DLD<HAD=NALIQ<LAD |
| Pretend play | 32.6 (N=164) | (10.3) | 44.6 (N=41) | (11.9) | 43.6 (N=52) | (15.2) | 39.7 (N=71) | (11.4) | 20.3*** | DLD<NALIQ<HAD=LAD |
| Engaging another child in play | 29.4 (N=158) | (10.9) | 45.5 (N=37) | (16.9) | 41.0 (N=50) | (16.8) | 35.4 (N=74) | (12.2) | 21.1*** | DLD<NALIQ<HAD=LAD |
| Understanding rules of games | 39.3 (N=122) | (9.9) | 52.0 (N=26) | (13.2) | 51.9 (N=30) | (18.3) | 45.3 (N=36) | (9.8) | 14.1*** | DLD<NALIQ<HAD=LAD |

[1]Includes only children who have achieved milestone.

***$p < 0.001$ (analysis of variance).

TABLE 5.15
**Delayed developmental milestones—percentage of children in each group who have not achieved milestone**

| | DLD | HAD | LAD | NALIQ | All |
|---|---|---|---|---|---|
| Mean age (mo) at interview | 49 | 58 | 60 | 56 | 54 |

**A: Total group**

| Milestone | (N=201) | (N=51) | (N=125) | (N=110) | (N=487) |
|---|---|---|---|---|---|
| Walking | | | | | |
|   at 18 mo (N=60)*** | 4.0 | 0.0 | 18.4 | 26.4 | 12.3 |
|   at interview (N=0) | — | — | — | — | — |
| Toilet trained (day bladder) | | | | | |
|   at 36 mo (N=231)*** | 29.9 | 43.1 | 70.4 | 55.5 | 47.4 |
|   at interview (N=98)*** | 11.0 | 11.8 | 37.6 | 20.9 | 20.1 |
| Toilet trained (day bowel) | | | | | |
|   >36 mo (N=253)*** | 34.3 | 52.9 | 75.2 | 57.3 | 52.0 |
|   at interview (N=117)*** | 14.0 | 11.8 | 46.4 | 22.7 | 24.0 |
| Pretend play | | | | | |
|   at 36 mo (N=225)*** | 24.4 | 70.6 | 68.8 | 49.1 | 46.2 |
|   at interview (N=93)*** | 5.0 | 15.7 | 45.6 | 16.4 | 19.1 |
| Engaged another child in play | | | | | |
|   at 36 mo (N=204)*** | 22.9 | 68.6 | 67.2 | 35.5 | 41.9 |
|   at interview (N=103)*** | 9.0 | 23.5 | 46.4 | 13.6 | 21.2 |
| Understood rules of games | | | | | |
|   at 48 mo (N=241)*** | 29.9 | 60.8 | 72.0 | 54.6 | 49.5 |
|   at interview (N=191)*** | 22.4 | 23.5 | 46.4 | 13.6 | 21.2 |

**B: Children with nonverbal IQ equivalent >50**

| Milestone | (N=201) | (N=51) | (N=55) | (N=76) | (N=383) |
|---|---|---|---|---|---|
| Walking | | | | | |
|   at 18 mo (N=28)*** | 4.0 | 0.0 | 9.1 | 19.7 | 7.3 |
|   at interview (N=0) | — | — | — | — | — |
| Toilet trained (day bladder) | | | | | |
|   at 36 mo (N=152)*** | 29.9 | 43.1 | 60.0 | 48.7 | 39.7 |
|   at interview (N=59)*** | 11.0 | 11.8 | 34.6 | 15.8 | 15.4 |
| Toilet trained (day bowel) | | | | | |
|   at 36 mo (N=173)*** | 34.3 | 52.9 | 69.1 | 51.3 | 45.2 |
|   at interview (N=68)*** | 13.9 | 11.8 | 40.0 | 15.8 | 17.8 |
| Pretend play | | | | | |
|   at 36 mo (N=157)*** | 24.4 | 70.6 | 67.3 | 46.1 | 41.0 |
|   at interview (N=47)*** | 5.0 | 15.7 | 38.2 | 10.5 | 12.3 |
| Engaged another child in play | | | | | |
|   at 36 mo (N=143)*** | 22.9 | 68.6 | 69.1 | 31.6 | 37.3 |
|   at interview (N=64)*** | 9.0 | 23.5 | 43.6 | 13.2 | 16.7 |
| Understood rules of games | | | | | |
|   at 48 mo (N=169)*** | 29.9 | 60.8 | 69.1 | 52.6 | 44.1 |
|   at interview (N=130)*** | 22.4 | 35.3 | 58.2 | 46.1 | 33.9 |

***Significant difference among groups ($\chi^2$, p <0.001).

severely impaired, nonetheless, because half as many LAD as HAD children were able to engage other children in play by the time of testing. Both autistic groups were also more impaired than the other groups in understanding the rules of games. Removal of the children with NVIQ equivalents below 50 did not greatly decrease the proportion who had not achieved these milestones (Table 5.15B).

LANGUAGE MILESTONES

Achievement of language milestones was of central interest to the study because delayed language acquisition is likely to be the presenting complaint of most parents of children in all groups (Tuchman *et al.* 1991*a*). Subject to the same caution regarding accuracy of report as for motor milestones, these data are presented in Tables 5.16 and 5.17. With the possible exception of age at babbling, all groups, compared to normal children, had severely delayed language development, supporting our expectation. There were differences among groups in reported age at achievement of all expressive milestones except babbling and intelligibility, yet analysis of variance revealed no significant difference between the DLD and HAD groups, or between the NALIQ and LAD groups, for reported ages at speaking single words, naming objects, and putting two words together. As one might expect, the two LIQ groups achieved these milestones significantly later than the DLD and HAD groups, with the LAD group generally most delayed. The DLD differed significantly from the HAD group, and the NALIQ from the LAD group, in the ages at which the children spoke in sentences and asked so-called 'wh–' questions (such as, in order of learning, 'what?', 'who?', 'where?', 'why?', 'when?', and 'how?').

The cut-offs for failure to achieve milestones chosen for Table 5.17 are more lenient than those in the well-validated Early Language Milestone Scale (Coplan 1989). That scale indicates that 90 per cent of normal children will have achieved polysyllabic babble by 10.5 months, first words by 17.5 months, two-word utterances by 23 months, and the ability to hold a conversation by 34.5 months. They can obey single-step commands without gestures by 13 months, and two-step commands by 24 months. By these criteria, the language of the children in our study is indeed severely delayed. The MacArthur Communicative Development Inventories (Fenson *et al.* 1991), which also depend on parental report, confirm this. They indicate that, while there is considerable variability in the age at which normal infants achieve language milestones, most infants comprehend some single words before 1 year, start to produce single words at 12–13 months, start to combine words by 18–20 months, and progress rapidly in their ability to speak in grammatical sentences between 20 and 36 months (Bates and Marchman 1988, Bates *et al.* 1992).

Except for babbling and single words, a significant number of children had not yet achieved these expressive milestones at the time of testing (Table 5.17A). Again, the LAD children stand out as the most likely to be severely delayed. The DLD and HAD groups and the LAD and NALIQ groups resembled one another in age at producing one-word utterances and short phrases, no doubt reflecting the role of mental retardation in language delay. There was no difference among groups as far as achieving intelligibility. In dramatic contrast, children in the HAD group were delayed by almost a year,

## TABLE 5.16
### Mean ages (months) at language development by diagnostic group[1]

| Milestone | Group | | | | | | F | Significant contrasts |
|---|---|---|---|---|---|---|---|---|
| | DLD Mean (SD) | | HAD Mean (SD) | LAD Mean (SD) | NALIQ Mean (SD) | | | |
| **A: Expressive Language** | | | | | | | | |
| Babbling | 9.1 (6.1) (N=145) | | 7.1 (3.1) (N=39) | 10.9 (12.0) (N=87) | 9.3 (7.1) (N=69) | | 2.2 | ns |
| Single words | 18.0 (8.3) (N=186) | | 17.0 (10.5) (N=49) | 20.4 (13.1) (N=109) | 21.2 (11.3) (N=94) | | 3.0* | DLD=HAD=LAD<NALIQ |
| Naming | 26.5 (9.7) (N=179) | | 26.4 (11.4) (N=45) | 32.1 (18.4) (N=87) | 31.7 (11.9) (N=82) | | 5.9*** | DLD=HAD<LAD=NALIQ |
| Phrases | 27.2 (9.4) (N=178) | | 29.0 (11.7) (N=44) | 36.0 (16.3) (N=82) | 33.7 (12.3) (N=86) | | 12.3*** | DLD=HAD<LAD=NALIQ |
| Sentences | 34.4 (8.9) (N=158) | | 39.1 (12.7) (N=37) | 47.9 (19.0) (N=50) | 39.7 (12.8) (N=74) | | 15.0*** | DLD<HAD=NALIQ<LAD |
| 'Wh-' questions | 37.7 (9.6) (N=142) | | 47.0 (10.7) (N=32) | 50.7 (14.8) (N=22) | 44.5 (13.5) (N=62) | | 14.3*** | DLD<NALIQ<HAD=LAD |
| Intelligibility | 29.9 (10.8) (N=153) | | 29.0 (12.3) (N=44) | 30.6 (17.2) (N=68) | 34.2 (11.3) (N=78) | | 2.4 | ns |
| **B. Receptive Language** | | | | | | | | |
| Discourse | 22.9 (9.9) (N=177) | | 35.8 (14.4) (N=38) | 39.3 (17.3) (N=76) | 29.2 (13.5) (N=89) | | 32.4*** | DLD<NALIQ<HAD=LAD |
| 1 step commands | 23.4 (9.4) (N=183) | | 33.0 (12.5) (N=44) | 37.4 (14.7) (N=107) | 30.6 (12.5) (N=95) | | 33.3*** | DLD<NALIQ=HAD<LAD |
| 2 step commands | 32.0 (9.6) (N=164) | | 42.5 (12.2) (N=37) | 47.3 (16.5) (N=54) | 42.3 (12.0) (N=80) | | 30.5*** | DLD<NALIQ=HAD<LAD |

[1]Includes only children who have achieved milestone.
*p<0.05; *** p<0.001.

81

TABLE 5.17
**Delayed language milestones—percentage of children in each group who have not achieved milestone**

| | DLD | HAD | LAD | NALIQ | All |
|---|---|---|---|---|---|
| Mean age (mo) at interview** | 49 | 58 | 60 | 56 | 54 |
| **A: Total group** | (N=201) | (N=51) | (N=125) | (N=110) | (N=487) |
| *Production milestones* | | | | | |
| Babbling | | | | | |
| at 12 mo (N=83) | 14.4 | 9.8 | 21.6 | 20.0 | 17.0 |
| at interview (N=34) | 5.0 | 5.9 | 9.6 | 8.2 | 7.0 |
| Single words | | | | | |
| at 18 mo (N=176)* | 31.8 | 25.5 | 39.2 | 45.5 | 36.1 |
| at interview* (N=13) | 1.0 | 2.0 | 6.4 | 1.8 | 2.7 |
| Naming | | | | | |
| at 24 mo (N=253)** | 47.8 | 39.2 | 64.0 | 51.8 | 52.0 |
| at interview*** (N=49) | 4.0 | 3.9 | 24.0 | 8.2 | 10.1 |
| Phrases | | | | | |
| at 24 mo (N=295)*** | 53.2 | 49.0 | 72.0 | 66.4 | 60.6 |
| at interview (N=54)*** | 4.0 | 2.0 | 26.4 | 10.9 | 11.1 |
| Sentences | | | | | |
| at 36 mo (N=271)*** | 40.3 | 49.0 | 82.4 | 56.4 | 55.7 |
| at interview (N=141)*** | 14.9 | 15.7 | 56.0 | 30.0 | 29.0 |
| 'Wh–' questions | | | | | |
| at 36 mo (N=323)*** | 52.2 | 76.5 | 82.4 | 69.1 | 66.3 |
| at interview*** (N=173) | 19.4 | 27.5 | 68.0 | 31.8 | 35.5 |
| Intelligibility | | | | | |
| at 30 mo (N=226)* | 39.3 | 43.1 | 54.4 | 51.8 | 46.4 |
| at interview (N=76)*** | 9.5 | 5.9 | 32.0 | 12.7 | 15.6 |
| *Reception milestones* | | | | | |
| Comprehension | | | | | |
| at 24 mo (N=237)*** | 30.9 | 64.7 | 73.6 | 45.5 | 48.7 |
| at interview (N=54)*** | 4.5 | 7.8 | 28.0 | 5.5 | 11.1 |
| 1 step commands | | | | | |
| at 24 mo (N=242)*** | 29.9 | 64.7 | 72.8 | 52.7 | 49.7 |
| at interview (N=19)* | 1.5 | 3.9 | 8.0 | 3.6 | 3.9 |
| 2 step commands | | | | | |
| at 36 mo (N=233)*** | 26.9 | 52.9 | 76.0 | 51.8 | 47.8 |
| at interview (N=89)*** | 7.0 | 7.8 | 46.4 | 11.8 | 18.3 |
| **B: Children with NVIQ equivalent >50** | (N=201) | (N=51) | (N=55) | (N=76) | (N=383) |
| *Production milestones* | | | | | |
| Babbling | | | | | |
| at 12 mo (N=54) | 14.4 | 9.8 | 14.6 | 15.8 | 14.1 |
| at interview (N=21) | 5.0 | 5.9 | 5.5 | 6.6 | 5.5 |
| Single words | | | | | |
| at 18 mo (N=124) | 31.8 | 25.5 | 30.9 | 39.5 | 32.4 |
| at interview (N=5) | 1.0 | 2.0 | 3.6 | 0.0 | 1.3 |
| Naming | | | | | |
| at 24 mo (N=186) | 47.8 | 39.2 | 61.8 | 47.4 | 48.6 |
| at interview (N=21)** | 4.0 | 3.9 | 16.4 | 2.6 | 5.5 |

| | | | | | |
|---|---|---|---|---|---|
| Phrases | | | | | |
| at 24 mo (N=216) | 53.2 | 49.0 | 67.3 | 61.8 | 56.4 |
| at interview (N=23)** | 4.0 | 2.0 | 16.4 | 6.6 | 6.0 |
| Sentences | | | | | |
| at 36 mo (N=187) | 40.3 | 49.0 | 78.2 | 50.0 | 48.8 |
| at interview (N=81)*** | 14.9 | 15.7 | 45.5 | 23.7 | 21.2 |
| 'Wh–' questions | | | | | |
| at 36 mo (N=240)*** | 52.2 | 76.5 | 85.5 | 64.5 | 62.7 |
| at interview (N=106)*** | 19.4 | 27.5 | 60.0 | 26.3 | 27.7 |
| Intelligibility | | | | | |
| at 30 mo (N=169) | 39.3 | 43.1 | 52.7 | 51.3 | 44.1 |
| at interview (N=38)* | 9.5 | 5.9 | 20.0 | 6.6 | 9.9 |
| *Reception milestones* | | | | | |
| Comprehension | | | | | |
| at 24 mo (N=163)*** | 30.9 | 64.7 | 69.1 | 39.5 | 42.6 |
| at interview (N=26)*** | 4.5 | 7.8 | 23.6 | 0.0 | 6.8 |
| 1 step commands | | | | | |
| at 24 mo (N=299)* | 73.1 | 82.4 | 90.9 | 79.0 | 78.1 |
| at interview (N=10) | 1.5 | 3.9 | 8.0 | 3.6 | 3.9 |
| 2 step commands | | | | | |
| at 36 mo (N=269)*** | 61.2 | 72.6 | 92.7 | 76.3 | 70.2 |
| at interview (N=47)*** | 7.0 | 7.8 | 46.4 | 11.8 | 18.3 |

*Significant difference among groups ($\chi^2$, p<0.05).
**Significant difference among groups ($\chi^2$, p<0.01).
***Significant difference among groups ($\chi^2$, p<0.001).

compared to the DLD group, when it came to asking questions. There was no significant difference between the ages at which children in the HAD and LAD groups achieved this milestone. Children in the NALIQ group asked questions seven months later than those in the DLD group but a full six months earlier than the verbal children in the LAD group. One needs to remember that these data pertain only to verbal children who had achieved these skills. Table 5.17A shows that fully two thirds of the LAD group did not yet ask questions, a proportion twice as high as that in the NALIQ group.

Age at achievement of comprehension most sharply distinguished HAD from DLD children, and LAD from NALIQ children (Table 5.16), that is, autistic from non-autistic children with relatively similar nonverbal cognitive skills. Again the LAD group was the most severely delayed. That this difference was not entirely attributable to cognitive incompetence was demonstrated by the persistence of differences even when children with NVIQ equivalents <50 were removed from the LAD and NALIQ groups (Table 5.17B). It was also shown by the similar proportions of children in the two AD groups whose comprehension was delayed.

In general, parents reported that there were many more children who lagged severely in achieving expressive than receptive milestones, reflecting the parents' impression that most children with communication disorders understand more than they can say. What may also have contributed to this finding is the much more lenient cut-offs we chose in

**TABLE 5.18**
**Reported loss of achieved skills: number and percentage of children who lost previously achieved skills[1]**

| Skill | Group | | | | | | | | | |
|---|---|---|---|---|---|---|---|---|---|---|
| | DLD | | HAD | | LAD | | NALIQ | | All | |
| | N | % | N | % | N | % | N | % | N | % |
| Walking | (N=197) | | (N=50) | | (N=120) | | (N=105) | | (N=472) | |
| | 0 | 0.0 | 1 | 2.0 | 0 | 0.0 | 1 | 1.0 | 2 | 0.4 |
| Single words*** | (N=186) | | (N=49) | | (N=109) | | (N=94) | | (N=438) | |
| | 6 | 3.2 | 10 | 20.4 | 32 | 29.4 | 5 | 5.3 | 53 | 12.1 |
| Sentences | (N=158) | | (N=38) | | (N=45) | | (N=61) | | (N=302) | |
| | 2 | 1.3 | 1 | 2.6 | 4 | 8.9 | 2 | 3.3 | 9 | 3.0 |
| Comprehension | (N=177) | | (N=38) | | (N=76) | | (N=89) | | (N=380) | |
| | 1 | 0.6 | 1 | 2.6 | 4 | 5.3 | 2 | 2.3 | 8 | 2.1 |
| Pretend play* | (N=164) | | (N=41) | | (N=52) | | (N=71) | | (N=328) | |
| | 0 | 0.0 | 2 | 4.9 | 2 | 3.9 | 0 | 0.0 | 4 | 1.2 |

[1]The N values in brackets indicate the numbers of children who had achieved skills and for whom data were available. See Tables 5.15 and 5.17 for the percentage of children in each group who had not yet achieved skills.
*Significant difference among groups ($\chi^2$, p<0.05).
***Significant difference among groups ($\chi^2$, p<0.001).

the questionnaire for achievement of receptive than expressive language. The LAD children again stand out as most severely delayed.

DEVELOPMENTAL REGRESSION

Many parents of autistic children state that their child's language underwent an unexplained insidious regression or that it stagnated for a period of months or even a year or more before resuming progress, always at a lower level than earlier (Kurita 1985, Tuchman et al. 1991b, Kurita et al. 1992). This usually happens between the ages of 1 and $2^1/_2$–3 years. Combining the individual group data presented in Table 5.18 indicates that 26.6 per cent of the parents of the autistic children reported regression in single words, compared to 3.9 per cent of the parents of children in the other two groups. Although many fewer parents reported regression of sentences, the most likely explanation is that the majority of autistic children had not yet achieved this milestone at the time of the regression. Surprisingly, these same parents rarely reported regression of comprehension and play, which clinical experience indicates usually accompanies language regression in autistic children (Volkmar and Cohen 1989, Rogers and DiLalla 1990). Parents did not volunteer that there was a temporal relation between the occurrence of language loss and that of seizures. As we did not ask about this specifically, and in view of our *a priori* exclusion of children with severe seizure disorders and resultant small number of children with seizures in the study (N=33), we have no data to evaluate a potential temporal link between seizure onset and language regression (Deonna 1991). The data do, however, confirm that regression of motor milestones does not accompany language regression

**TABLE 5.19**
**Children's habilitation**

|  | DLD (N=201) % | HAD (N=51) % | LAD (N=125) % | NALIQ (N=110) % | All (N=487) % |
|---|---|---|---|---|---|
| (Mean age (mo) at interview) | (49) | (58) | (60) | (56) | (54) |
| *Type of habilitation* |  |  |  |  |  |
| None (N=107) | 25.9 | 13.7 | 20.8 | 20.0 | 22.0 |
| Speech + language therapy (N=359) | 73.6 | 80.4 | 72.8 | 71.8 | 73.7 |
| Sign language (N=97)*** | 13.9 | 9.8 | 29.6 | 24.6 | 19.9 |
| Special school (N=269)*** | 42.3 | 68.6 | 68.8 | 57.3 | 55.2 |
| Behavior modifying drug |  |  |  |  |  |
|   in the past (N=43)*** | 1.5 | 15.7 | 18.7 | 8.3 | 8.9 |
|   at time of interview (N=41) | 11.9 | 6.3 | 12.6 | 13.2 | 11.9 |

***Significant difference among groups ($\chi^2$, p<0.001).

**TABLE 5.20**
**Mean age (mo) at start of habilitation**

|  | DLD (N=201) | HAD (N=51) | LAD (N=125) | NALIQ (N=110) | All (N=487) |
|---|---|---|---|---|---|
| (Mean age (mo) at interview) | (49) | (58) | (60) | (56) | (54) |
| *Type of habilitation* |  |  |  |  |  |
| Speech + language therapy (N=359) | 38.0 | 39.9 | 37.6 | 33.9 | 37.4 |
| Sign language (N=97) | 37.7 | 36.0 | 42.0 | 44.0 | 41.0 |
| Special school (N=269) | 37.7 | 43.6 | 38.5 | 38.0 | 38.7 |

No reliable age difference among groups at start of habilitation (ANOVA).

(Table 5.18), suggesting that regression is unlikely to be caused by a progressive brain degeneration.

HABILITATION

We inquired whether the children had attended a specialized preschool, had received individual speech and language therapy, had been exposed to sign language to supplement oral language, or had been prescribed behavior modifying medications. As one might have predicted, the two autistic groups were most likely to have received behavior modifying drugs (Table 5.19), although, surprisingly, there was little difference among groups in the number of children taking these drugs at the time they were evaluated.

Table 5.19 shows that there was no difference among groups in the number of children receiving speech and language therapy. Fewer children in the HAD group had been exposed to sign language, presumably because they were more likely to be verbal and to have adequate phonology than the other groups. The fact that the two AD groups were the most likely to be enrolled in a specialized preschool indicates that their disabilities were least likely to go unnoticed. The DLD children were less apt to be in a specialized preschool than the other three groups, but this may be in part an artifact in that they were younger (49 months *vs* 58 months) and that a number of them were recruited to the study at the time they came for the evaluation required for entry into a specialized program. Mean age at the start of habilitation did not differ among groups (Table 5.20).

DISCUSSION

Most of the significant differences among the four groups as far as achievement of walking, toilet training, play, and language comprehension and expression were in the direction of the DLD group being least delayed and the LAD group most delayed. A notable exception was the ability to engage another child in play, where the HAD children were almost as impaired as those in the LAD group.

• *Play.* Children with DLD, compared to matched normal controls, have been stated to be deficient in symbolic play (Udwin and Yule 1983), and mothers in our study tended to agree, a finding that was not confirmed in the formal play session of this study (see Chapter 9). Parents of DLD children reported better play than those of NALIQ children, in agreement with the observation of the neurologists (Chapter 6) and the results of the formal play analysis. A small study comparing play in DLD and NALIQ children indicated that there is a correlation of capacity for symbolic play and expressive language ability in NALIQ but not DLD children (Sarimski *et al.* 1985), a finding disputed by others who did find a correlation between linguistic ability and play behavior in DLD (Lombardino *et al.* 1986, Roth and Clark 1987).

According to their parents, less than a third of children in either autistic group could play symbolically at 3 years, whereas half of the NALIQ group had achieved this milestone. Inasmuch as mental retardation cannot be invoked to explain delay in the HAD group, markedly delayed and inadequate ability to play symbolically is indeed a good marker for autism (Wulff 1985) (see Chapter 9).

• *Walking and toilet training.* As a group, DLD children in this study did not walk late, conflicting with findings of Haynes and Naidoo (1991) who reported that of the DLD children in their study only 44 per cent walked by 14 months and one third walked at 18 months or later, clearly later than British norms indicating that only 25 per cent of children walk later than 14 months. Haynes and Naidoo found no correlation between age at walking and receptive or expressive language skill, or intelligence. They also provided data on achievement of toilet training: 75 per cent of the DLD children in their cohort had daytime bladder and bowel continence by age 3 years—figures identical to ours— which they interpreted as indicating mild delay, with, surprisingly, an inverse relation between age at achievement of bladder and bowel control and social class.

Our study indicates that, as expected, age at walking and achievement of toilet training is correlated with IQ, but that autism presents a special obstacle for toilet training inasmuch as both autistic groups were more delayed than their comparison groups. Tsai *et al.* (1981) reported that only 15 per cent of autistic girls, who were likely to be more severely affected than boys, were toilet trained at 3½ years, compared to 40 per cent of the boys. Toilet training may take over two years and can persist as a major problem in autism into adult life, especially in mentally retarded nonverbal individuals (Dalrymple and Ruble 1992).

Some but not all of the developmental findings in the present study parallel those in a large study carried out by Jacobson and Ackerman (1990) who compared intelligence with competence for gross motor skills, toilet training and language in 5- to 12-year-old autistic (N=213) and mentally retarded (N=1469) children. They divided the children in both groups into four cognitive levels ranging from mild to severe mental retardation. As expected, the proportion of children achieving competence in all three skills declined with increasing severity of intellectual impairment. In contrast to our findings, for both motor skill and toilet training their autistic sample was superior to the mentally retarded one. Motor skill was high in the autistic group, only 20 per cent of the severely mentally retarded children being considered incompetent, as compared to 68 per cent in the non-autistic severely retarded group.

• *Language*. Jacobson and Ackerman's study underlines that both autistic and mentally retarded children at all levels of cognitive competence are significantly delayed, and much more so than for adaptive motor skills. They reported no difference between autistic and mentally retarded groups in overall verbal competence, whereas parents of our LAD children reported considerably more delay and less verbal competence than those of children in the NALIQ group.

Language development, including speech intelligibility, was delayed in all groups in our study, with the LAD group showing increasingly severe impairments as higher levels of linguistic development failed to be attained. The parents' reports confirmed our hypothesis that all four groups would be delayed, indicating why failure to speak at the expected age is the most frequent presenting complaint in all three groups (DLD, AD and NALIQ) of preschool children.

There is less information on the development of language in NALIQ children than in DLD and AD children. Kamhi and Johnston (1982) reported that mentally retarded children do not have the same types of language deficits as DLD children. In our study, the NALIQ children lagged about half a year behind the DLD group in achievement of milestones beyond single words.

The development of language in the HAD group followed a quite similar timetable to that of the DLD group, with greater lag apparent for higher linguistic achievement such as producing sentences and, especially, asking questions. The fact that about a third of the LAD children were still at the single word stage and three quarters were still not producing sentences at a mean age of 5 years is consonant with reports of others (*e.g.* Baltaxe and Simmons 1975; Bartak *et al.* 1975, 1977; Cohen *et al.* 1976) and confirms the severity of their language impairment. Echolalia and the use of learned scripts, a hallmark of autistic language (Prizant and Rydell 1984, Wetherby and Prizant 1985), were reported by parents of both AD groups significantly more often than by parents of the other groups. However, echolalia was reported by parents of nearly half of the DLD and NALIQ children as well, more often than observed by the neurologists (see Table 6.9, p. 112). In general, parents reported less severe impairment of comprehension than of production, but they confirmed that comprehension was disproportionately affected in the two AD groups. More severely delayed comprehension in the HAD than in the DLD group needs emphasis and may have contributed to HAD children's disproportionate difficulty asking and answering 'wh–' questions.

• *Regression of language.* The proportion of parents of AD children in this study who reported loss of language skills (26.6 per cent) was similar to that of parents of autistic children evaluated clinically by one of the investigators in another study (28 per cent) (Tuchman *et al.* 1991*a,b*). Most of the parents in that study stated that not only their children's language but also their sociability and play underwent regression. It is somewhat surprising, therefore, that very few parents of autistic children in the present study who reported language regression in their children reported regression of sociability and play.

• *Habilitation.* The observation that the AD and NALIQ children were more likely to be in school than those with DLD at the time of the evaluation may be in part a function of the fact that they were older on average. It is also more appropriate for those DLD children who are more mildly affected to be receiving speech and language therapy outside of a preschool setting than would be the case for the more pervasively affected AD and NALIQ groups. It is somewhat surprising that a third of the parents of autistic children and more than 40 per cent of those of NALIQ children reported that their child was not attending a specialized school program in the face of US Public Law 94-142 which was fully in effect at the time of the study and which mandates free public education for all disabled children.

• *Medications.* The finding that an almost equal number of children in all four groups were receiving behavior modifying drugs was unexpected, albeit that past use of a variety of these drugs had been higher in the AD group. Unexpectedly, 12 per cent of the DLD children, who were only 49 months old on average, were stated to be receiving behavior modifying drugs, in most cases methylphenidate, at the time we examined them. The sole indication for methylphenidate in young children is attention deficit disorder (ADD), but whether one can legitimately conclude that children taking this medication actually have ADD as a co-morbid condition is uncertain. Behavioral co-morbidity is an important issue in developmentally delayed children. Beitchman and colleagues (1986*a*, 1987, 1988) report that there is an increased prevalence of ADD in children with DLD. Investigators have reported an increased prevalence of other behavior disorders in the DLD population (Baker and Cantwell 1987), as well as a high prevalence of language disorders among children seen in psychiatric consultation (Kotsopoulos and Boodoosingh 1987). In a clinic population of children being investigated for mental retardation, 75 per cent had behavior problems of some sort, of whom 26 per cent were frankly autistic or had some autistic behaviors (Kaminer *et al.* 1984). The term 'pervasive developmental disorder' for children on the autistic spectrum was chosen precisely because involvement of such a wide variety of behaviors is its characteristic feature, in contrast to the specific disorders where behavioral co-morbidity, although frequent, is not the rule.

*Aberrant behaviors*

According to DSM III-R, what characterizes children on the autistic spectrum, in contrast to other developmentally impaired children, is their aberrant social skills, affect and language, their impoverished play, their rigidity and their stereotypies. Although in our study several persons rated the children's behavior during the course of the evaluation, the testing situation was mostly highly structured and often brought out either the best or the worst in the children. Parents, who have seen their children in the broadest range of circumstances, are often the best reporters of their children's typical behaviors.

We reviewed several questionnaires [*e.g.* the HBS (Appendix 5), the Vineland Adaptive Behavior Scales (Sparrow *et al.* 1984*a*) and the Childhood Autism Rating Scale (CARS—Schopler *et al.* 1986)] to select the questions to put in the parental questionnaire for this study. We added some additional items based on our clinical experience to prepare a list of behaviors which we felt would capture children with autistic behaviors (see section IID of the History Questionnaire in Appendix 3). We asked parents whether the behaviors were observed occasionally or often, and whether or not they were still present at the time of the evaluation.

FINDINGS

There were 32 behavioral items in the questionnaire. Parents of DLD children endorsed a mean of 2.1 (SD 3.1) items, those of HAD children 8.3 (SD 5.7) items, those of LAD children 10.9 (SD 6.5) items, and those of NALIQ children 4.1 (SD 4.8) items. These differences were highly significant (F=94.9, p<0.0001). *Post hoc* analysis indicated that all groups were significantly different from one another. We then compared the mean number of checked items in the AD groups (10.2, SD 6.4) and non-AD groups (2.8, SD 3.9), this difference again being highly significant (p<0.0001). These overall results indicate that the questions were successful in picking out autistic children from their non-autistic counterparts, including those with subnormal NVIQs.

We then grouped behaviors into broad categories and listed the mild–moderate and severe responses as a single (abnormal) category (Tables 5.21–5.26). In most cases, responses of the parents of the autistic children differed sharply from those of the two other groups but did not differentiate HAD from LAD children. Parents of NALIQ children gave positive responses to the questions somewhat more often than those of the DLD group, but did so much less often than those of the AD children.

All the aberrant behaviors characteristic of autistic children were reported by parents: impaired sociability, labile affect, resistance to change, unusual fears, attentional deficits and poor play skills, as well as echolalia and use of scripts by verbal autistic children. A few questions did differentiate the two autistic groups. HAD children were somewhat more likely than LAD children to have temper tantrums, whereas LAD children were much more likely to laugh and cry without provocation. Stereotypies were reported most frequently by the parents of LAD children; parents of NALIQ children also reported stereotypies, but only half as often as those of the LAD children.

Impaired play strongly discriminated autistic from non-autistic children (Table 5.24). Over 70 per cent of the parents of LAD children reported that they manipulated toys rather than playing with them, but it is noteworthy that almost 50 per cent of parents of HAD children gave the same report. The low percentage (19 per cent) of LAD children

**TABLE 5.21**
**Parents' view of child's behavior: sociability\*\*\***

|  | DLD (N=201) % | HAD (N=51) % | LAD (N=125) % | NALIQ (N=110) % |
|---|---|---|---|---|
| *Problem behaviors* |  |  |  |  |
| Stares, tunes out | 15.9 | 52.0 | 65.6 | 24.6 |
| Remote from family members | 8.5 | 31.4 | 56.8 | 10.9 |
| Unaware mother's departure | 7.0 | 21.6 | 34.4 | 10.9 |
| Ignores affection | 7.5 | 33.3 | 46.4 | 13.6 |
| Dislikes interactive games | 12.9 | 56.9 | 72.8 | 28.2 |
| (Mean number out of 5) | (0.5) | (1.9) | (2.8) | (0.9) |

\*\*\*All differences among groups significant ($\chi^2$, p<0.001).

**TABLE 5.22**
**Parents' view of child's behavior: mood and affect\*\*\***

|  | DLD (N=201) % | HAD (N=51) % | LAD (N=125) % | NALIQ (N=110) % |
|---|---|---|---|---|
| *Problem behaviors* |  |  |  |  |
| Nervous, anxious | 15.4 | 41.2 | 37.6 | 20.0 |
| Needs to carry a prop | 9.0 | 17.7 | 40.0 | 15.6 |
| Excessive fears | 18.4 | 49.0 | 56.0 | 30.0 |
| Catastrophic reactions | 9.5 | 41.2 | 51.2 | 19.1 |
| Unprovoked rages, aggression | 11.9 | 33.3 | 33.6 | 20.0 |
| Tantrums | 35.8 | 70.6 | 63.2 | 40.9 |
| Difficult to comfort | 11.5 | 43.1 | 44.8 | 20.0 |
| Unprovoked laughing/crying | 6.0 | 37.3 | 62.4 | 16.4 |
| Labile mood | 9.0 | 31.4 | 41.6 | 20.9 |
| (Mean number out of 8) | (1.3) | (3.6) | (4.3) | (2.0) |

\*\*\*All differences among groups significant ($\chi^2$, p<0.001).

**TABLE 5.23**
**Parents' view of child's behavior: language\*\*\***

|  | DLD (N=201) % | HAD (N=51) % | LAD (N=125) % | NALIQ (N=110) % |
|---|---|---|---|---|
| *Character of language* |  |  |  |  |
| Decreased coo + babble\*\* | 21.4 | 25.5 | 30.4 | 33.6 |
| Uses scripts\*\*\* | 41.4 | 75.0 | 75.4 | 52.8 |
| Echolalic, doesn't respond to questions\*\*\* | 48.1 | 85.4 | 86.0 | 48.4 |
| [% nonverbal—no data for items 2 and 3] | [10] | [6] | [54] | [17] |
| (Mean number out of 3) | (1.1) | (1.8) | (1.5) | (1.2) |

\*\*Differences among groups significant ($\chi^2$, p<0.01).
\*\*\*Differences among groups significant ($\chi^2$, p<0.001).

**TABLE 5.24**
**Parents' view of child's behavior: abnormalities of play\*\*\***

|  | DLD (N=201) % | HAD (N=51) % | LAD (N=125) % | NALIQ (N=110) % |
|---|---|---|---|---|
| *Character of play* | | | | |
| Absent or manipulative only | 20.9 | 49.0 | 72.8 | 40.0 |
| Lines up, spins toys | 22.9 | 70.6 | 80.8 | 35.5 |
| Prefers puzzles, blocks | 28.9 | 60.8 | 55.2 | 32.7 |
| Prefers machines to toys | 30.4 | 54.9 | 64.0 | 40.0 |
| One line pretend play | 13.3 | 51.4 | 37.0 | 15.7 |
| (Mean number out of 5) | (1.2) | (2.9) | (3.0) | (1.7) |

\*\*\*All differences among groups significant ($\chi^2$, p<0.001).

**TABLE 5.25**
**Parents' view of child's behavior: attention deficits, rigidity\*\*\***

|  | DLD (N=201) % | HAD (N=51) % | LAD (N=125) % | NALIQ (N=110) % |
|---|---|---|---|---|
| *Attentional abnormalities* | | | | |
| Underactive | 6.0 | 5.9 | 17.6 | 10.0 |
| Extra long attention span | 13.9 | 45.1 | 50.4 | 15.5 |
| (Mean number out of 2) | (0.2) | (0.5) | (0.7) | (0.3) |
| *Rigidity* | | | | |
| Upset by change | 22.9 | 60.8 | 61.6 | 27.3 |
| Upset by interruption | 30.0 | 70.6 | 64.0 | 31.8 |
| Repetitive activities | 6.5 | 45.1 | 57.6 | 19.1 |
| (Mean out of 3) | (0.6) | (1.7) | (1.8) | (0.8) |

\*\*\*All differences among groups significant ($\chi^2$, p<0.001).

with one-line pretend play is attributable to the fact that 57 per cent of these children were reported not to have developed any pretend play at the time of testing. HAD children who had developed at least some pretend play tended to be repetitive, to produce again and again the few pretend scenarios they had learned—perhaps a form of perseveration and delayed 'echolalia in play'. Pica and mouthing were reported by close to half of the parents of LAD children (Table 5.26). They were more frequent in NALIQ than in HAD children, probably because severe mental retardation predisposes to these behaviors in autistic as well as non-autistic children.

Lack of response to pain was reported twice as often among LAD children as in any other group. The cause of behavioral improvement with fever is unknown, but this observation was made more frequently in autistic than in non-autistic children.

Intelligent autistic children regularly have uneven cognitive skills, and some of them have such remarkably developed, albeit narrow skills, that these extraordinary skills earn them the title of 'savants' (Obler and Fein 1988, Treffert 1989). We asked parents

**TABLE 5.26**
**Parents' view of child's behavior: stereotypies, other features\*\*\***

|  | DLD (N=201) % | HAD (N=51) % | LAD (N=125) % | NALIQ (N=110) % |
|---|---|---|---|---|
| *Stereotypies* |  |  |  |  |
| Flapping, touching, etc. | 13.0 | 56.9 | 76.8 | 28.2 |
| Flipping switches, etc. | 17.9 | 39.2 | 64.8 | 40.9 |
| (Mean number out of 2) | (0.3) | (1.0) | (1.4) | (0.7) |
| *Other features* |  |  |  |  |
| Pica, mouthing | 10.5 | 23.5 | 46.4 | 29.1 |
| Unaware of pain | 9.5 | 21.6 | 42.4 | 19.1 |
| Behavior improves with fever[1] | 6.8 | 32.5 | 22.0 | 14.6 |
| (Mean number out of 3) | (0.2) | (0.5) | (0.9) | (0.5) |

\*\*\*All differences among groups significant ($\chi^2$, p<0.01).
[1]Number of children with data: 337.


**TABLE 5.27**
**Parents' report of child's special abilities**

| Salient ability | DLD (N=201) % | HAD (N=51) % | LAD (N=125) % | NALIQ (N=110) % |
|---|---|---|---|---|
| Memory\*\*\* | 21.4 | 70.6 | 44.0 | 23.6 |
| Music\*\* | 11.4 | 27.5 | 23.2 | 12.7 |
| Puzzles, spatial skills\*\*\* | 13.4 | 35.3 | 26.4 | 9.1 |
| Numbers, dates\*\*\* | 8.0 | 45.1 | 13.6 | 4.6 |
| Fine motor skills\*\* | 9.0 | 21.6 | 14.4 | 4.6 |
| Writing letters or numbers\*\* | 3.0 | 25.5 | 9.6 | 3.6 |
| Other\*\*\* | 11.9 | 31.4 | 17.6 | 7.3 |

\*\*Significant difference among groups ($\chi^2$, p<0.01).
\*\*\*Significant difference among groups ($\chi^2$, p<0.001).


whether they felt that their child had unusually well developed abilities in memory, mathematics, recognition of letters and numbers, music or motor skills. Data in Table 5.27 show that parents of autistic children, especially those in the HAD group, were more likely than parents of DLD and NALIQ children to think their child had special abilities. Parents of children in the HAD group were especially likely to report an excellent memory and interest in numbers and puzzles, and parents of almost half of the LAD children were impressed with their child's memory. The figures indicate that parents often thought that their child had several unusual skills, but the data were not collected in such a way as to enable us to determine whether the parents thought these skills were exceptional relative to the child's other abilities or relative to normal children.

In summary, our study emphasizes that parents of AD children strongly endorsed the views of their children's behaviors which were used by teachers, psychiatrists and other investigators to classify the children into autistic and non-autistic groups for this study (see Chapter 8). The important corollary of this finding is that any clinician who evaluates developmentally disabled children will be well advised to include questions about typical autistic behaviors in routine history taking to avoid missing a diagnosis with important genetic, educational and prognostic implications.

DISCUSSION

The data from our study indicate clearly that questions to parents regarding aberrant behaviors are a most, perhaps the most, efficient and reliable means for determining that a child with inadequate communication skills is autistic, rather than only language impaired or mentally retarded. The questions need to address sociability with both adults and peers, the effectiveness of verbal and nonverbal communication skills, and the child's preferred activities and interests. In preschool children, questions about play and attentional skills, especially joint attention, are essential and revealing. The DSM and WHO criteria for PDD have long recognized this but it bears emphasizing for physicians and other professionals who provide primary care for young children and who may not routinely ask this type of question.

## Summary

There were a number of items in the histories that discriminated DLD children from AD children and from NALIQ children. Positive family histories, pointing to a substantial genetic contribution to etiology, were prevalent in both DLD and AD children. They suggested that these disorders were more likely to be distinct than variants of a single underlying condition. The histories were compatible with continuity of DLD with reading and spelling deficit. The prevalence of NALIQ, DLD and learning deficits, but not AD, was somewhat higher in families with low SES than in others. While it is likely that SES factors interact with genetic and acquired biological factors in the genesis of developmental problems in some individuals, the strength of this interaction needs further investigation.

Length of pregnancy, complications of pregnancy and delivery, and birthweights did not differentiate the groups, except that the NALIQ children were somewhat more likely to be small at birth. Children in both low NVIQ groups, especially the NALIQ group, were slightly more likely to have experienced difficulties in the neonatal period, including asphyxia, abnormal movements, and poor tone and nursing. Because we lacked a comparison group of normal children, we cannot weigh the potential contribution of perinatal factors to the developmental disorders of the children in our study, but their overall prevalence was low and few mothers reported severe problems.

Acquired deleterious events did not seem to play a major etiological role in the vast majority of the children and did not occur selectively in any group, with the possible exception of encephalitis or meningitis which, although rare, occurred disproportionately (6/9 cases) in LAD children. There was no group difference in the frequency of ear infections, head injuries or hospitalizations.

No doubt the exclusion from the study of children with definable brain anomalies and of those with acquired lesions causing overt sensorimotor deficits and frequent seizures contributed to the paucity of clearly acquired etiologies. Epilepsy was correlated with low NVIQ, with infantile spasms occurring most frequently in the LAD group (7 per cent). The prevalence of seizures was highest in the LAD group but was increased over normal expectation in all except the HAD group. Sleep problems also occurred differentially: children in the two autistic groups were more likely to have difficulty falling asleep. Sleep problems were reported in over a third of LAD children, who were the group most likely to awaken early and have multiple sleep problems.

Age of walking and other motor milestones were delayed in the two low NVIQ groups. These children were also delayed in daytime toilet training, and many of them (especially the LAD children) had not yet achieved training at a mean age of 5 years. Children in the two autistic groups showed later onset of pretend play, play with other children, and understanding the rules of a game than those in their comparison groups. Removal of children with NVIQs <50 did not alter these findings substantially.

Children in all groups had significantly delayed language milestones, and children in both low NVIQ groups were more delayed than children in the other two groups. Among expressive milestones, single words, naming objects and putting two words together did not differentiate autistic from their comparison non-autistic children. The two autistic groups were more delayed than the non-autistic groups in asking 'wh–' questions and in speaking in sentences. Many children in all groups (least for DLD, most for LAD) did not yet have these skills, a lack that was not attributable to children with an NVIQ <50. Achievement of comprehension milestones differentiated autistic from non-autistic children more strongly than did expressive milestones. It is doubtful that ear infections, which occurred in all groups but by no means in all children, played a major role in the delayed language acquisition of the children in the study.

Many more parents of autistic children (21 per cent) reported regression in language skills than did parents of non-autistic children (4 per cent). Most often, this was a loss of language at the single word level. Surprisingly few parents in any group reported regression of play, social or motor skills, possibly because these were less salient than mutism.

Language regression, preceding or following the development of seizures or, in some cases, without seizures but with an epileptiform EEG, is the hallmark of the Landau–Kleffner syndrome (Landau and Kleffner 1957). A proportion of children with this syndrome develop severe behavior disorders, and in some cases, frankly autistic ('psychotic') behaviors (Rapin 1995). The question of whether the abnormal behavior is entirely attributable to loss of language with severely compromised comprehension, or whether it a consequence of a convulsive disorder affecting limbic brain structures like the amygdala as well as the temporal auditory neocortex (Deonna 1991), or whether the language disorder, the autistic behaviors and the seizures are all symptoms of the underlying brain dysfunction (Rapin 1985) remains an open question.

Parental reports of impaired play and abnormal behaviors characteristic of autistic children discriminated AD from non-autistic groups so strongly as to make them mandatory questions in the evaluation of all children with inadequate language acquisition.

Parents of autistic children endorsed autistic behaviors in all domains much more often than parents of non-autistic children. Few behaviors differentiated the HAD from the LAD children significantly, but the LAD children tended to show more severe behavioral deficits on most items.

The developmental history data do not support preterm birth or perinatal difficulties as differential causes for any of the syndromes under study. The data do support diffuse brain involvement in the low NVIQ groups, who showed more language and motor delays and more seizures, although demographic data also support the contribution of sociocultural deprivation to such delays. Autistic children, relative to the cognitively matched non-autistic children, had more severe difficulties in language comprehension, development of social and pretend play, sleep problems, seizures—notably infantile spasms—and regression in language skills. The provocative finding that six out of the nine cases of encephalitis/meningitis occurred in the LAD group suggests one possible etiological mechanism for this devastating and presumably diffuse brain dysfunction.

## Clinical implications

One of the most important findings of our study, and of many others, is that genetic factors are more likely than deleterious perinatal or postnatal events to play an etiological role in DLDs and in autism unassociated with overt structural brain pathology, and perhaps also in mental retardation of unknown etiology. The data support evidence from genetic studies of language disorders, reading disability and autism pointing to distinct genetic etiologies of DLD and AD, and to a significantly high prevalence of learning disabilities in the families of children with DLD. The demographic data in Chapter 4 indicate, once again, that socioeconomic deprivation is significantly associated with low NVIQ, and probably also with learning disability. There is an inextricable relation of genetic and environmental influences on developmental skills and on their disorders.

Clearly, after one has gathered adequate data on the pregnancy, delivery, and neonatal and postnatal events, relevant items on which to focus are acquisition of language milestones, adequacy of social skills and, especially in preschool children, level of play. Clinical experience and research by investigators of early development indicate that pointing, showing and imitating are preludes to later verbal and social abilities and, therefore, that it is critical to ask whether the child acquired these preverbal skills in timely fashion. Inadequacies in these skills, especially if combined with stereotypies and deficient play, point to a diagnosis of AD rather than DLD or mental retardation.

Although inadequate verbal skills are ubiquitous in virtually all developmentally impaired preschool children, and although mental retardation complicates AD in many children, a history of unusual behaviors must be taken seriously because they are such potent evidence for a diagnosis of AD. A competent developmental history must include questions relevant to AD. An important question, not asked in this study, is whether a young child with minimal expressive language points not just to request, but to draw another's attention. Failure of joint attention (Mundy *et al.* 1990) and lack of understanding of what others mean or are thinking are hallmarks of autism (Frith 1993). These questions must be asked of parents of intelligent children with atypical behaviors, even if they did not speak late and if they speak clearly and fluently, in some cases with a rich vocabulary, otherwise one will overlook mild autistic features that may, nonetheless, create severe problems for such children and their families.

Detecting LAD preschool children by inspection offers little difficulty for the experienced clinician because the typical profile of stereotypies and other repetitive behaviors, disinterest in sustained play, impaired sociability and joint attention, flat or excessively labile affect, and severely deficient communication skills are readily apparent. The situation may be much more difficult in the case of HAD children whose overlearned verbal scripts may be used to such good effect as to not be recognized as such. Some HAD children will have learned the basic functions of certain toys so that impoverishment of their pretend play may not be apparent to a casual observer and may require searching questioning of the parents to bring it out.

In the main, answers to questions about autistic behaviors from questionnaires such as the one used in this study or one of the others such as the Childhood Autism Rating Scale (CARS—Schopler *et al.* 1986), supplemented by observation of the child's spontaneous play with age-appropriate representational toys, are likely to identify autistic children more reliably than observations in the unnatural and usually highly structured circumstances of an initial clinical assessment.

Questions about sleep problems are important both because adequate management will be helpful to the families of autistic children with such problems and because they may provide clues on the pathophysiology of autism.

Asking specifically about loss of language and cognitive and social milestones is also critical because this loss is reported so much more often in AD children than in DLD or NALIQ children. If one elicits such a history, one needs to inquire about seizures and previous EEGs. If the regression is a recent one, one should recommend an all night—or at least a prolonged—sleep EEG, even if there is no history of clinical seizures, looking either for focal spikes or for electrical status epilepticus in sleep or continuous spikes and waves during slow sleep (Boel and Casaer 1989, Jayakar and Seshia 1991, Deonna *et al.* 1993, Perez *et al.* 1993). One also needs to ask about a history of infantile spasms or other seizure types. Although what to do in the face of an unequivocally paroxysmal EEG without clinical seizures is controversial, the current trend is to treat children who have a paroxysmal EEG and loss of language, with or without autistic regression, with anticonvulsants like sodium valproate or ethosuximide, or with ACTH or steroids (Marescaux *et al.* 1990, Lerman *et al.* 1991). This is an area where research is sorely needed and where collaborative studies will be required if one is to accumulate a sufficient number of cases to draw reliable conclusions about the indications and efficacy of such treatments. The burden of identifying children between ages 1 and 3 years who are undergoing regression is clearly on the shoulders of family doctors and pediatricians; such children need to be referred promptly for study rather than reassuring parents or accusing them of being overanxious when they raise questions about their child's language.

Our study indicates that American physicians are surprisingly prone to prescribe behavior modifying medications, especially stimulants, to preschool children with developmental disabilities and behavior problems. It does not provide data on the use of antipsychotic drugs in autism. Most studies to date of the efficacy of a variety of drugs for attention deficit with hyperactivity and of psychotropic drugs in autism have been carried out in school-age rather than preschool children. This is clearly another unmet need, and as a result, prescription in the clinic is still very much a hit or miss affair because indications, if any, for pharmacotherapy are largely missing for very young children.

# 6
# NEUROLOGICAL EXAMINATION

*I. Rapin*

The purposes of a medical and neurological examination of a child with a known neurological or developmental condition are to determine the type of disorder and what parts of the nervous system are affected (localization), and to look for findings that might disclose the cause (etiology) of the person's illness or disorder. In order to make a diagnosis, a neurologist depends not only on the findings from the medical and neurological examination but also on the historical data and, in some cases, on ancillary laboratory tests to confirm or disprove the diagnostic hypothesis derived from the historical data and examination.

In a child with a developmental problem, the medical examination focuses on the search for findings pointing to a genetic condition, for example the skin lesions of neurofibromatosis, and unusual facial features or minor hand anomalies suggesting a malformative syndrome like those due to an intrauterine infection or the fetal alcohol syndrome, or, more often, a syndrome of genetic, developmental or unknown cause. Rarely, the medical evaluation discloses findings suggestive of a postnatal condition, for example lead poisoning, or a systemic disease such as hypothyroidism.

The classic neurological examination relies heavily on the mental status and on the pattern of sensorimotor deficits in the limbs and cranial nerves to determine what parts of the nervous system are affected. Like all medical evaluations, the neurological examination is hypothesis-driven, and the detail with which any part of it is carried out depends on the problem that has brought the particular patient to the physician, on the history, and on the findings in the general medical examination. To avoid overlooking unsuspected abnormalities, every patient undergoes a brief screening routine neurological examination as well.

Research on large patient cohorts requires a standardized examination to ensure that uniform data are collected from every subject. For the purpose of this study, the neurologists discussed how best to carry out a reliable neurological examination in hard-to-test preschool children. Inasmuch as cooperation in performing certain tasks would not necessarily be attainable, it was important to have items requiring only observation of functional skills (see below). Because the project was concerned with developmentally disabled children, the examination emphasized the mental status, language and communication. A short period of play with representational toys was a required part of the examination because this type of play fosters conversation and is an economical way to obtain a representative sample of a young child's behavioral and communicative repertoire.

A number of investigators (*e.g.* Denckla 1985, Deuel 1992) have developed standardized neurological examinations suitable for school-age children with learning disabilities that focus on fine motor performance and the presence of mirror movements and over-flow, so-called 'neurological soft signs', most of which are permissible in preschool children. Few standardized neurological examinations are suitable for assessing pre-school children, especially those with developmental problems. Interest in quantitative neurological examinations is on the increase, driven in part by the need to assess the effects of drug trials and other therapies across institutions and for evaluating develop-ment longitudinally in survivors of perinatal intensive care units (*e.g.* Amiel-Tison and Stewart 1989).

In designing the examination for this study, the neurologists consulted the examina-tion of Touwen and Prechtl (1979), the neurological examination forms used in the Collaborative Perinatal Project (kindly provided by Dr Karin Nelson), and the quantita-tive neurological examination for adults developed by Potvin and Tourtellotte (1985).

## Method

For this study, the pediatric neurologists developed a standard neurological examination appropriate for preschool and young school-age children without a gross motor deficit (children with gross motor deficits were excluded from the study), yet one that would not overlook subtle evidence of generalized or lateralized sensorimotor deficits, and that emphasized the mental status, language and oromotor function. In a cooperative child, the examination took about 30 minutes, including a five minute period of play with representative toys.

The form (Appendix 4) provided an opportunity to score 'no data' for each item, but did not distinguish explicitly failure to administer the item from unwillingness or in-ability to perform. The neurologist's decision would necessarily be judgmental in such cases: failure to complete the item might have resulted from a motor or sensory deficit, notably apraxia, lack of comprehension of what was wanted, inattentiveness, resistance, lack of motivation or other behavioral difficulty. Neurologists were instructed to score as severely abnormal any child who manifestly could not do a test because of severe motor disability, lack of comprehension, mental retardation or autistic withdrawal.

Each item in the examination was scored on a three-point ordinal scale: 0 = normal; 1 = mild to moderately abnormal; 2 = very abnormal or unable to perform at all. These scores were used to develop summary scores for each neurological system or functional category; the summary scores were devised so as not to give excessive weights to functional areas such as the motor system with many measures, compared to those with only a few such as comprehension of language. Summary scores were calculated by dividing the sum of scores in a functional area by the number of component scores (excluding items with no data). Summary scores provided an index of impairment which ranged between 0.0 (perfectly normal on all measures of that functional area) and 1.0 (severely abnormal on all measures). These summary scores provided a continuous measure of level of deficit or abnormality in each area expressed in a common metric that enabled comparisons across domains. For presentation of frequencies of abnormal scores in this chapter, we collapsed the 0 to 2 scale to a normal/abnormal form, *viz.* normal = 0, abnormal = 1 or 2. Scores are presented across the four clinical groups

**TABLE 6.1**
**Appearance and general examination**

| Abnormality | N with data | Groups | | | | |
|---|---|---|---|---|---|---|
| | | DLD (N=201) % | HAD (N=51) % | LAD (N=125) % | NALIQ (N=110) % | All (N=487) % |
| Major anomaly | 481 | 1.5 | 2.0 | 0.8 | 1.9 | 1.5 |
| Minor anomaly* | 481 | 15.4 | 5.9 | 9.0 | 24.3 | 14.8 |
| Middle ear problem | 486 | 11.4 | 17.7 | 19.2 | 19.3 | 15.8 |
| Head <2 centile** | 454 | 1.6 | 2.1 | 3.4 | 16.0 | 5.3 |
| Head >98 centile | 454 | 5.8 | 8.3 | 4.3 | 7.0 | 5.9 |

*Significant difference among groups ($\chi^2$, $p<0.05$).
**Significant difference among groups ($\chi^2$, $p<0.01$).

discussed in earlier chapters: DLD—developmental language disorder (N=201), HAD—high-functioning autistic disorder (N=51), LAD—low-functioning autistic disorder (N=125), and NALIQ—non-autistic, low NVIQ (N=110).

We prepared an examiner manual and held training sessions for all neurologists who evaluated children in the study. In order to enhance and evaluate inter-examiner reliability, each neurologist was asked to use the standardized examination to score videotaped examinations given by the other physicians. In addition, the neurologists also scored four neurological examinations live which were then reviewed.

In most cases, neurologists were not blind to the type of child they were examining because, with the exception of the Bronx site, sites were to recruit, in addition to NALIQ children, children with either DLD or AD. At sites where the neurologists went over the history form with the parent, they also had access to historical data. No neurologist had access to any of the formal test data, and they did not discuss diagnoses with other investigators before carrying out their examinations.

## Findings
### General physical examination
The neurologists performed a brief medical examination, looking for unusual features, major or minor malformations, skin lesions, and evidence of acute or chronic illness (Table 6.1). The higher prevalence of physical anomalies in the NALIQ group was accounted for in part by the nine children (8.1 per cent of the NALIQ group) with Down syndrome. Overall, 15 per cent of children had one or more minor anomalies such as somewhat unusual facial features or external ears, and minor finger anomalies like clinodactyly. A specific diagnosis was made in four autistic children after the inception of the study: fragile X syndrome (Simko *et al.* 1989) in two unrelated boys and Cornelia de Lange syndrome (Jones 1988) in a pair of monozygotic twins.

As stated in Chapter 4, all children had to pass a screening pure tone audiogram at a threshold of 20 dB or better binaurally at 1000 and 2000 Hz and 25 dB or better binaurally at 500 and 4000 Hz. The neurologists examined the tympanic membranes to make sure that the child did not have an acute ear infection or fluid behind the drum. Only 1 per cent had active otitis or a perforated drum; the remainder of those with abnormalities had ceruminosis, or thickened or retracted drums.

## Neurological examination

### HEAD SIZE

Head circumference was measured and compared to the Nellhaus norms (1968). 5 per cent of the children had a head circumference below the second centile (microcephaly). This was four times more common in the NALIQ group than in the LAD group (Table 6.1). Inasmuch as microcephaly is a well recognized correlate of subnormal intelligence, this finding is noteworthy because, paradoxically, the mean NVIQ equivalent of the NALIQ group was nine points higher than that of the LAD group (55 *vs* 46), suggesting different biological causes for the depressed IQ in these two groups of children. Macrocephaly (a head circumference above the 98th centile), was present in 6 per cent of the cohort and was most prevalent, although not significantly so, in the HAD group.

### SENSORIMOTOR EXAMINATION

A typical neurological examination comprises many more motor than sensory items. So as not to give undue weight to motor functions assessed with multiple measures, and also to deal with missing data, items were grouped by function and summary scores were expressed as the ratio of the sum of individual scores over the total number of items assessed. Ratio scores thus ranged from 0 to 1; the fewer the problems within an area, the closer the score was to 0. The data were evaluated by analysis of covariance, co-varying age and NVIQ equivalent since these are important determinants of motor skill. Scores on tests of lateralized function were summed separately for the left and right sides. The items included in the sensorimotor examination are listed in Table 6.2.

• *Motor examination.* Because some children were unable to cooperate with examiners' requests, the examination included a number of motor items that could be scored entirely by observation. These included gait, muscle tone, the presence of abnormal movements or posture, overall motor skills, eye and facial movements, and drooling. Other items depended on the child's ability to cooperate, *e.g.* jumping, hopping, imitating hand and mouth movements, drawing, building with blocks, and repeating syllables. There were separate scores for gross and fine motor skills. The four groups differed significantly with regard to both gross and fine motor findings (Table 6.3). As one would expect, LAD and NALIQ children, presumed to have more diffuse brain dysfunction, performed less well than DLD and HAD children. The children in the LAD group performed significantly worse than those in the NALIQ group, even though NVIQ equivalent was controlled. Analysis of covariance showed that children in the HAD group had better gross motor skills, but inferior fine motor skills, than children in the DLD group. There was no difference in the gross and fine motor skills of children in the HAD and NALIQ groups.

LAD children were more likely not to perform tasks than children in the other three groups. For example, while 90 per cent of DLD and HAD children and 84 per cent of the

**TABLE 6.2**
**Items of the sensorimotor examination**

| Gross motor items | Fine motor items |
|---|---|
| Gait | Finger-to-nose |
| Gait on toes | Patting |
| Gait on heels | Apposing index to thumb |
| Jumping | Apposing fingers to thumb |
| Hopping (> age 5 yrs) |   sequentially (> age 5 yrs) |
| Tandem gait (> age 5 yrs) | Pile 1 inch (2.5 cm) blocks |
| Standing on one foot (> age 5 yrs) | Copy block pattern |
| | Drawing |
| *Type of motor deficit* | |
| Spasticity | *Sensory examination* |
| Rigidity | Touching one spot on body |
| Hypotonia | Touching both sides of body |
| Weakness |   simultaneously |
| Tremor | |
| Choreoathetosis | *Cranial nerves*[1] |
| Dystonia | Confrontation fields |
| Tics | Visual acuity ≥ 20/40 |
| Stereotypies | Nystagmus and eye movements |
| Apraxia | Facial movements |

[1]Excluding oromotor findings.

NALIQ children had data on toe-walking, only 52 per cent of LAD children imitated toe-walking. Similarly, while 93–96 per cent of DLD, HAD and NALIQ children drew, only 70 per cent of LAD children did so. Neurologists were instructed to score children whom they felt were incapable of performing tasks as severely deficient (score 2). As discussed earlier, there were many potential reasons for failure to perform, including inability to initiate or imitate a movement on command (apraxia), lack of verbal comprehension because of mental retardation or severe receptive language disorder, resistance and refusal to cooperate, distractibility, lack of motivation, and anxiety; when uncertain, neurologists may have been inconsistent and assigned scores of no data rather than assigning a score of 2. Providing separate scores for 'wouldn't do' and 'couldn't do' might have minimized ambiguity, even though making this distinction is a matter of judgment. Marking this distinction would be desirable in future studies.

Neurologists were asked to rate the children's particular types of motor deficit, based on their overall observations. These are summarized in Table 6.4, which reports frequencies of children with deficits (whether mild/moderate or severe/profound). As children with 'hard' motor deficits were excluded from the study, the data pertain only to children considered to have less obvious 'soft' motor findings. A negligible number of children had mild spasticity, weakness, dystonia, rigidity and tics. Tremor, recorded in 6 per cent of the children, was in some probably benign familial tremor. Only 2 per cent of the children were felt to have a mildly spastic gait, most of them in the LAD and NALIQ groups. Testing of individual tendon stretch reflexes was used by the neurologists to assess motor status and lateralization but was not entered into the data base.

**TABLE 6.3**
**Mean sensorimotor scores[1]**

| Function | Group | | | | F | Significant contrasts[2] |
|---|---|---|---|---|---|---|
| | DLD<br>Mean (SD) | HAD<br>Mean (SD) | LAD<br>Mean (SD) | NALIQ<br>Mean (SD) | | |
| Gross motor | 0.35 (0.21)<br>(N=201) | 0.34 (0.23)<br>(N=51) | 0.59 (0.22)<br>(N=125) | 0.52 (0.24)<br>(N=109) | 67.0*** | DLD=HAD=NALIQ<LAD |
| Fine motor | 0.21 (0.16)<br>(N=201) | 0.28 (0.26)<br>(N=51) | 0.67 (0.25)<br>(N=125) | 0.49 (0.23)<br>(N=109) | 131.1*** | DLD<HAD=NALIQ<LAD |
| Sensory | 0.12 (0.21)<br>(N=165) | 0.01 (0.06)<br>(N=29) | 0.13 (0.32)<br>(N=41) | 0.11 (0.27)<br>(N=69) | 2.3* | DLD=HAD=LAD=NALIQ |
| Cranial nerves[3] | 0.01 (0.08)<br>(N=199) | 0.03 (0.10)<br>(N=51) | 0.02 (0.10)<br>(N=124) | 0.05 (0.14)<br>(N=109) | 4.5*** | DLD=HAD=LAD<NALIQ |

[1]ANCOVA, with age and NVIQ equivalent covaried. (NVIQ equivalent = ratio of nonverbal mental age to chronological age based on Stanford–Binet and Bayley scores. See Chapter 4 for details.) Scores are expressed as the ratio of the sum of scores over total number of items scored. Scores range from 0 to 1: the closer to zero, the better the score.
[2]Least mean square group comparisons.
[3]Exclusive of oromotor findings which are detailed in Tables 6.5 and 6.6.
*p<0.05, ***p<0.001.

**TABLE 6.4**
**Types of motor deficits[1]**

| Abnormality | N with data | Group | | | | |
|---|---|---|---|---|---|---|
| | | DLD (N=201) % | HAD (N=51) % | LAD (N=125) % | NALIQ (N=110) % | All (N=487) % |
| Spastic gait | 486 | 0.5 | 0.0 | 4.0 | 3.7 | 2.1 |
| Spasticity (supine) | 486 | 0.6 | 2.0 | 5.6 | 5.5 | 3.5 |
| Rigidity | 486 | 0.5 | 0.0 | 2.4 | 0.9 | 1.0 |
| Hypotonia*** | 486 | 12.9 | 25.5 | 24.0 | 33.0 | 21.6 |
| [severe hypotonia] | [5] | [0.0] | [0.0] | [1.6] | [2.8] | [1.0] |
| Weakness | 486 | 0.4 | 0.0 | 2.4 | 1.8 | 1.4 |
| Tremor | 486 | 8.5 | 3.9 | 3.2 | 7.3 | 6.4 |
| Choreoathetosis | 486 | 0.0 | 0.0 | 0.0 | 0.0 | 0.0 |
| Dystonia | 484 | 0.0 | 2.0 | 1.6 | 1.8 | 1.0 |
| Limb apraxia*** | 486 | 16.9 | 29.4 | 75.2 | 56.9 | 42.2 |
| [severe limb apraxia] | [130] | [8.9] | [9.8] | [63.2] | [25.7] | [26.7] |
| Tics | 486 | 0.0 | 0.0 | 0.0 | 0.9 | 0.2 |
| Stereotypies*** | 483 | 2.0 | 41.2 | 65.3 | 13.0 | 24.8 |
| [severe stereotypies] | [30] | [0.0] | [3.9] | [21.0] | [1.9] | [6.2] |

[1]Neurologists' summary impressions. The data represent the percentage of children in each group scored as having either mild–moderate or severe–profound deficit.
***Significant difference among groups ($\chi^2$, $p<0.001$).

The neurologists detected no significant right/left difference in gross or fine motor skills in any of the groups, therefore these data are not presented. This finding is not surprising because patients with known lateralized brain lesions were excluded from the study. It may be the case, however, that the standard neurological examination is insensitive to minor right/left differences inasmuch as performance on the Annett Pegboard (see Chapter 7) disclosed a significant though small group difference in dexterity: the DLD group was significantly below average with the right hand, the HAD group below average with both hands but worse with the right than the left, while the two LIQ groups were severely deficient with both hands.

Three motor deficits stand out as significantly frequent and discriminating: hypotonia, limb apraxia and stereotypies (Table 6.4). Defining hypotonia is difficult in preschool children whose joints are much more supple than those of older children and adults. Nonetheless, there was a clear trend for hypotonia to be reported twice as often in the AD and NALIQ groups as in the DLD group. Not one of the DLD or HAD children was severely hypotonic, as compared to 2 per cent of the LAD and 3 per cent of the NALIQ group. The NALIQ group included nine children with Down syndrome, who are characteristically hypotonic; recalculating the prevalence of hypotonia in the NALIQ group after removing these nine children reduced hypotonia from 33 per cent to 28 per cent and reduced the level of significance across groups from $p<0.001$ to $p<0.01$.

Apraxia is defined as the inability to imitate movements, manipulate objects appropriately or carry out a complex activity requiring a sequence of motor acts despite adequate comprehension of verbal commands, and lack of a motor deficit or of mental retardation sufficiently severe to preclude the performance of the target task. According to the neurologists' clinical impression rather than a formal test for apraxia, apraxia was considerably less prevalent in the DLD group than in the other three groups. Like hypotonia, limb apraxia was most prevalent in the two LIQ groups, but it predominated among children in the LAD group. As in the case of hypotonia, HAD children were twice as likely to be apraxic as DLD children.

The neurologists reported stereotypies in 25 per cent of the children. Stereotypies—such as rocking from one foot to the other; hand flapping; rubbing; twiddling of fingers, hair or clothing; shaking a string; running around aimlessly; jumping or tensing of the body when excited; and self-abuse—were almost entirely confined to the two autistic groups, and were more common in the LAD (65 per cent) than in the HAD group (41 per cent). Notably, only 2 per cent of the DLD children and 13 per cent of the NALIQ children had stereotypies, none of them scored as severe. Thus, although stereotypies were not pathognomonic of or always present in AD, their existence was a strong marker for this condition.

We investigated how well neurologists and parents agreed on the prevalence and severity of stereotypies (see Chapter 5). Mothers reported repetitive behaviors in 37.3 per cent of the children, compared to the neurologists' observation of 24.8 per cent. According to the mothers 110 children had very frequent repetitive behaviors, whereas the neurologists observed severe stereotypies in only 30 children. Perhaps this discrepancy between mothers' reports and neurologists' observations is due to the very much longer observation time available to parents than to neurologists. It may also be that the structured situation of the neurological examination was not conducive to the emergence of stereotypies which, like tics and other abnormal involuntary movements, are strongly affected by situational variables: abnormal movements tend to decrease while persons are involved in other activities and to increase during unstructured times and in stressful situations.

• *Sensory examination.* For this examination the children were required to report, eyes closed, whereabouts on their bodies the examiner had touched them with one finger or with two fingers simultaneously on both sides of the body. This part of the examination proved to be both insensitive and unreliable (Table 6.3). So many children were untestable (196 for single stimulation, 299 for double simultaneous stimulation) that we would not include it again in a study of this age group. Failure to perform was not limited to the AD and NALIQ groups: 16 per cent of the DLD children did not report single stimuli and 32 per cent double simultaneous stimuli. However, both autism and LIQ contributed to untestability: for single stimuli, 41 per cent of HAD, 77 per cent of LAD and 77 per cent of NALIQ children were untestable. For double simultaneous stimuli, the figures were 61 per cent for HAD, 89 per cent for LAD and 66 per cent for NALIQ children.

• *Cranial nerves.* Visual acuity no worse than 20/40 was measured by presenting calibrated 20/20 cards* depicting line drawings of a house, an apple and an umbrella, at a

---

*Flash-Card Vision Test for Children, The New York Association for the Blind Optical Aids Service, 36–02 Northern Boulevard, Long Island, NY 11101, USA.

**TABLE 6.5**
**Items of the oromotor examination**

| Drooling | Tongue |
|---|---|
| | Move in and out |
| **Jaw** | Move side to side |
| Move up and down | Tuck into cheek |
| Move sideways | Click and 'tsk' |
| Jaw jerk | |
| | **Diadochokinesis** (>5×) |
| **Lips** | Pa-pa-pa... |
| Purse | Ta-ta-ta... |
| Kiss | Ke-ke-ke... |
| | Pa-ta - pa-ta... |
| **Palate** | Pa-ta-ka... (> age 5 years) |
| Elevates when saying ah... | |

distance of 3 m (10 feet). The child was asked to name the item or point to a matching card. Overall, 26 percent of the children were untestable on this simple task—66 per cent of the LAD and 46 per cent of the NALIQ, as opposed to 7 per cent of the DLD and 15 per cent of the HAD children. We relied on reports of previous ophthalmological examinations to rule out a gross refractive error in untestable children.

The neurologists evaluated confrontation visual fields by any effective method, such as the child pointing to or grabbing the examiner's wiggling finger, imitating the raising of a finger on the appropriate side, pointing to a salient toy brought into the peripheral visual field from behind, or turning the head and eyes toward the moving finger or object. Eye and facial movements were observed informally during the course of the examination. No attempt was made to look at the eyegrounds. Summary results of examinations of cranial nerve function, excluding oromotor findings, are shown in Table 6.3. Abnormal cranial nerve findings were infrequent and did not discriminate among groups, with the exception of mild strabismus, which was slightly more common in children in the NALIQ group.

• *Oromotor examination.* The neurologists paid particular attention to examining oromotor function because we were interested in its relation to prominent expressive language deficits. Items in the examination of oromotor function are listed in Table 6.5.

Results of this examination are detailed in Table 6.6. Once again, the LAD children were most deficient, with the exception of drooling in the NALIQ group. The scores of children in the DLD and HAD groups differed only for tongue movements. These data must be considered in the context of the unequal prevalence of missing data. For example, while 95 per cent of the DLD, 91 per cent of the HAD, and 81 per cent of the NALIQ children provided data, only 48 per cent of the LAD children did so for a task as easy as sticking out their tongue five times, a movement almost certainly in their motor repertoire.

Syllable repetition is a test that is very sensitive to deficits in phonological programming. Children who could not repeat single or sequential syllables were scored as

**TABLE 6.6**
**Mean oromotor scores[1]**

| Function | Group | | | | | | | F | Significant contrasts[2] |
|---|---|---|---|---|---|---|---|---|---|
| | DLD | | HAD | | LAD | | NALIQ | | |
| | Mean (SD) | | Mean (SD) | | Mean (SD) | | Mean (SD) | | |
| Drooling | 0.11 (0.27) (N=194) | | 0.10 (0.25) (N=51) | | 0.11 (0.26) (N=123) | | 0.26 (0.37) (N=109) | 5.0*** | DLD=HAD=LAD<NALIQ |
| Jaw | 0.24 (0.31) (N=201) | | 0.22 (0.29) (N=51) | | 0.64 (0.39) (N=125) | | 0.46 (0.33) (N=109) | 37.4*** | DLD=HAD=NALIQ<LAD |
| Lips | 0.18 (0.32) (N=201) | | 0.21 (0.34) (N=51) | | 0.66 (0.43) (N=125) | | 0.37 (0.40) (N=109) | 38.3*** | DLD=HAD=NALIQ<LAD |
| Tongue | 0.23 (0.27) (N=201) | | 0.35 (0.31) (N=51) | | 0.74 (0.33) (N=125) | | 0.55 (0.34) (N=109) | 72.2*** | DLD<HAD=NALIQ<LAD |
| Palate | 0.08 (0.27) (N=201) | | 0.18 (0.39) (N=51) | | 0.58 (0.50) (N=125) | | 0.18 (0.38) (N=109) | 31.7*** | DLD=NALIQ<HAD<LAD |
| Diadochokinesis | 0.32 (0.32) (N=201) | | 0.25 (0.34) (N=51) | | 0.72 (0.36) (N=125) | | 0.52 (0.37) (N=109) | 37.2*** | DLD=HAD=NALIQ<LAD |

[1]ANCOVA with age and nonverbal IQ equivalent covaried. Scores are expressed as the ratio of the sum of scores over total number of items scored. Scores range from 0 to 1. The closer to zero, the better the score.
[2]Least mean square group comparisons.
***p<0.001, analysis of covariance.

severely impaired. Syllable repetition is the only task where the HAD children obtained a (nonsignificantly) better score than the DLD children. Many intelligent verbal autistic children do not have phonological deficits once they start to speak (Tager-Flusberg 1981, 1989), contrary to many DLD children who are likely to continue to make phonological errors for much longer after they start to express themselves verbally. Better performance of the HAD group is consonant with their better fluency and intelligibility than children in the other groups, and with the verbosity of some children in that group (see below). The relation between oromotor deficit and phonology is discussed later.

MENTAL STATUS

Because this study was concerned with disorders of higher cerebral function, the mental status part of the examination was expanded beyond the more usual brief conversation and observation of the child's behavior that take place while the rest of the neurological examination is carried out. The neurologists were instructed to engage the child in a brief play period and to score the child's alertness and attention, cognition, language, affect and social skills. Items of the mental status were deliberately placed at the end of the form with the expectation that the neurologists would score mental status items based on their entire interaction with the child.

• *Play.* To assess mental status the neurologists observed the children's play with representational toys and talked to them as they played. Each neurologist had a doll house with furniture, small wooden dolls and cars on a table when the child entered the room; the child was encouraged to play with these toys or others such as a tea set or toy airport. Observing the child's play with the toys revealed whether he recognized their symbolic value and could 'pretend' with them. It provided an opportunity to assess the child's affect and conversational and other interpersonal skills. After a few minutes of play, the child was more likely to be willing to cooperate with such tasks as building with blocks, writing, walking and the more formal aspects of the examination.

Neurologists were asked to rate the child's play as to whether it was imaginative, mainly manipulative, or absent. Results are summarized in Table 6.7. Data were available on 95 per cent of the children. There was a dramatic difference between the DLD group, with 17 per cent judged mildly–moderately deficient and only a single child (0.5 per cent) judged severely deficient, and the other groups. The AD children were the most likely of all the groups to be judged incompetent players. As expected, the children in the LAD group were the most deficient, both in terms of the total number judged deficient (109 or 92 per cent) and those judged severely deficient (57 or 48 per cent). Although play was judged inadequate in almost half of the NALIQ children, it was judged severely deficient in only 9 per cent. Inasmuch as fully 63 per cent of the HAD group were poor players, albeit only 8 per cent severely so, deficient play was a marker for autism and not LIQ. Autistic children often manipulated toys in a stereotyped way rather than playing with them. Stereotyped use of toys was most striking in the LAD children but was often present in more subtle ways in the HAD children who lined up or classified toys rather than playing with them imaginatively.

These findings illustrate that even a brief clinical appraisal of play with representa-

**TABLE 6.7**
**Mental status abnormalities[1]**

| Abnormality | N with data | DLD (N=201) % | HAD (N=51) % | LAD (N=125) % | NALIQ (N=110) % | All (N=487) % |
|---|---|---|---|---|---|---|
| [Mean age at test (mo)] | | [49] | [58] | [59] | [56] | [56] |
| [Mean NVIQ equivalent[2]] | | [102] | [103] | [46] | [55] | [77] |
| *Play* | | | | | | |
| Deficient play*** | 461 | 17.1 | 63.3 | 92.4 | 45.5 | 47.5 |
| *Attention, activity* | | | | | | |
| Underaroused** | 479 | 0.6 | 4.0 | 9.9 | 6.5 | 5.0 |
| Hypoactive*** | 482 | 6.5 | 5.9 | 20.2 | 9.3 | 10.6 |
| Hyperactive*** | 482 | 13.1 | 43.1 | 65.3 | 39.8 | 35.7 |
| Distractible*** | 484 | 20.0 | 60.0 | 94.4 | 60.6 | 52.5 |
| *Mood, affect* | | | | | | |
| Flat, depressed*** | 477 | 16.1 | 35.3 | 61.2 | 23.6 | 31.2 |
| *Social skills* | | | | | | |
| Withdrawn*** | 473 | 17.4 | 44.0 | 74.2 | 24.3 | 36.2 |
| Uncooperative*** | 482 | 27.5 | 64.0 | 96.7 | 63.3 | 57.1 |
| Inappropriately interactive*** | 480 | 7.0 | 51.0 | 78.5 | 26.9 | 34.2 |
| Intrusive | 473 | 1.5 | 2.0 | 5.8 | 4.7 | 3.4 |

[1]The data are presented as the percentage of children in each group whom neurologists scored as having mild–moderate or severe deficit.
[2]NVIQ equivalent = ratio of nonverbal mental age to biological age, based on Stanford–Binet and Bayley scores (see Chapter 4).
**Significant difference among groups ($\chi^2$, p<0.01).
***Significant difference among groups ($\chi^2$, p<0.001).

tional toys should draw clinicians' attention, especially if there are also stereotypies, because these easily observable characteristics are easy ways to spot potentially autistic children from their non-autistic communication-impaired peers.

We examined how well the neurologists' views of the children's play corresponded to their mothers' impressions. We had asked the mothers whether their child's play was limited to mouthing, banging, throwing or inspecting toys, whether the child disliked play requiring a partner, *e.g.* ball playing or games necessitating turn-taking, whether the child used toys inappropriately, such as lining up, pulling back and forth, spinning wheels, or flipping pages of books, and whether the child preferred puzzles and blocks to more imaginative play (see Chapter 5). Neurologists and mothers were in fairly good agreement: mothers responded 'no' to these questions in about 62 per cent of cases, and neurologists reported that 53 per cent of children played in an age-appropriate way. Agreement was only partial, however, because mothers reported severely deficient play in 32 per cent of the children whom the neurologists scored as playing adequately, and adequate play in 22 per cent of those who played very poorly according to the neurologists. Disagreement about play was not limited to any one group of children. Assuming that mothers may be more reliable observers because they have access to a much larger sample of play than the neurologists, the findings suggest that the neurologists' sample of play was too short, or that some of the neurologists may have been insensitive to less than adequate play, or, perhaps, that mothers of only children may have lacked a sufficient base of comparison for judging the adequacy of their child's play (for a quantitative evaluation of the children's play, see Chapter 9).

• *Alertness and arousal, attention and activity level.* Neurologists were required to rate the children's alertness, arousal and attention as normal or decreased, and their activity level as either increased or decreased. Table 6.7 shows that three times as many children were judged inattentive and hyperactive as opposed to underaroused and hypoactive. Again, the prevalence of abnormalities, especially inattentiveness, was highest in the LAD children and lowest in the DLD group. The LAD group also had the largest proportion of children (20 per cent) who were judged to be hypoactive.

Children with attention deficit hyperactivity disorder (ADHD) are often reported to have poorly regulated sleep, to fall asleep late and to wake up early. This was confirmed across the entire sample in this study inasmuch as there was a clear relationship between the neurologists' score for distractibility/hyperactivity and the parents' report of difficulty falling asleep and waking up early in the morning ($\chi^2$, p<0.01 and p<0.02 respectively). Hyperactivity and frequent nighttime awakenings appeared unrelated, and there was no consistent relation between age, sleep disturbances and hyperactivity. We did not ask parents whether they viewed their child as hyperactive or distractible, so were unable to make a direct comparison between the parents' and neurologists' views.

• *Affect.* The neurological examination form had only one item dealing with affect, which did not clearly separate lack of affect from negative affect. As one would expect, the two autistic groups, especially the LAD group, were significantly more likely to have a flat affect or to be withdrawn or tearful than the other two groups.

• *Social skills.* The children's ability to interact with the examiner, the appropriateness of the interaction, and their ability to cooperate were evaluated. There were clear differences between groups (Table 6.7), with the DLD children having the lowest prevalence of deficits and those in the LAD group the highest. Virtually all the LAD children were scored as moderately (26 per cent) or severely (71 per cent) uncooperative. Social withdrawal and inappropriate social skills were considerably higher in the autistic than in the non-autistic children.

LANGUAGE AND COMMUNICATION

Professionals inexperienced at assessing the many aspects of developing child language can be taught to attend to specific dimensions of children's expressive language, as well as to their comprehension. Table 6.8 shows the dimensions of language listed on the neurological examination form, including amount of speech, its intelligibility (phonology) and fluency, whether the child made syntactic errors, had word finding difficulty, and could engage in meaningful conversation, whether the melody and rhythm of language were appropriate (prosody), and whether the child made errors often seen in

**TABLE 6.8**
**Dimensions of language scored by the neurologists**

*Expression*
- Amount of speech: either
    - (a) normal
    - (b) too little, or
    - (c) too much
- Fluency
- Melody and rhythm (prosody)
- Intelligibility (phonology)
- Sentence structure (syntax)
- Naming to confrontation (vocabulary, word retrieval)
- Communicative use (pragmatics): either
    - (a) normal
    - (b) too little initiating and responding, or
    - (c) intrusively inappropriate
- Use of facial expression and gestures to supplement speech: either
    - (a) normal
    - (b) increased to supplement inadequate speech, or
    - (c) too little in the face of inadequate speech
- Aberrant language (immediate or delayed echolalia, perseveration, pronominal reversal, referring to self by name)

*Comprehension*
- Pointing to object named
- Comprehension of simple commands
- Comprehension of 'wh–' questions

verbal autistic children such as perseveration, echolalia, and referring to self by name or as 'you'.

Children's conversation with a parent is often more representative of their skills than that with a stranger who may bombard the child with a stream of questions that elicit mostly yes/no or single word answers. The neurologists were therefore instructed to enter into the child's play and to encourage the parent(s) (or the teacher in the case of children seen with a teacher rather than a parent) to do so as well. They were to ask open-ended questions requiring higher level comprehension and formulation, such as 'why', 'who' or 'how' questions ('wh–' questions). The neurologists also asked the child to point to a series of ten standard objects that they named and to carry out single- and two-level commands.

• *Amount of language.* Results of the neurologists' assessments of the children's language are shown in Table 6.9. Formal analysis of language transcripts from the 20 minute play sessions obtained for quantitative evaluation of spontaneous language, sociability and play indicated that, overall, 8 per cent of the children were nonverbal and another 14 per cent had a vocabulary of fewer than 25 words (see Chapter 7). The neurologists agreed with the formal analyses inasmuch as they reported that 23 per cent of all the children were essentially nonverbal, including over half of the LAD children. They also re-

111

TABLE 6.9
Language abnormalities[1]

| Abnormality | N with data | Group | | | | |
|---|---|---|---|---|---|---|
| | | DLD (N=201) % | HAD (N=51) % | LAD (N=125) % | NALIQ (N=110) % | All (N=487) % |
| *Expression*[2] | | | | | | |
| Too little speech*** | 478 | 68.0 | 55.8 | 87.9 | 76.2 | 73.6 |
| [Little or no speech][2]*** | [110] | [10.1] | [5.9] | [55.3] | [17.9] | [23.0] |
| Too much speech*** | 478 | 1.5 | 25.5 | 8.1 | 3.8 | 6.3 |
| Fluency[2] | 361 | 46.7 | 27.3 | 50.0 | 44.3 | 44.3 |
| Melody + rhythm[2]*** | 347 | 17.0 | 61.4 | 63.3 | 28.9 | 32.0 |
| Intelligibility[2]* | 369 | 67.4 | 43.7 | 69.1 | 65.9 | 64.2 |
| Sentence structure[2]* | 353 | 3.1 | 66.7 | 90.2 | 81.9 | 76.8 |
| Naming[2]*** | 344 | 14.6 | 26.7 | 50.0 | 23.2 | 23.0 |
| Decreased use of speech for communication*** | 477 | 45.4 | 51.0 | 73.4 | 51.9 | 54.7 |
| Inappropriate use of speech for communication*** | 477 | 1.5 | 31.4 | 21.8 | 5.7 | 10.9 |
| Increased use of gestures to supplement speech | 443 | 17.7 | 10.6 | 22.6 | 21.4 | 19.0 |
| Decreased use of gestures to supplement speech*** | 443 | 0.5 | 6.4 | 49.1 | 9.2 | 14.7 |
| Echolalia[2]** | 368 | 10.1 | 64.6 | 80.0 | 21.2 | 32.1 |
| *Comprehension* | | | | | | |
| Pointing*** | 445 | 3.2 | 14.0 | 71.3 | 24.2 | 26.6 |
| Commands*** | 466 | 23.1 | 55.1 | 86.6 | 49.5 | 48.5 |
| Questions*** | 446 | 42.6 | 74.5 | 92.9 | 72.6 | 65.3 |

[1]The data are presented as the percentage of children in each group whom the neurologists scored as having mild–moderate or severe–profound deficits.
[2]Nonverbal children (N=37 or 7.6% of the entire sample) and those with less than 25 single words (N=73 or 15.0% of sample) are listed separately (in parentheses); they are included in the total percentage with deficits but are not included among children scored for fluency, melody and rhythm of language, intelligibility, sentence structure, naming, and echolalia.
*Significant difference among groups ($\chi^2$, p<0.05).
**Significant difference among groups ($\chi^2$, p<0.01).
***Significant difference among groups ($\chi^2$, p<0.001).

ported that fewer than a third of the LAD children used gestures (or signs) to supplement their inadequate verbal expression, as opposed to 40 per cent of nonverbal DLD children.
• *Expression.* Nonverbal children could be scored only on their use of gestures to communicate. Among autistic children, those in the LAD group were the most likely to have severely deficient speech and nonverbal communication, and those in the HAD group were least likely of all the children to be dysfluent and poorly intelligible. The HAD group also was the only one with a significant number of verbose and intrusive children. A majority of children in all groups were judged to have deficient syntax.

We examined the relation of oromotor function to intelligibility and to general motor skill, keeping in mind that there were 174 children who could not be scored on both variables, either because they spoke too little or because they were unable to cooperate with the oromotor examination. One might have anticipated that oromotor function would be related to general motor skills; surprisingly, analysis of variance disclosed no significant relationship. With regard to the relation between oromotor function and intelligibility, although this was highly significant, only half of the children with adequate oromotor skills were poorly intelligible, and only 30 per cent of those judged intelligible were reported to have impaired oromotor function. These findings suggest that programming of phonology and control of oromotor movements may be dissociable skills, at least in some children.

We sought to determine how much severe mental retardation contributed to oromotor dysfunction and overall expressive competence by dividing the entire sample into two groups, children with NVIQ equivalents <50 and 50. There was no significant relation between NVIQ equivalent and oromotor function overall, whereas of the 44 children considered to have adequate expression, 95 per cent had NVIQ equivalents >50 and 5 per cent <50, a significant and expected difference.

The naming task was included as part of the neurological examination for expressive language because children with communication disorders often have word finding deficits and small vocabularies. Unfortunately, naming the ten objects listed on the form was an insufficiently sensitive task for many children in the DLD group. This was not the case for children in the other groups: a quarter of those in the HAD and NALIQ groups and half those in the LAD group had difficulty. Provided that lack of motivation is not at fault, this finding suggests that naming deficits may be more prevalent in AD than in non-AD children.

Verbal autistic children in both the HAD and LAD groups were twice as likely as the NALIQ children and three times as likely as the DLD children to speak with aberrant prosody (pitch, rhythm and melody of speech). These observations highlight once again that high-pitched, sing-song, overprecise or wooden speech should strongly suggest that a child may be autistic.

Typically, pragmatics is more deficient in AD children than in other children with impaired communication. According to the neurologists, whereas the use of speech was decreased in half or more of the children in all groups—especially in their ability to initiate or sustain a conversation—inappropriate production of speech for communication was prevalent only in the two AD groups. A minority of children in all groups were judged to have increased their gestures to accompany and supplement speech. Children in the LAD group stood out by their failure to attempt to communicate by means of gestures; this was notable because they were the group with by far the largest proportion of nonverbal or minimally verbal children.

Although the neurologists reported that aberrant language was frequent, especially in the autistic groups, immediate echolalia seems to have been the main feature to which they were sensitive (Table 6.10). They reported delayed echolalia (the use of scripts), pronominal reversal, the child referring to himself by name, and perseveration so infrequently that no conclusion can be drawn regarding their relative prevalence in the four groups.

**TABLE 6.10**
**Aberrant language features\*\*\***

| Abnormality | Group | | | | |
|---|---|---|---|---|---|
| | DLD (N=194) % | HAD (N=44) % | LAD (N=80) % | NALIQ (N=98) % | All (N=416) % |
| None of those listed | 90.7 | 36.4 | 36.3 | 69.4 | 69.5 |
| Immediate echolalia | 9.3 | 40.9 | 52.5 | 25.5 | 24.7 |
| Delayed echolalia | 0.0 | 9.1 | 5.0 | 0.0 | 1.9 |
| Pronominal reversal | 0.0 | 0.0 | 0.0 | 0.0 | 0.0 |
| Refers to self by name | 0.0 | 4.6 | 0.0 | 1.0 | 0.7 |
| Refers to self as you | 0.0 | 0.0 | 1.2 | 0.0 | 0.2 |
| Perseverates | 0.0 | 9.1 | 5.0 | 4.1 | 2.9 |

\*\*\*Significant difference among groups ($\chi^2$, p<0.001).

**TABLE 6.11**
**Neurologists' summary impressions[1]**

| Abnormality | N with data | Group | | | | |
|---|---|---|---|---|---|---|
| | | DLD (N=201) % | HAD (N=51) % | LAD (N=125) % | NALIQ (N=110) % | All (N=487) % |
| Sensorimotor\*\*\* [moderate ; severe] | 469 | 23.9 [23.9 ; 0.0] | 11.8 [11.8 ; 0.0] | 31.4 [28.0 ; 3.4] | 47.6 [40.8 ; 6.8] | 29.6 [27.3 ; 2.3] |
| Oromotor\*\*\* [moderate ; severe] | 394 | 51.5 [46.2 ; 5.3] | 26.7 [26.7 ; 0.0] | 37.9 [21.8 ; 16.1] | 61.3 [45.2 ; 16.1] | 48.0 [38.3 ; 9.6] |
| Expressive language\*\*\* [moderate ; severe] | 469 | 88.3 [56.6 ; 31.6] | 86.3 [56.9 ; 29.4] | 96.7 [17.5 ; 79.2] | 90.2 [52.9 ; 37.3] | 90.6 [45.8 ; 44.8] |
| Receptive language\*\*\* [moderate ; severe] | 457 | 38.6 [31.7 ; 6.9] | 70.6 [52.9 ; 17.7] | 93.1 [30.2 ; 62.9] | 64.4 [50.5 ; 13.9] | 61.7 [37.9 ; 23.8] |
| Cognition\*\*\* [moderate ; severe] | 435 | 7.9 [7.9 ; 0.0] | 15.7 [15.7 ; 0.0] | 64.4 [35.7 ; 28.6] | 69.5 [60.0 ; 9.5] | 34.9 [26.4 ; 8.5] |
| Autistic behaviors\*\*\* [moderate ; severe] | 473 | 4.0 [4.0 ; 0.0] | 75.5 [52.9 ; 21.6] | 90.8 [40.8 ; 50.0] | 22.1 [20.2 ; 1.9] | 37.6 [22.2 ; 15.4] |

[1]Percentage of children in group scored as having mild–moderate and severe–profound deficit.
\*\*\*Significant difference among groups ($\chi^2$, p<0.001).

In summary, a decreased amount of language, which was poorly intelligible and syntactically incorrect, was prevalent in all groups. Oromotor skill and intelligibility were often dissociated. Autistic children had impaired prosody and communicative use of language and were more likely to be echolalic and to produce aberrant language than those in the non-autistic groups. The HAD children were least likely to be unintelligible and dysfluent; in fact a quarter of them were stated to be verbose chatterboxes, and a third seemed to chatter in order to speak rather than to communicate. HAD children had more difficulty naming than did DLD children.

• *Comprehension.* Like the naming of ten objects to assess word-finding and vocabulary, pointing to ten items turned out to be an inadequately sensitive way to assess comprehension (Table 6.9). Only the two LIQ groups had significant numbers of children (71 per cent among the LAD and 24 per cent among the NALIQ) who had difficulty with the task. In general, neurologists reported that children had more difficulty answering 'wh–' questions than following commands. This finding is hardly surprising because obeying commands does not require a verbal response. The open-ended 'wh–' questions the neurologists were instructed to ask not only required a verbal answer but are the last to be acquired in normal language development (Brown 1973). The DLD group was the least impaired on both these measures, although almost half had difficulty responding to 'wh–' questions. Children in the LAD group were severely impaired in all three gauges of comprehension; in fact, only 7 per cent were judged able to answer questions.

The problem of determining how much of the communication disorder of the LAD children was due to a specific language disorder and how much to their lack of co-operation and negativistic behavior remains unanswered. Furthermore, mental retardation contributed as well, judging from the large number of children in the NALIQ group whose comprehension was deficient. What is noteworthy is that of the children in the HAD group, 93 per cent of whom were at least somewhat verbal and a quarter of whom were reported to be fluent, verbose, and to have adequate syntax, over half obeyed commands inadequately, and three quarters were impaired for understanding 'wh–' questions.

SUMMARY IMPRESSIONS

The neurologists' scores on each of the 120 items of the examination represented their view of every area of the child's function. The form also asked them to provide summary statements representing their overall impression of the child along the six dimensions listed in Table 6.11. They were to decide whether, overall, they considered the child normal or near normal, mildly to moderately impaired, or severely to profoundly impaired. They were told they were not required to score as abnormal children whom they had scored as abnormal in one or another of the items of the detailed examination if their overall impression was that the abnormality was trivial. Thus their overall impression tended toward leniency. The form gave the neurologists no opportunity to score No Data for their summary impressions. For the most part they acceded to this injunction, except for the oromotor item where they failed to provide a score for 93 children (30 per cent of the children in the LAD group, 12–16 per cent in the other three groups). The neurologists, quite appropriately, were unwilling to score oromotor function in children who had not cooperated with the test. They also failed to score 52 children (11 per cent of the sample) for cognitive competence, presumably because they were undecided.

Despite the *a priori* exclusion of children with 'hard' neurological findings, 30 per cent of the children were judged to have a sensorimotor deficit, overwhelmingly of a mild–moderate severity, mostly apraxia. Oromotor deficits were reported in 48 per cent of the children (not counting the 19 per cent without a score). The HAD group was least likely to have children with sensorimotor or oromotor deficits.

115

Neurologists's impressions were not always consistent with the formal diagnoses assigned to the children: they considered 8 per cent of DLD and 16 per cent of HAD children to have mild mental retardation, and 4 per cent of DLD and 22 per cent of NALIQ children to be on the autistic spectrum. The neurologists were undecided about cognitive ability in 11 per cent of the children, half of them in the AD group. They did not detect intellectual subnormality in 36 per cent of LAD and 31 per cent of NALIQ children. Thus they were more likely to overlook mental retardation than to overdiagnose it. These findings highlight the importance of supplementing the qualitative assessment of higher cognitive functions made by a neurologist in the office with quantitative evaluations based on standardized tests, even when the neurologist, as was the case in this study, is forced to examine a child with a standard and relatively detailed examination.

**Discussion**

As stated in the introduction to this chapter, the purpose of the general examination was to look for clues regarding etiology, and the two main purposes of the neurological examination were to define the extent and type of neurological dysfunction and, hopefully, to gain some insight as to what parts of the nervous system might be dysfunctional.

*Etiology*

The physical examination turned out to provide essentially no help for establishing an etiological diagnosis. This lack of sensitivity was in part a consequence of the deliberate exclusion of children with diseases associated with autism and learning disabilities, for example neurofibromatosis and tuberous sclerosis, and of children with overt motor deficits and known structural brain lesions.

Many findings in our study are similar to those in the Collaborative Perinatal Project (CPP) (Broman *et al.* 1987). In the CPP, both major and minor malformations were more prevalent in the mentally retarded groups, and more prevalent in the severely retarded children than in those whose IQ fell between 50 and 69. Even borderline children, with IQs between 70 and 89, tended to have significantly more malformations than the children with average (90–119) and above average (≥120) IQs. In the CPP, mean head circumference at birth and at 7 years was significantly correlated with cognitive outcome at 7 years. In the present study, a small head circumference was not necessarily characteristic of LIQ: although prevalent in the NALIQ group it was not so in the LAD group in which the mean NVIQ was lower; furthermore, there was a trend for the prevalence of enlarged head circumferences to be highest in the HAD group. These findings raise the possibility of a distinct biological basis for AD, distinct from LIQ without autistic features.

Given that one has selected children without overt brain lesions or clear diagnoses, the etiology of the developmental disorders is generally unknown, with genetics probably playing a significant part (Rapin 1994). Among 82 children in a British school for severely language disordered children, Robinson (1987) reported that nine (11 per cent) had prenatal etiologies (three each having a chromosome abnormality, a cleft palate or a diagnosable syndrome), 4 per cent had a history of a perinatal problem, and 12 per cent had an acquired, presumably causal abnormality, half of them the Laudau–Kleffner syndrome (Landau and Kleffner 1957, Rapin *et al.* 1977, Deonna 1991), an epileptic disorder associated with loss of language whose etiology is unknown. Robinson found that 40 per cent of the children had a family member with a history of delayed language acquisition, in 28 per cent of cases an affected sibling, figures only slightly higher than the 23 per cent of affected siblings reported in our study (see Chapter 5).

As for autism, Steffenburg (1991) reviewed the presumed etiologies in all 35 cases of autism and 17 of 'autistic-like' conditions in Göteborg, Sweden and its surrounding county. She reported that, with exhaustive review of all medical records and tests, she had identified signs of neurological dysfunction in 81 per cent of children with autism of unknown etiology and 93 per cent of those with known syndromes. This high figure reflects in part the inclusion of cases with deafness, fragile X syndrome, tuberous sclerosis and known structural brain lesions that were excluded from our study. Both the Robinson and the Steffenburg studies support genetic etiology in a sizeable proportion of children with DLD and AD (see also Pennington and Smith 1983, Folstein and Piven 1991, Cardon *et al.* 1994, Piven and Folstein 1994).

*Value of the neurological examination*
The purpose of the neurological examination in evaluating children with developmental disorders of brain function is to detect the presence and assess the medical significance of so-called 'soft signs' such as minor anomalies, unusual facial features and mild sensorimotor deficits. Another role is to exclude unexpected 'hard' findings (which constituted *a priori* exclusionary criteria for this study) that might point to an overt structural anatomic lesion or to progressive brain pathology. The mental status examination used in this study provided a clinical check on the findings obtained by formal tests of language and cognition and the opportunity to examine in a standard clinical way a large cohort of young children with well documented developmental conditions.

In the present study, the neurological examination identified a number of abnormalities, especially in the motor and mental status parts of the evaluation, but it did little to indicate what parts of the nervous system were dysfunctional. As might be expected, LIQ children with and without autistic features, whose intellectual subnormality is likely to signal more pervasive brain pathology than that of non-LIQ children with more circumscribed developmental problems, had the higher prevalence of abnormalities such as microcephaly, deficits in gross and fine motor coordination and oromotor skills, and abnormalities of mental status. A notable finding was the lack of microcephaly, presumed to reflect inadequate brain growth or an exogenous insult to the immature brain, in DLD and in autism. The finding of macrocephaly in a proportion of AD, particularly HAD, children is a strong argument against 'brain damage' as an important etiology for autism, at least in children selected not to have overt evidence for structural or metabolic brain lesions. This finding is not unique to this sample (Bailey *et al.* 1993), but here head size differences had imaging correlates (Filipek *et al.* 1992) that suggest atypical brain development, possibly with lack of the normal pruning of redundant cells or connections that marks optimal maturation of the nervous system (Rosen *et al.* 1990).

In the CPP, minor neurological abnormalities on examination at 7 years were 15–20 times more prevalent in the severely retarded group, and five times more prevalent in the mildly retarded group, than in the average group. These figures are higher than those in the present study which excluded children with 'hard' neurological signs such as cerebral palsy. The CPP found even more dramatic differences in the prevalence of dyskinesia and ataxia in these same groups. The CPP does not provide data on oromotor function such as drooling, which was a prevalent motor deficit in our sample.

MOTOR ABNORMALITIES

Turning first to the motor abnormalities, this study highlighted three that deserve much closer scrutiny, especially in autistic children, than they have so far been given. These are hypotonia, stereotypy and apraxia.

Hypotonia is well known in Down syndrome, and the nine children with Down syndrome in the NALIQ group may have contributed to the high prevalence of hypotonia in that group. Whether in Down syndrome it reflects a collagen abnormality resulting in hyperlaxity of joints and muscles or it has a neurological basis is not known. There is no evidence for anterior cell or peripheral nerve abnormality in Down syndrome or in those children with obvious central nervous system abnormalities who are labelled as having hypotonic cerebral palsy. Hypotonia is a classic sign of cerebellar dysfunction or dysgenesis. The cause of hypotonia in children without classic cerebellar signs or evidence of cerebellar dysgenesis or disease but with clear signs of cerebral dysfunction is not understood. Whether in autism hypotonia is a non-specific finding or it is related to reported pathological (Bauman 1992a, Bauman and Kemper 1994) and MRI (Courchesne 1991, Courchesne et al. 1994) evidence of cerebellar pathology remains to be determined.

Stereotypies are often referred to as self-stimulation, which is conjectural, or they are attributed to many autistic children's high level of anxiety, which is also conjectural. The thought that stereotypies may represent a movement disorder, presumably of basal ganglia origin and involving dopaminergic pathways, has been given very little consideration even though stereotypies may respond to some of the same medications as tics. There were a few children in this study in whom stereotypies were not easily distinguished from tics; the hypothesis that Tourette syndrome and AD may be related genetically has been proposed recently (Comings and Comings 1991, Sverd 1991). In older autistic persons who have been on psychotropic drugs, the differential diagnosis between stereotypies and akithesia and tardive dyskinesia may also pose serious difficulty (Meiselas et al. 1989). Inasmuch as stereotypies may persist in AD into adulthood, albeit often in miniaturized form in high-functioning autistic persons, further study of these abnormal movements and their neurological basis is in order (Bauman 1992b). There is also a need to study the relation of self-injurious behaviors, perseveration and stereotypy, all of which are common in AD and suggest involvement of striatal and limbic circuits.

Apraxia, the inability to imitate movements or program complex motor acts despite willingness to cooperate, adequate attention and intelligence, ability to understand commands, and lack of weakness, spasticity or abnormal movements suggests left parietal,

118

mesial frontal or prefrontal deficit in adults with acquired brain lesions (Watson *et al*. 1992). Inability to imitate gestures is notorious in autism (DeMyer *et al*. 1972, Bartak *et al*. 1975). Ascribing lack of imitation entirely to apraxia in severely affected LAD children is hazardous because of their multiple disabilities. Yet the neurologists reported that both moderate and severe apraxia were much more common in the LAD than in the NALIQ group and that moderate apraxia was almost twice as prevalent in the children with HAD than DLD.

There is a resurgence of interest in apraxia in nonverbal autistic persons in whom it has been blamed for inability to communicate using a communication board or keyboard without the help of another person acting as a 'facilitator' (Biklen 1990). Although this claim has now been virtually disproved (*e.g.* Cummins and Prior 1992, Eberlin *et al*. 1993), it does highlight the need for a more rigorous evaluation of apraxia in autism.

MENTAL STATUS

Assessment of mental status is an integral part of the neurological examination and therefore neurologists in the present study were required to rate children's behavior, language and play. The CPP, in which fully 18 per cent of the severely mentally retarded children could not be tested reliably with formal IQ measures, relied on ratings of behavior during testing sessions to assess cognition and personality. The behaviors rated in the CPP were more numerous but quite similar to those in this study. They included fearfulness, verbal communication, attention span, dependency, assertiveness, self-confidence, activity level, impulsivity, separation anxiety, frustration tolerance, goal orientation, hostility, emotionality and atypical staring. All were highly correlated with IQ.

In the CPP, summary ratings of behavior were the largest and most consistent discriminators between severely mentally retarded children and all other groups. Behavior was rated as severely impaired in three quarters of the severely retarded group and in one quarter of the mildly retarded group. Language age was below 3 years at 7 years in the severely retarded children, but their mean score for free drawing of a human figure was 60, suggesting that language was more severely impaired than nonverbal skills in that group. [All IQ measures used as criteria in the CPP were Full Scale (Wechsler Intelligence Scales for Children—WISC) IQs; separate Verbal and Performance IQs were not provided. Many of the severely retarded group were untestable with the WISC.] The most discriminating variables between the mildly retarded and non-retarded groups were short attention span, poor goal orientation and decreased verbal communication. These findings in the CPP suggest that at least some of their severely retarded children may have fulfilled criteria for LAD in the present study and some of the borderline children may have had language disorders.

The CPP 7 year examinations were carried out in the mid- to late 1960s and early '70s, a time when autism was still widely considered a psychiatric disorder. Autism is not mentioned as such, but it is noteworthy that 7 per cent of severely retarded White children had a 'history of treatment for mental illness' (Broman *et al*. 1987), a feature reported in less than 1 per cent of the mildly retarded group, 1 per cent of the borderline group, and 0.5 per cent of the average and above average groups. Among Blacks less than 1 per cent of all groups had been treated for mental illness, perhaps reflecting access to care rather than severity of morbidity.

## Summary of data from the neurological examination

### Mental status

The mental status findings were, by and large, consonant with clinical features found in the literature: a high proportion of children in all groups were judged to have too little speech, impaired production of syntax, and at least mildly impaired language comprehension. Specific to autism, but not retardation, were deficient representational play, flat or depressed mood, inappropriate or uncooperative social behavior, poor melody of speech, and echolalia. Occurring primarily in the HAD children were too much speech and normal language fluency.

On the mental status examination, most children in both autistic groups (especially the LAD children) were judged deficient in representational play; the NALIQ children were intermediate, and few of the DLD children were judged deficient. Few children showed hypoactivity; this was most prevalent in the LAD children. Many more children were judged hyperactive and distractible; this was most prevalent in the LAD group and least prevalent in the DLD group. The two autistic groups were most likely, and the DLD group least likely, to show depressed or flat affect. Uncooperative, withdrawn or inappropriate social behavior was most marked in the two autistic groups, especially the LAD children.

Neurologists rated the children on several aspects of language. About half the LAD children, and a quarter of the NALIQ children, had little or no speech, but a majority of even the HAD and DLD children were rated as having too little speech. Only the HAD group had a significant number of children rated as having too much speech. A majority of children in all groups were judged to have deficient syntax, and half or more of the children in all groups, except the HAD, were judged to have poor fluency and intelligibility. In contrast, echolalia and impaired melody and rhythm of speech were most marked in the two autistic groups. Severely impaired comprehension was characteristic of both autism and LIQ (only the DLD children had low rates of severely impaired comprehension). Many children in all groups had difficulty answering 'wh–' questions or following commands; the two autistic groups were most impaired, and the DLD children least impaired, in these areas.

The neurologists' summary impressions were in generally good agreement with data from other sources related to autistic behavior and language. The main inconsistency in the overall impressions was the under-detection of intellectual subnormality in about a third of the LIQ children, and failure to detect autism in a quarter of HAD children. The neurologists also rated almost a quarter of the NALIQ children as having autistic behaviors.

### Physical and sensorimotor examination

In this study, twice as many children as would be expected by chance had head sizes larger than the 98th centile or smaller than the 2nd centile. The small head sizes occurred most often in the NALIQ children and there was a trend for large heads in the HAD group. Sensory testing was difficult, but when it could be done, sensory abnormalities were rare, as was dysfunction of cranial nerves, oromotor dysfunction excepted.

The two LIQ groups (NALIQ and LAD) showed most impaired gross and fine motor skills, even with NVIQ covaried. No significant difference in right/left motor skill was observed. A negligible number of children showed mild spasticity, weakness, dystonia, rigidity and tics; most of these were in the two LIQ groups. Occurring more frequently were hypotonia, lowest in the DLD group, and limb apraxia (highest in the two LIQ groups, and almost twice as frequent in HAD as in DLD children), and stereotypies (much more prevalent in the two autistic groups, especially the LAD group, uncommon in the NALIQ and DLD groups). On measures of oromotor function, again almost all the children in the two LIQ groups had severe deficits, and a significant number, especially in the LAD group, were untestable; but mild to moderate deficits were very common in the DLD group and somewhat common in the HAD group.

Most important is the fact that the sensorimotor neurological examination did not point to specific sites or sides of dysfunction for children in the different clinical groups, with the possible exception of the basal ganglia in the genesis of stereotypies, and perhaps the cerebellum in the genesis of hypotonia, both of which were most prevalent in the autistic sample.

**Clinical implications of findings**
Together, the CPP and the present study indicate that the role of the physician is important but limited for making a specific diagnosis in preschool children with developmental disorders of higher cerebral function without obvious cause or evidence of gross brain pathology. Even a detailed medical and neurological evaluation is likely to add limited data to the child's evaluation. When dealing with the developmental disorders of brain function, it is the history and the results of age-appropriate standardized psychological and language tests and behavioral questionnaires that are most likely to be informative (Brunquell *et al.* 1991). Yet, clinical evaluation of the mental status, including play, contributes an important and independent check on the results of these tests. The yield of EEGs, especially if obtained during sleep, for localizing brain dysfunction in DLD and AD may be somewhat higher than usually appreciated, even in the absence of clinical seizures (Tuchman *et al.* 1991*a,b*; Echenne *et al.* 1992). Neuroimaging studies rarely contribute etiological information in the absence of physical or sensorimotor neurological findings but, ultimately, they may provide critical information on the neurological basis of the developmental disorders of brain function (Filipek *et al.* 1992).

Evaluation of the medical and genetic history and findings on examination of the child guide the physician's choice of ancillary tests such as neuroimaging, electrophysiological and newer genetic tests. Such tests are unlikely to alter the prescription for habilitation of the child but they may be essential for excluding a treatable condition, for example hypothyroidism, and for detecting a condition with genetic implications like fragile X syndrome. It will remain the physician's role to interpret the biological implications of the findings, subtle or not, from the aggregate of the investigations so as to provide the parents with the assurance that no biological cause requiring medical intervention, including psychopharmacological medication, has been overlooked.

The classic neurological examination is of course important, especially for ruling out unsuspected evidence for a structural brain lesion or specific systemic condition, but its contribution to the diagnosis of developmental disorders is modest. It is the mental status that is most informative and supplements historical information and data derived from quantitative neuropsychological tests. Physicians' clinical assessment of language and communicative skill supplements the test data because it focuses on behavior and communication in a naturalistic setting, provided it is systematic. Evaluation of comprehension is inferential inasmuch as it depends entirely on what the child does or says in response to a verbal request or a question: a child who does not carry out a command or respond to a question or a comment may be inattentive or oppositional, or lack motivation or comprehension. Physicians can judge whether children produce only single words or grammatically correct sentences (syntax), whether they are intelligible (phonology) and can name objects they are shown (word retrieval, richness of the vocabulary), and whether they can enter into a meaningful conversation (pragmatics), initiating as well as responding, staying on topic, and using language to request and comment rather than speaking to themselves without regard to their conversational partner. In addition, observers can attend to abnormalities like echolalia and perseveration that characterize the language of verbal autistic children. Our results do suggest that formal testing is often a necessary supplement to the neurologist's office evaluation to detect mild to moderate (and sometimes even severe) degrees of intellectual deficit.

# 7
# LANGUAGE AND
# NEUROPSYCHOLOGICAL FINDINGS

*D. Fein, M. Dunn, D.A. Allen, D.M. Aram, N. Hall, R. Morris and B.C. Wilson\**

The importance of defining language and neuropsychological functions in autism and DLDs is clear, yet there is little agreement on the extent to which they can be used to differentiate the two sets of disorders. Among the key questions addressed by our project were: What are the typical linguistic and cognitive profiles found within each of the four groups? Are there particular profiles that suggest membership in a particular diagnostic group? Do the data suggest one or more key language or neuropsychological deficits for either diagnostic group or for a significant number of individuals within a diagnostic group? Is the underlying factor structure of cognitive and linguistic abilities similar in the AD, DLD and NALIQ groups, or do different relationships among cognitive functions exist within the groups? Finally, for the children with significant behavioral impairments, are there specific cognitive impairments that are highly correlated with specific behavioral abnormalities and is there a correlation between severity of cognitive impairment and severity of behavioral disorder, or are the two domains largely independent? This chapter will present results relevant to the questions concerning characteristic group profiles; results pertaining to individual differences, within-group variability and the relationship between behavior and cognition will be presented in later papers.

Much is known about aspects of cognition and language in DLD and AD but there have been few direct comparisons (for examples, see Lincoln *et al.* 1988, Cantwell *et al.* 1989). In past efforts to elucidate cognitive patterns and key deficits, cognitive functioning has largely been explored separately and with different approaches in AD and DLD children. The differential diagnosis between DLD and AD, especially HAD, is often difficult, particularly in preschool children. Documenting similarities and differences, as well as specific variables or cognitive and linguistic patterns that optimally differentiate the groups, is an essential need which this study attempts to fill.

Findings include descriptive statistics for all measures across the four groups of children (DLD, HAD, LAD, NALIQ); results also include factor structure of the battery for the entire sample and for each of the four groups.

**Method**
Measures discussed in this chapter have been described in Chapter 4 and listed in Table 4.19 (pp. 46–47).

*D. Fein and M. Dunn assumed major responsibility for this chapter; other participating investigators are listed alphabetically.

**Findings**

The results are presented in three sections. The first two sections contrast data from the four groups in the study (DLD, HAD, LAD, NALIQ). These data are presented by area of language and cognitive function. Key variables within each domain of function were selected based on their theoretical interest and adequate reliability for all groups. Group means and significant differences will be presented in tables and figures and discussed in the text; non-significant differences and changes in significance with covariation of age, SES and NVIQ will be discussed in the text.

Inasmuch as the DLD and HAD groups are well matched for NVIQ, and the use of standard scores takes chronological age (CA) into account, covarying age, SES and NVIQ generally did not affect the significance of differences between the HAD and DLD groups, and in most cases will not be reported here. Where covariation changed differences between the LAD and the NALIQ groups, who differ somewhat in NVIQ, they are presented.

The last section will present the results of several factor analyses, showing the structure of the cognitive battery for the total sample, and within each group of children.

*Group differences in verbal functions*

Following are results of major language variables studied in all groups. The language test results presented below address the groups' functioning on composite language tests, receptive language tests and expressive language tests, followed by a summary of the overall findings for the four groups. In reviewing the results of language tests and analyses of the children's spontaneous language, one needs to remember that 8 per cent of the DLD, 4 per cent of the HAD, 53 per cent of the LAD, and 24 per cent of the NALIQ groups were nonverbal or essentially nonverbal. The fact that the children with the poorest expressive language were not included must be kept in mind when interpreting comparisons among the groups as they comprise different numbers of children, depending on the task: deficits will be minimized in groups encompassing many nonverbal or untestable children.

STANDARDIZED LANGUAGE MEASURES

• *Composite language tests*. Three composite language measures were administered to all four groups: the Test of Early Language Development (TELD), the Verbal Reasoning domain subtests of the Stanford–Binet (S-B), and the Communication domain of the Vineland*. Mean scores for each of these measures across the four groups are presented in Table 7.1 and Figure 7.1. Figure 7.1 shows that, in general, the DLD group scored the highest, followed in order by the HAD, NALIQ and LAD groups. The profiles of the DLD and NALIQ groups were essentially flat and parallel, with the NALIQ group achieving lower scores than the DLD group, as one might anticipate given their NVIQ differences. The HAD group and the (testable children in the) LAD group were parallel

*See Chapter 4 for a discussion of floor effects and of the use of the Sequenced Inventory of Communicative Development and Bayley Scales of Infant Development in very low-functioning LAD and NALIQ children.

124

# TABLE 7.1
## Verbal scores by group

| Task[1] | Group | | | | | | | F | p[2] | Significant group contrasts |
|---|---|---|---|---|---|---|---|---|---|---|
| | DLD | | HAD | | LAD | | NALIQ | | | |
| | Mean (SD) | | Mean (SD) | | Mean (SD) | | Mean (SD) | | | |
| Test of Eearly Language Development (SS: Mean=100, SD=16) | 79.26 (13.59) (N=201) | | 70.55 (13.74) (N=51) | | 61.88 (7.01) (N=125) | | 65.45 (9.95) (N=110) | 23.88 | 0.0001 | DLD=HAD>NALIQ>LAD |
| Stanford–Binet Verbal Reasoning Area (SS: Mean=100, SD=16) | 91.07 (12.96) (N=201) | | 77.94 (17.63) (N=51) | | 45.18 (15.90) (N=125) | | 60.09 (21.94) (N=110) | 217.73 | 0.0001 | DLD>HAD>NALIQ>LAD |
| Stanford–Binet Vocabulary (SS: Mean=50, SD=8) | 44.57 (8.54) (N=201) | | 40.39 (9.07) (N=51) | | 27.60 (5.97) (N=125) | | 32.89 (9.02) (N=110) | 125.44 | 0.0001 | DLD>HAD>NALIQ>LAD |
| Stanford–Binet Comprehension (SS: Mean=50, SD=8) | 45.39 (6.30) (N=201) | | 37.02 (7.65) (N=51) | | 27.99 (4.78) (N=125) | | 33.23 (7.96) (N=110) | 201.51 | 0.0001 | DLD>HAD>NALIQ>LAD |
| Stanford–Binet Absurdities (SS: Mean=50, SD=8) | 43.98 (10.13) (N=201) | | 34.96 (9.44) (N=51) | | 27.92 (4.26) (N=125) | | 31.66 (7.74) (N=110) | 110.01 | 0.0001 | DLD>HAD>NALIQ>LAD |
| Peabody Picture Vocabulary Test (SS: Mean=100, SD=16) | 86.09 (18.09) (N=199) | | 72.20 (19.43) (N=49) | | 46.32 (14.11) (N=118) | | 61.18 (19.15) (N=101) | 132.80 | 0.0001 | DLD>HAD>NALIQ>LAD |
| Expressive One-Word Picture Vocabulary Test (SS: Mean=100, SD=16) | 87.46 (19.94) (N=199) | | 88.84 (19.68) (N=49) | | 60.72 (14.56) (N=117) | | 70.48 (17.29) (N=104) | 61.44 | 0.0001 | DLD=HAD>NALIQ>LAD |
| McCarthy Verbal Fluency (SS: Mean=100, SD=16) | 86.62 (20.63) (N=167) | | 60.56 (14.95) (N=27) | | At basal (N=66) | | 69.60 (16.97) (N=63) | 55.78 | 0.0001 | DLD>NALIQ>HAD=LAD |
| Vineland Communication Domain (SS: Mean=100, SD=16) | 78.90 (12.15) (N=197) | | 79.70 (20.39) (N=50) | | 52.70 (13.32) (N=125) | | 63.29 (12.16) (N=103) | 111.88 | 0.0001 | DLD=HAD>NALIQ>LAD |

[1]SS = standard score.
[2]Least square means ANOVA without covariates.

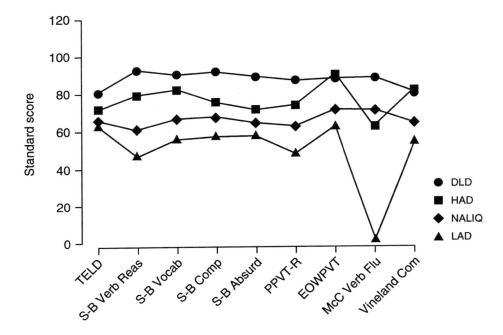

**Fig. 7.1.** Verbal scores by group.

The verbal tasks ranked the groups according to their mean NVIQ and dichotomized along AD/non-AD dimensions, with the AD lower than their NVIQ comparison groups. A salient finding was that both autistic groups had selective impairment for Verbal Fluency on the McCarthy and relative strength on the Expressive One-Word Picture Vocabulary Test (EOWPVT).

TELD = Test of Early Language Development; S-B = Stanford–Binet; Verb Reas = Verbal Reasoning; Vocab = Vocabulary; Comp = Comprehension; Absurd = Absurdities; PPVT-R = Peabody Picture Vocabulary Test—Revised; McC Verb Flu = McCarthy Verbal Fluency; Vineland Com = Vineland Composite.

to each other and again ranked by their NVIQs, but their profiles were markedly different from those of the non-autistic groups: both had a small peak on the Expressive One-Word Picture Vocabulary Test (EOWPVT) and a large dip on the McCarthy Verbal Fluency test (word retrieval) where the LAD group was at basal. Thus the verbal tasks dichotomized the autistic from the non-autistic children. The autistic groups also obtained lower scores than their comparison groups.

Looking more closely at the TELD results in Table 7.1, whereas the difference between the DLD and HAD unadjusted means did not reach significance, covariation for age, SES and NVIQ made this difference significant. The unadjusted mean of the NALIQ group was significantly higher than that of the LAD group, even after covariation.

Figure 7.1 indicates that the overall Verbal Reasoning area scores from the S-B discriminate more strongly between the four groups than the TELD but maintain the same rank order; this is reflected by significant differences among three out of four clinical groups (Table 7.1). Covariation does not change the pattern of significant differences; the NALIQ children remain higher scoring than the LAD children. On the S-B verbal subtests of Vocabulary, Comprehension and Absurdities, the DLD children are less than 1 SD below normal, while the HAD children are between 1 and 2 SD below normal, with the lowest performance in explaining pictured absurdities. Overall, on these measures of verbal reasoning which require both receptive and expressive linguistic skills and the production of connected discourse, the DLD children as a group are only minimally impaired, as compared to the HAD children who are significantly impaired but score significantly better than the NALIQ children, who in turn score better than the LAD children.

The third composite measure of overall language functioning, the Communication domain of the Vineland, involves parents' evaluation of their child's level of communication in the areas of receptive, expressive and written language. The DLD and HAD groups did not differ significantly; both were higher than the NALIQ group, who were higher than the LAD group; covariation did not change these results. An explanation for the unexpected lack of significant differences between the DLD and HAD groups may be found in examination of the subdomain scores in Receptive, Expressive and Written Communication discussed below.

• *Receptive language functioning.* Since standard scores are not available for subdomains of the Vineland, to obtain an index of receptive functioning on the Communication subdomains, receptive mental age (MA) equivalents were divided by the CA for each child. Group means were: DLD = 84, HAD = 73, LAD = 36, NALIQ = 62. An alternative approach for analyzing the subdomain scores was to covary the raw scores for NVIQ as well as for age. This revealed that the NALIQ children were most competent, followed by the DLD children, followed by the HAD children, followed by the LAD children, with all groups significantly different from each other.

An additional measure of receptive language abilities, the Peabody Picture Vocabulary Test—Revised (PPVT-R), a test of comprehension of single word vocabulary, was administered to all subjects. The means, presented in Table 7.1, revealed that the DLD children scored almost 1 SD below the normative mean, but significantly higher than the HAD children, followed by the NALIQ and LAD children, with all the groups significantly different from one another. Covariation did not change the pattern of results; LAD children remained lower than the NALIQ children. Both autistic groups, therefore, were deficient relative to their comparison groups. The PPVT-R standard scores were very similar to the MA/CA ratios on the Vineland Receptive subdomain (see Table 7.1), suggesting that functional use of receptive skill is closely related to single word receptive competence for all groups.

• *Expressive language tests.* On the Expressive subdomain of the Vineland, the MA/CA ratios were: DLD = 69; HAD = 65; LAD = 32; NALIQ = 47. These were all lower than the Receptive ratios, suggesting that, according to parental report, the functional use of expressive language is more impaired than that of receptive language. Covariation of NVIQ and age on analysis of raw scores indicated that the NALIQ, HAD and DLD children were not significantly different from one another, and that all were more competent than the LAD children.

The EOWPVT was administered to all groups as a second expressive language measure. In contrast to receptive vocabulary, as measured by the PPVT-R, the DLD and HAD children did not differ on single word expressive vocabulary skills (Table 7.1, Fig. 7.1); both groups were almost 1 SD below average, and both were higher than the NALIQ children, who were higher than the LAD children. Covarying by age, SES and NVIQ raised the NALIQ children to the level of the DLD and HAD groups, but the LAD children remained lower than the other groups. The relative standing of the groups on EOWPVT was identical to that on the Expressive subdomain of the Vineland, but scores were higher than on the Vineland, suggesting that functional use of expressive capacity is more impaired than expressive naming skills.

On the McCarthy Verbal Fluency subtest, few of the LAD children were able to perform the task and the others were assigned a score of 0.1. A substantial difference is observed between the DLD children (86.62) and the HAD children (60.56); even the NALIQ children (69.60) were significantly higher than the HAD children (see Table 7.1 and Fig. 7.1). This measure of rapid categorical word retrieval, therefore, represents an area of mild dysfunction for the DLD children and an area of severe dysfunction for the HAD and LAD children.

• *Between-test comparisons.* The relationship between Receptive Lexical (PPVT-R) and Expressive Lexical (EOWPVT) is notable. The DLD children achieved equivalent scores on the two tests, and the NALIQ children had a 9 point higher standard score on Expressive Vocabulary. The autistic groups, on the other hand, had greater discrepancies, with the HAD children exhibiting a mean Expressive Vocabulary standard score 17 points higher than Receptive, and the LAD children showing a mean Expressive standard score 14 points higher than their Receptive mean.

The relative performance of the DLD and HAD groups on the Vineland Written Communication subdomain appears to explain the lack of difference between the two groups on the composite score of the Vineland Communication domain. On the Written Communication subdomain, the deficit of the autistic children relative to the DLD children on the Receptive subdomain was reversed (raw scores: DLD = 1.90, HAD = 8.12, LAD = 1.62, NALIQ = 0.94). With and without covariation, the HAD group was superior to the other three groups; the very low scores of the other three groups made comparisons among them questionable. The MA/CA ratio for this subdomain was DLD = 69 and HAD = 91; the LAD and NALIQ scores were too low to be meaningful. These findings suggest that the HAD children are age-normal in regard to written language and show superior written to spoken communication skills. The findings for the DLD group point to significant impairment in letter skills, although many of the children in this group were not yet in school and the findings may thus reflect lack of experience. Hence, the lack of difference between the DLD and HAD groups on the overall Vineland Communication domain appears to be attributable to the superiority of the DLD children in receptive language, in combination with the superiority of the HAD children in written language.

Overall, the results of comparisons among the four groups on selected standardized measures of language suggested that, as a group, the DLD children showed relatively even deficits across both receptive and expressive skills, with all scores falling slightly less than 1 SD below norms; functional expressive language and written language skills may show more significant impairment. HAD children, in contrast, demonstrated a more uneven pattern on standardized measures of language, with strengths in written language and confrontation naming and deficits (relative to their own skills and relative to the DLD children) in language comprehension, formulated output of connected speech, verbal reasoning and rapid naming within a category. The NALIQ children exhibited an even pattern of language skills, with most standard scores falling within the 60–65 range. The LAD children were lower than the NALIQ children on every language measure, even when NVIQ and age were covaried. Given the floor effect, it is difficult to detect a pattern among their consistently low scores.

SPONTANEOUS LANGUAGE ANALYSIS

Analysis of the spontaneous language sample derived from the videotaped play session with an adult described in Chapter 9 provided data that could not be obtained through formal language measures. This included assessment of a child's conversational abilities, and errors committed when the child was engaged in interpersonal discourse (see Chapter 4 for details of the procedures and measures used). Several key variables, presented here, were analyzed for differences between the four clinical groups and a normal control group[1]. Tables 7.2, 7.3 and 7.4 present the results of these intergroup comparisons among verbal children[2]. Results of covarying age and SES were examined for these five groups; as with the other language and neuropsychological data, differences between the four clinical groups were also examined after additional covariation of NVIQ.

*Children's discourse functions* from the pragmatic analysis were rated, using the system described in Appendix 4.1. Table 7.2 shows the percentage of utterances in which the child assumed the discourse role of initiation, topic continuation, responding and immediate repetition (echoing) of the prior utterance (of either self or adult). There was no significant group difference in the percentage of utterances in which the children initiated a conversation with the adult during play. The numbers were low for all groups, suggesting either a reluctance of all children to initiate a conversation with the adult in this setting, or involvement in ongoing play and conversation that precluded initiating new conversations; different factors may have been operating in the different groups. Covarying age and SES for the five groups and NVIQ for the four clinical groups brought out no group differences.

The LAD group produced significantly fewer continuations of a previous topic than children in the other groups; no other difference was significant. When age and SES

---

[1]The provision of a group of normally developing children was required for comparisons of the conversational language and play of the four *a priori* groups inasmuch as there are no standardized norms for these skills in preschool children.

[2]It is important to keep in mind that 8 per cent of DLD and 4 per cent of HAD children were nonverbal, compared to 53 per cent of LAD and 24 per cent of NALIQ children, and that transcriptions were available for 64 per cent of DLD, 63 per cent of HAD, 33 per cent of LAD, 50 per cent of NALIQ and 100 per cent of normal children.

**TABLE 7.2**

**Spontaneous language: pragmatic discourse function**

| Variable | Group | | | | | | | | | | F | p[1] | Significant group contrasts |
|---|---|---|---|---|---|---|---|---|---|---|---|---|---|
| | DLD (N=128) | | HAD (N=32) | | LAD (N=41) | | NALIQ (N=55) | | Normal (N=46) | | | | |
| | Mean | (SD) | Mean | (SD) | Mean | (SD) | Mean | (SD) | Mean | (SD) | | | |
| Initiations (%) | 9.54 | (15.33) | 8.34 | (5.23) | 12.49 | (8.65) | 11.22 | (17.27) | 8.02 | (6.68) | 0.90 | ns | |
| Continuations (%) | 36.31 | (15.44) | 35.88 | (17.62) | 29.02 | (15.97) | 35.40 | (13.98) | 40.89 | (13.92) | 3.34 | 0.01 | Normal=DLD=HAD=NALIQ LAD<all groups |
| Responses (%) | 50.87 | (17.89) | 43.83 | (20.63) | 34.85 | (20.06) | 45.98 | (14.92) | 49.98 | (14.57) | 7.13 | 0.0001 | Normal=DLD=HAD=NALIQ DLD>HAD,NALIQ LAD<all groups |
| Echoes/repetitions (%) | 11.20 | (25.33) | 15.09 | (22.54) | 19.07 | (16.99) | 16.80 | (25.58) | 2.20 | (4.76) | 4.11 | 0.003 | Normal<all groups DLD=HAD=NALIQ DLD<LAD |

[1]Least square means ANOVA without covariates.

**TABLE 7.3**
**Spontaneous language: error analysis**

| Variable | Group | | | | | | | | | | | F | $p^1$ | Significant group contrasts |
|---|---|---|---|---|---|---|---|---|---|---|---|---|---|---|
| | DLD (N=128) | | HAD (N=32) | | LAD (N=41) | | NALIQ (N=55) | | Normal (N=46) | | | | | |
| | Mean | (SD) | Mean | (SD) | Mean | (SD) | Mean | (SD) | Mean | (SD) | | | | |
| Meaning errors (%) | 12.74 | (8.37) | 15.86 | (7.26) | 19.24 | (16.11) | 15.60 | (8.71) | 8.75 | (7.71) | 7.62 | 0.0001 | Normal<all groups DLD<LAD |
| Structural errors (%) | 22.81 | (11.65) | 23.66 | (13.25) | 26.52 | (15.62) | 23.38 | (10.87) | 11.67 | (7.71) | 10.55 | 0.0001 | Normal<all groups DLD=HAD=LAD=NALIQ |
| Pragmatic errors (%) | 4.12 | (3.76) | 5.75 | (5.35) | 9.31 | (9.40) | 4.73 | (2.82) | 2.55 | (2.57) | 12.35 | 0.0001 | Normal=DLD DLD=HAD=NALIQ LAD>all groups |
| Total errors (%) | 39.45 | (17.02) | 45.28 | (19.99) | 53.30 | (29.85) | 43.70 | (19.22) | 22.97 | (15.94) | 14.20 | 0.0001 | Normal<all groups DLD=HAD=NALIQ LAD>DLD,NALIQ |

[1]Least square means ANOVA without covariates.

131

**TABLE 7.4**

**Spontaneous language: Lingquest analysis of morphology and syntax**

| Variable | Group | | | | | F | $p^1$ | Significant group contrasts |
|---|---|---|---|---|---|---|---|---|
| | DLD<br>Mean (SD) | HAD<br>Mean (SD) | LAD<br>Mean (SD) | NALIQ<br>Mean (SD) | Normal<br>Mean (SD) | | | |
| Mean length of utterances (MLU) | 2.59 (1.27)<br>(N=185) | 2.76 (1.56)<br>(N=46) | 1.02 (1.13)<br>(N=116) | 2.00 (1.35)<br>(N=94) | 3.90 (0.77)<br>(N=43) | 53.26 | 0.001 | Normal>all groups<br>DLD=HAD>NALIQ<br>LAD<all groups |
| Form Classes (%) | 32.86 (11.42)<br>(N=149) | 31.77 (14.78)<br>(N=36) | 26.92 (11.99)<br>(N=26) | 33.43 (12.58)<br>(N=60) | 43.60 (9.39)<br>(N=43) | 10.01 | 0.001 | Normal>all groups<br>DLD=HAD=NALIQ<br>DLD, NALIQ>NALIQ<br>HAD=LAD |
| Verb Forms (%) | 26.90 (9.04)<br>(N=149) | 26.38 (11.52)<br>(N=36) | 21.91 (9.84)<br>(N=27) | 28.19 (17.70)<br>(N=60) | 35.07 (6.69)<br>(N=43) | 6.67 | 0.001 | Normal>all groups<br>DLD=HAD=NALIQ<br>DLD, NALIQ>LAD<br>HAD=LAD |

[1]Least square means ANOVA without covariates.

were covaried, the LAD children were still lower than all other groups, but the normal children's superiority over the NALIQ children reached significance. The only significant difference, when NVIQ was covaried for the four clinical groups, was that the LAD children produced fewer continuations than the NALIQ group.

The LAD was the only clinical group to respond less than the normal children in terms of proportion of utterances that were responses to the adults' initiations; the DLD children showed significantly higher rates of responding than the HAD children, with the LAD children significantly less likely to respond than all other groups; the scores of DLD children remained significantly higher than those of the two AD groups even when age and SES were covaried. Additional covariation of NVIQ did not alter the significantly lower score of the LAD group compared to the two non-autistic groups.

The normal children showed a very low percentage of utterances that were echoes (repetitions) of a prior utterance, with all clinical groups showing more echolalia than the normal children. The DLD children produced fewer echoes than the LAD group, but they did not differ from the HAD and NALIQ groups. Covarying for age, SES and NVIQ did not alter the pattern of results.

*Error analyses* were performed on each child's transcript for errors in meaning, structure and pragmatics as described in Appendix 4.1. Group comparisons of the percentage of utterances containing each of these types of errors, plus the percentage of utterances containing any of these errors, are shown in Table 7.3.

The normal children made fewer meaning errors than the children in all four clinical groups; among the clinical groups, the LAD children made more errors than the DLD children. When age and SES were covaried, the normal children remained lowest in errors, the DLD children were lower in errors than the other clinical groups, and the NALIQ children were lower in errors than the LAD children. When NVIQ was also covaried, the DLD children made fewer errors than children in the two autistic groups, who did not differ from each other; the LAD children made significantly more errors than NALIQ children.

With respect to structural errors, the normal children made fewer errors than children in the four clinical groups, who did not differ from each other. Covarying age and SES preserved the superiority of the normal children over the children in the four clinical groups. The LAD children made significantly more errors than the DLD and NALIQ children but their error rate was equivalent to that of the HAD group. Covarying NVIQ in addition did not change the pattern of group differences.

The LAD children produced more utterances containing pragmatic errors than the other groups, who did not differ from each other. When age and SES were covaried, adjusted means for errors were significantly lower in the normal group than in any clinical group, and significantly higher in the LAD group than in any other group. The DLD and NALIQ children were almost equivalent; only the DLD children's superiority over the HAD children reached significance. When NVIQ was also covaried, these relationships were preserved except that the HAD–LAD difference was no longer significant.

Combining utterances containing any errors in meaning, structure or pragmatics, the normal children produced the fewest flawed utterances. The LAD children produced more utterances with errors than the DLD and NALIQ children. When age and SES were covaried, the DLD group had significantly fewer errors than the two autistic groups; covarying NVIQ did not alter this pattern of results.

Thus, it appears that discourse errors are sensitive to diagnosis along two dimensions: clinical group *vs* normal, and autistic *vs* non-autistic. The normal children committed fewer errors in meaning, structure and communicative use than any of the clinical groups.

*Analysis of morphology and syntax* was performed using the Lingquest system (Mordecai *et al.* 1985) as described in Appendix 4.1. The program includes computerized counts of parts of speech (form classes) used and different verb forms used, as well as computation of mean length of utterance (MLU) in morphemes. The results of these analyses are shown in Table 7.4.

The normal children used a significantly higher percentage of the 81 different form classes identified by the Lingquest program than any of the clinical groups. The DLD, HAD and NALIQ groups did not differ in this respect. Both non-autistic groups used a higher percentage of forms than the LAD group, while the two autistic groups were equivalent.

The patterns of group similarities and differences in verb form use were identical to those seen in the parts of speech form classes. Covarying for age and SES did not change the group differences significantly for either form class or verb form analysis, suggesting that these two linguistic dimensions tap closely related functions.

Finally, MLUs, defined by average number of morphemes in an utterance, were computed. The normal children had the longest utterances, significantly longer than those of the DLD and HAD children, who did not differ from each other; they also had longer utterances than the NALIQ children, who in turn had longer utterances than the LAD children (who were more likely than any other group to be nonverbal). Covarying age and SES did not affect the pattern of results. Covarying NVIQ among the four clinical groups left only the LAD children lower than the DLD and NALIQ children. The adjusted means were highest for the NALIQ children, indicating that their MLUs were the highest of the four groups relative to their NVIQ scores.

SUMMARY OF LANGUAGE FINDINGS

On the major language variables presented, the DLD group show a relatively flat profile of scores, all approximately 1 SD below the normal mean. Exceptions are that functional use of receptive language is about equivalent to formal measures of receptive language, but functional use of expressive language may be more impaired than indicated by formal language tests, and capacity for written language may be beginning to show deficits, although the children are too young to make this a robust finding. In addition, selected verbal memory tests indicate greater impairment than other language tests (see memory section).

The HAD children show a more uneven pattern of tested language skills, with particular deficits in functions requiring formulated output of connected speech, verbal reasoning, comprehension and rapid naming, and relative strengths in single word confrontation naming and written language. As with the DLD children, functional use of receptive language is about equivalent to formal measures of receptive language, but functional use of expressive language is significantly below almost all expressive test scores.

When the DLD and the HAD children were compared, they did not differ on single word expressive vocabulary and on functional use of expressive skills, but the HAD children were significantly more impaired on all measures of comprehension, functional use of receptive skills, fluency, formulated output and verbal reasoning. The HAD children scored higher than the DLD children on acquisition of written language skills.

The NALIQ children showed a more even pattern of language skills, with most functions at about a standard score of 60–65. The LAD children were lower than the NALIQ children on every language measure, even when NVIQ and age were covaried; it was difficult to detect a specific profile because their standard scores were very low on all tests.

Thus, the NALIQ and DLD children had relatively even patterns of performance. The HAD children had preserved acquisition of written language and confrontation naming, but severely affected comprehension and production of formulated output. The extent of the comprehension deficit was the language factor that most strongly differentiated the autistic from the non-autistic groups.

The spontaneous language sample analyses presented here indicate that the normal children performed better, with fewer errors, longer utterances and a richer variety of forms than any of the clinical groups. Verbal LAD children, who comprised only 47 per cent of that group, were universally poorer in their performance than the DLD and NALIQ groups but were equivalent to the HAD children on several measures. It is clear, at least in the language dimensions reported here, that all of the clinical groups are language impaired relative to the children in the normal control group.

*Group differences in neuropsychological functions*
VISUOSPATIAL AND QUANTITATIVE FUNCTIONS

S-B nonverbal subtest standard scores were not appropriate for covariation of age and NVIQ, since age is already taken into account in the standard score, and the subtests themselves were used in the computation of NVIQ. Results of these tests are given in Table 7.5 and depicted in Figure 7.1.

The pattern of nonverbal scores shown in Figure 7.1 differs rather dramatically from that of verbal scores that can be seen in Figure 7.2. As stated earlier, the verbal profiles dichotomized the groups according to the autistic/non-autistic dimension, with the verbal profiles ranked according to mean NVIQ, except for the HAD group which scored lower than the DLD group despite their identical mean NVIQs. In contrast, the nonverbal scores divided the children into two groups on the dimension of NVIQ: the DLD and HAD groups vs the NALIQ and LAD groups, with the LAD group slightly lower than the NALIQ group, reflecting their 10 point lower NVIQ. The same dichotomous pattern was repeated for the Seguin Formboard test results. Scores on the Hiskey–Nebraska Picture Identification subtest were the highest for each group, suggesting a possible inflation of norms on this test, but not invalidating the group comparisons.

**TABLE 7.5**
**Visuospatial and quantitative scores by group**

| Task[1] | Group | | | | F | p²[2] | Significant group contrasts |
|---|---|---|---|---|---|---|---|
| | DLD Mean (SD) | HAD Mean (SD) | LAD Mean (SD) | NALIQ Mean (SD) | | | |
| Stanford–Binet Abstract Visual Reasoning Area (SS: Mean=100, SD=16) | 100.25 (12.98) (N=201) | 99.92 (16.07) (N=51) | 47.09 (15.24) (N=125) | 55.78 (16.70) (N=110) | 451.44 | 0.0001 | DLD=HAD>NALIQ>LAD |
| Stanford–Binet Pattern Analysis (SS: Mean=500, SD=8) | 51.89 (6.21) (N=201) | 49.90 (8.61) (N=51) | 27.98 (7.34) (N=125) | 31.53 (7.66) (N=110) | 387.40 | 0.0001 | DLD=HAD>NALIQ>LAD |
| Stanford–Binet Copying (SS: Mean=50, SD=8) | 48.25 (7.27) (N=201) | 49.31 (10.21) (N=51) | 28.39 (4.42) (N=125) | 31.86 (5.84) (N=110) | 309.05 | 0.0001 | HAD=DLD>NALIQ>LAD |
| Stanford–Binet Quantitative (SS: Mean=50, SD=8) | 45.64 (11.51) (N=201) | 48.20 (8.86) (N=51) | 30.54 (5.97) (N=125) | 32.07 (6.41) (N=110) | 112.20 | 0.0001 | HAD=DLD>NALIQ=LAD |
| Hiskey–Nebraska Picture Identification (SS: Mean=100, SD=16) | 111.50 (24.29) (N=198) | 110.20 (23.59) (N=50) | 71.82 (26.78) (N=99) | 80.58 (23.17) (N=98) | 76.90 | 0.0001 | DLD=HAD>NALIQ>LAD |
| Seguin Formboard (N correct) | 8.54 (1.91) (N=196) | 9.05 (2.39) (N=51) | 6.16 (3.83) (N=122) | 6.03 (3.67) (N=105) | 76.90 | 0.0001 | DLD=HAD>NALIQ=LAD |

[1]SS = standard score.
[2]Least square means ANOVA without covariates.

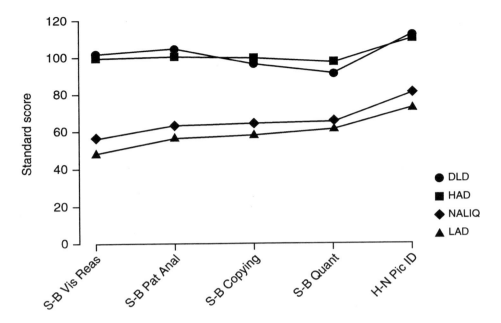

**Fig. 7.2.** Visuospatial and quantitative scores by group.

Figure shows rather a flat profile of visuospatial and quantitative scores in all four groups which were dichotomized by their NVIQ scores: the DLD and HAD groups with NVIQ ≥80 obtained uniformly higher scores than the NALIQ and LAD children with NVIQ <80.

S-B = Stanford–Binet; Vis Reas = Visual Reasoning; Pat Anal = Pattern Analysis; Quant = Quantitative; H-N Pic ID = Hiskey–Nebraska Picture Identification.

In summary, the DLD and HAD children did not differ on any measure of visuospatial or quantitative skill, and both groups were within the normal range on each measure. The LAD and NALIQ children were rather evenly deficient, with the LAD children lower than the NALIQ children on all tests except the S-B Quantitative subtest and the Seguin Formboard.

SHORT-TERM MEMORY AND ATTENTION FUNCTIONS

Scores on tests of memory are shown in Table 7.6 and Figure 7.3, grouped into subtests of verbal memory, followed by those of visual memory. There are no specific tests of attention because there are none that are satisfactory for use in such young children; however, many investigators consider that memory and attention are linked and, for example, view Memory for Digits as a measure of attention.

On Memory for Digits from the S-B, the performance of all groups was significantly impaired. The HAD group was superior to the other three groups, who, because of low scores and high variability, were not different from each other. Even the HAD group, however, was about 2 SD below the normal mean. Examination of raw scores on this

**TABLE 7.6**

**Attention and memory scores by group**

| Task[1] | Group | | | | | | | F | p[2] | Significant group contrasts |
|---|---|---|---|---|---|---|---|---|---|---|
| | DLD Mean (SD) | | HAD Mean (SD) | | LAD Mean (SD) | | NALIQ Mean (SD) | | | |
| Stanford–Binet Short Term Memory Area (SS: Mean=100, SD=16) | 78.35 (21.57) (N=201) | | 80.47 (18.63) (N=51) | | 45.15 (16.00) (N=125) | | 55.29 (20.01) (N=110) | 93.26 | 0.0001 | HAD=DLD>NALIQ>LAD |
| Stanford–Binet Memory for Digits (SS: Mean=50, SD=8) | 29.50 (9.65) (N=201) | | 35.10 (13.60) (N=51) | | 27.58 (6.72) (N=125) | | 28.87 (8.31) (N=110) | 8.26 | 0.0001 | HAD>DLD=NALIQ=LAD |
| Stanford–Binet Memory for Sentences (SS: Mean=50, SD=8) | 40.22 (8.84) (N=201) | | 40.78 (8.09) (N=51) | | 27.56 (5.31) (N=125) | | 30.83 (7.10) (N=110) | 92.50 | 0.0001 | HAD=DLD>NALIQ>LAD |
| McCarthy Verbal Memory II (SS: Mean=100, SD=16) | 89.08 (15.88) (N=173) | | 77.41 (21.08) (N=34) | | 62.31 (13.16) (N=80) | | 72.95 (16.45) (N=88) | 55.54 | 0.0001 | DLD>HAD=NALIQ>LAD |
| Stanford–Binet Bead Memory (SS: Mean=50, SD=8) | 36.36 (12.53) (N=201) | | 31.31 (10.08) (N=51) | | 26.61 (3.07) (N=125) | | 27.60 (5.07) (N=110) | 37.44 | 0.0001 | DLD>HAD>NALIQ=LAD |
| Hiskey–Nebraska Visual Attention Span (SS: Mean=100, SD=16) | 112.65 (27.63) (N=189) | | 96.93 (22.70) (N=41) | | 60.59 (20.33) (N=71) | | 79.78 (27.86) (N=72) | 79.16 | 0.0001 | DLD>HAD>NALIQ>LAD |

[1]SS = standard score.

[2]Least square means ANOVA without covariates.

138

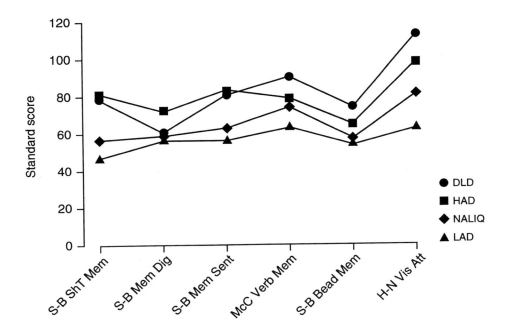

**Fig. 7.3.** Short-term memory and attention scores by group.

This figure illustrates the short-term memory deficits of children in the DLD group, especially in rote memory (Memory for Digits), and nonverbal sequencing (Bead Memory) deficits in all the groups. The scores on the other visual memory task (Hiskey–Nebraska Visual Attention Span), which requires sequential memory of verbally codable material, preserved the ranking of the children by NVIQ and the relative inferiority of the HAD compared to the DLD children. Increasing the semantic structure of the material to be remembered (S-B Memory for Sentences and McCarthy Verbal Memory II) helped the DLD children and to a lesser degree the NALIQ children but was of no help to the two AD groups. The superiority of the HAD groups, compared to the other three groups, on Memory for Digits illustrates their relative strength in rote verbal memory

S–B = Stanford–Binet; ShT Mem = Short-term Memory; Mem Dig = Memory for Digits; Mem Sent = Memory for Sentences; McC Verb Mem = McCarthy Verbal Memory II; Bead Mem = Bead Memory; H-N Vis Att = Hiskey–Nebraska Visual Attention Span.

task (DLD = 1.78, HAD = 2.94, LAD = 0.55, NALIQ = 0.84) reveals that many low-functioning children were totally unable to do the task, but that even the DLD children, who were high-functioning and could do the task, had very low digit memory spans.

On Memory for Sentences from the S-B, the DLD and HAD children obtained equivalent scores and both were more than 1 SD lower than normal; both were superior to the NALIQ children, 61 per cent of whom could do the task, and who were in turn superior to the LAD children, 39 per cent of whom were able to achieve interpretable mean scores above 0. These relationships were preserved with covariation.

On the McCarthy Verbal Memory II (memory for a story), the DLD children were only mildly impaired, and were superior to the HAD children. The NALIQ children also performed better than the LAD children. Covariation preserved these relationships.

On Bead Memory from the S-B, the DLD children were superior to the HAD children, but both groups were significantly impaired on this task (see standard scores on Table 7.6). These groups were superior to the NALIQ and LAD children, most of whom were unable to do this task.

On the Hiskey–Nebraska (H-N) Visual Attention Span subtest, Figure 7.3 suggests a greater spread of mean scores than with other measures. When scores were adjusted for NVIQ and age, the DLD children remained superior to the rest of the groups (as can be seen in Table 7.6, their mean score is above average), and the other groups become equivalent. The somewhat above average scores of the DLD children and average scores of the HAD group suggest that H-N norms may be somewhat inflated. The NALIQ and LAD children had deficient performance, explained by their lowered overall NVIQ. If the H-N norms are adjusted downward by about 10 points, the DLD children become average, and the HAD children are about 1 SD below average.

The overall S-B standard scores for the Short-term Memory Area, a composite that encompasses verbal (Memory for Digits and for Sentences) and visual (Bead Memory) task disclosed no difference between HAD and DLD children, who both functioned about 1.5 SD below average; both were superior to the NALIQ children, who were superior to the LAD children. These relationships were preserved with covariation. The lack of difference between the HAD and DLD children is explained by the equivalent performance of the groups on sentence memory, HAD superiority on digit memory, and DLD superiority on bead memory. The superiority of the NALIQ children over the LAD children is attributable to their superior performance on sentence memory, the only memory task within the competence of both low-functioning groups.

To summarize, the DLD children showed significant problems with tests of short-term memory and attention, even in the visual domain. They had significant difficulty with a visual memory task that required preserving a sequence of objects (Bead Memory), although they performed normally on another short-term memory task (H-N Visual Attention Span). Their verbal memory was impaired, only slightly on tasks where the semantic structure could assist them (stories and sentences), but severely on non-meaningful verbal rote memory (digit span). The HAD children also performed normally on one visual memory task (H-N) and poorly on the visual memory task that stressed the recall of sequences (Bead Memory). They were mildly impaired on memory for sentences, but moderately impaired on memory for a story and for digits. In direct comparisons of the DLD and HAD children, the DLD children were superior on both of the visual memory tasks. With verbal material, the DLD children were superior on memory for a story, the groups were equivalent on memory for sentences, and the HAD children were superior on digit span. Thus, as the semantic structure of the material increases, the DLD children enjoy an increasing advantage.

On tasks that the lower-functioning children could do, covarying NVIQ revealed that the LAD children were equivalent (for their NVIQ) to the NALIQ children on visual memory, but lower than the NALIQ children on semantic memory (sentences and stories).

140

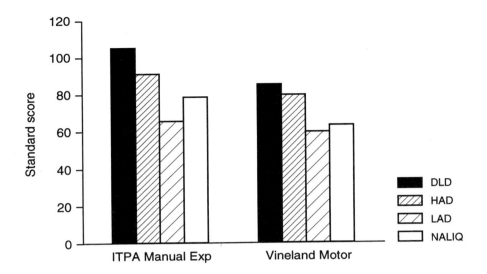

**Fig. 7.4.** Standard scores for praxis and overall motor skill.

The results of the ITPA Manual Expression subtest illustrate that the two AD groups were inferior to their non-AD counterparts, and that the LIQ (NVIQ <80) groups were more impaired than the groups with NVIQ ≥80. This indicates that both NVIQ and autism contributed to the distribution of scores. The Vineland Motor Domain showed the effect of NVIQ, with the HAD but not LAD groups inferior to their counterparts.

Thus, the DLD children were revealed to have significant short-term memory deficits affecting sequential material in both auditory and visual modalities, and both autistic groups had special deficits in the recall of semantically organized material.

MOTOR FUNCTIONS

Table 7.7 lists the motor scores of children in the four groups and Figure 7.4 displays measures of praxis and parents' perceptions of the children's overall motor competence. There was no significant difference between means for the Handedness Ratio [(R/R+L) × 100]*. On the ITPA Manual Expression subtest (a measure of praxis), the DLD children had an average mean score (*i.e.* equal to that of the normal population) and were superior to the HAD children, who were mildly impaired, a result to be taken cautiously because the HAD sample is small. The HAD children were superior to the NALIQ children, who were superior to the LAD children. When NVIQ was covaried, the DLD children remained superior to the HAD children, and the NALIQ children remained superior to the LAD children, but the two autistic groups and the two non-autistic groups were no longer different from each other, suggesting that lowered raw scores were independently contributed to by low NVIQ and by autism.

*This score indicates the strength of handedness: a strongly right-handed child would obtain a score of 100.

**TABLE 7.7**

**Motor scores by group**

| Task[1] | Group | | | | | $F$ | $p$[2] | Significant group contrasts |
|---|---|---|---|---|---|---|---|---|
| | DLD Mean (SD) | HAD Mean (SD) | LAD Mean (SD) | NALIQ Mean (SD) | | | | |
| Handedness ratio [(R/R+L) × 100] | 76.61 (26.88) (N=188) | 69.29 (33.45) (N=48) | 68.98 (32.72) (N=113) | 72.68 (29.22) (N=99) | | 1.87 | ns | |
| Vineland Motor Domain (SS: Mean=100, SD=16) | 84.62 (17.11) (N=190) | 79.14 (15.40) (N=37) | 58.85 (14.08) (N=87) | 62.13 (13.33) (N=84) | | 74.40 | 0.0001 | DLD>HAD>NALIQ=LAD |
| ITPA Manual Expression (SS: Mean=100, SD=16) | 103.87 (20.99) (N=79) | 90.41 (23.02) (N=17) | 64.07 (17.49) (N=41) | 78.37 (22.81) (N=41) | | 36.10 | 0.0001 | DLD>HAD>NALIQ>LAD |
| Annett Pegboard time—right hand (seconds) | 24.68 (10.95) (N=177) | 23.55 (17.87) (N=47) | 32.88 (21.97) (N=72) | 35.53 (20.44) (N=75) | | 10.67 | 0.0001 | HAD=DLD>LAD=NALIQ |
| Annett Pegboard time—left hand (seconds) | 25.56 (9.71) (N=176) | 24.09 (13.20) (N=47) | 32.42 (17.34) (N=67) | 40.21 (21.39) (N=76) | | 20.54 | 0.0001 | HAD=DLD>LAD>NALIQ |
| Seguin Formboard time (seconds) | 52.76 (34.90) (N=196) | 51.73 (43.24) (N=51) | 118.77 (101.42) (N=121) | 124.91 (100.79) (N=107) | | 30.39 | 0.0001 | DLD>NALIQ,LAD HAD>NALIQ,LAD DLD=HAD>NALIQ=LAD |

[1]SS = standard score.

[2]Least square means ANOVA without covariates.

142

On the Vineland Motor domain, which is concerned with the acquisition of functional motor skills in everyday life, all groups scored below average. The DLD children showed a small but significant superiority over the HAD children; both were superior to the two lower-functioning groups who, once again, did not differ. When adjusted for age and NVIQ, the only significant difference was that DLD children remained superior to the two lower-functioning groups. As described earlier, because subdomain standard scores are not available we divided the children's MA equivalents on subdomains by their CAs in order to obtain a rough index of functioning. On Gross Motor functioning, the ratios were: DLD = 83, HAD = 71, LAD = 54, NALIQ = 58. Covarying MA equivalents for age and NVIQ confirmed that the difference between the DLD and HAD children is significant, and suggested that the low performance of the LAD and NALIQ children is not solely attributable to their low NVIQ equivalent; the only significant finding in the analysis of covariance was that the DLD children were superior to the other three groups.

On Fine Motor functioning, the ratio of MA/CA ratios were: DLD = 90, HAD = 81, LAD = 52, NALIQ = 56. These ratios are very close to the Gross Motor ratios for the lower-functioning groups, but are higher than the Gross Motor ratios for the HAD and DLD children. Analysis of raw scores covaried for age and NVIQ resulted in only one significant difference, that the DLD children were superior to the LAD children.

Two measures of motor speed were derived: time to complete the Annett Pegboard and time to complete the Seguin Formboard. Results are displayed in Table 7.7 and Figure 7.5. On the Annett Pegboard, the HAD children equalled the DLD children for each of the hands; both were superior to the LAD children. The LAD children were faster than the NALIQ children for the left hand, but equivalent for the right hand. Co-variation of age and NVIQ left only the NALIQ group inferior in performance to the other groups. Examination of raw scores reveals that the two high-functioning groups were slightly (between 0.5 and 1 s) faster with the right hand, while the NALIQ children were much faster with the right hand, and the LAD children were slightly (0.5 s) faster with the left hand. Comparing these performances with the Annett norms, the DLD children are average with their left hands and 1 SD below average with their right hands, the HAD children are 1 SD below average with their left hands and 2 SD below average with their right hands, and both low-functioning groups are severely deficient with both hands.

On time to complete the Seguin Formboard, the DLD and HAD groups were equivalent, and were much faster than the two lower-functioning groups, who did not differ. When raw scores were covaried for age and NVIQ, only the HAD children remained faster than the LAD children.

To summarize, no group differences in handedness were found. Both autistic groups had significant difficulties with a test of praxis, compared to their NVIQ comparisons; the DLD children showed normal praxis. On two measures of motor speed, when NVIQ was covaried, only the NALIQ children remained significantly inferior to the other groups. There were trends for the HAD children to be slower than the DLD children, and both of these groups showed relative impairments (compared to norms) of the right

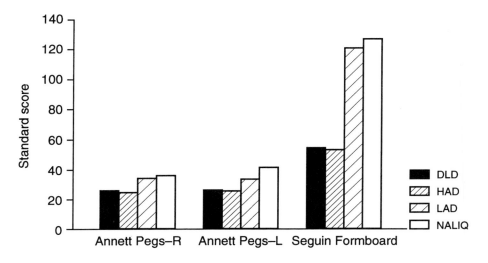

**Fig. 7.5.** Timed motor tasks.

The two LIQ groups were slower than the higher functioning groups on the Annett Pegboard (R = right hand; L = left hand). This is one of the only tasks where the LAD children (those who could perform the task) were superior to the NALIQ children for the left hand only. The Seguin Formboard strongly discriminates the groups along the NVIQ dimension.

hand. On parent report of acquisition of functional motor skills, all groups were deficient on both gross and fine motor areas, with the two high-functioning groups somewhat worse on gross than fine motor functioning.

Thus, the DLD children as a group had normal praxis and left hand motor speed, mild impairment in right hand motor speed and in acquisition of functional motor skills. The HAD children showed mildly impaired praxis and left hand motor speed, and moderate impairment in right hand motor speed and in acquisition of functional motor skills. Thus, the HAD children showed a pattern of impairments more marked but very similar to that of the DLD children. The LAD children were impaired on all motor skills. They were worse than the NALIQ children on praxis, equivalent on right hand motor speed and acquisition of functional skills, and better on left hand motor speed. The NALIQ children had motor speed and acquisition of functional motor skills which were lower than those of the other non-autistic (DLD) group, even when taking into account their lower NVIQs.

*Factor analyses*

A group of 15 cognitive variables were selected to be factor analyzed. They were selected on the basis of their being well-established and standardized measures with satisfactory reliabilities and good representation of all cognitive functions tested. As with any such analyses, the results would no doubt be somewhat different with another selection of tests. An SAS principal component factor analysis was run, with Promax

**TABLE. 7.8**
**Factor structure for the whole sample**

| Task | Factor 1 | Factor 2 |
|---|---|---|
| Stanford–Binet Vocabulary | 0.87 | –0.31 |
| Stanford–Binet Comprehension | 0.88 | –0.31 |
| Peabody Picture Vocabulary Test | 0.85 | –0.29 |
| Test of Early Language Development | 0.78 | –0.28 |
| Expressive One-Word Picture Vocabulary Test | 0.80 | –0.38 |
| Stanford–Binet Pattern Analysis | 0.86 | –0.47 |
| Stanford–Binet Copying | 0.85 | –0.45 |
| Stanford–Binet Quantitative | 0.67 | –0.45 |
| Hiskey–Nebraska Picture ID | 0.71 | –0.35 |
| Hiskey–Nebraska Visual Attention | 0.73 | –0.37 |
| Stanford–Binet Memory for Sentence | 0.81 | –0.33 |
| McCarthy Verbal Memory II | 0.71 | –0.18 |
| Annett Pegboard—right hand | –0.30 | 0.91 |
| Annett Pegboard—left hand | –0.33 | 0.91 |
| Seguin Formboard time | –0.53 | 0.77 |

rotation, allowing the factors to be correlated. The analyses were also run with Varimax rotation, and for each analysis the results were extremely close to the Promax rotation, which will be reported here. The number of factors was selected based on Eigen values of 1, and a scree test for each analysis confirmed the number of factors.

WHOLE SAMPLE

The factor analysis for the entire sample of children (N=487) is presented in Table 7.8. Two clearly interpretable factors emerge: all cognitive tests load on Factor 1, and the three measures of motor speed load on Factor 2. The collapsing of all cognitive variables onto one factor may be due to the different factor structures within the group making up the sample.

DLD SAMPLE

The factor analysis for the DLD children (N=201) is shown in Table 7.9. In order of magnitude of correlations, the tests loading highly on Factor 1 are the S-B Vocabulary and Memory for Sentences subtests, the EOWPVT, S-B Comprehension, the TELD, McCarthy Verbal Memory II (memory for a story), and the PPVT. This factor represents all the language tests.

Factor 2 contains the three measures of motor speed. Loading highly on Factor 3 are the S-B Quantitative, Copying and Pattern Analysis subtests, and the PPVT. Except for the PPVT (which has the smallest loading on this factor), this factor represents visuo-spatial skills.

Factor 4 has high loadings for H-N Visual Attention and Picture Identification, and S-B Pattern Analysis, and seems to represent an additional visual factor having more to do with attention to visual detail.

**TABLE 7.9**
**Factor structure for the DLD group**

| Task | Factor 1 | Factor 2 | Factor 3 | Factor 4 |
|---|---|---|---|---|
| Stanford–Binet Vocabulary | 0.81 | –0.18 | 0.06 | 0.28 |
| Stanford–Binet Comprehension | 0.69 | –0.01 | 0.13 | 0.37 |
| Peabody Picture Vocabulary Test | 0.55 | –0.18 | 0.56 | 0.43 |
| Test of Early Language Development | 0.69 | –0.34 | 0.28 | 0.31 |
| Expressive One-Word Picture Vocabulary Test | 0.74 | –0.50 | 0.28 | 0.16 |
| Stanford–Binet Pattern Analysis | 0.23 | –0.08 | 0.71 | 0.57 |
| Stanford–Binet Copying | 0.29 | –0.15 | 0.72 | 0.20 |
| Stanford–Binet Quantitative | –0.05 | –0.31 | 0.77 | 0.04 |
| Hiskey–Nebraska Picture ID | 0.34 | –0.03 | 0.28 | 0.79 |
| Hiskey–Nebraska Visual Attention | 0.20 | –0.15 | 0.17 | 0.86 |
| Stanford–Binet Memory for Sentences | 0.76 | –0.14 | 0.03 | 0.15 |
| McCarthy Verbal Memory II | 0.56 | –0.12 | 0.26 | 0.11 |
| Annett Pegboard—right hand | –0.24 | 0.87 | –0.15 | 0.02 |
| Annett Pegboard—left hand | –0.21 | 0.92 | –0.21 | –0.06 |
| Seguin Formboard time | –0.20 | 0.74 | –0.35 | –0.27 |

**TABLE 7.10**
**Factor structure for the HAD group**

| Task | Factor 1 | Factor 2 | Factor 3 | Factor 4 |
|---|---|---|---|---|
| Stanford–Binet Vocabulary | 0.41 | –0.16 | 0.85 | 0.22 |
| Stanford–Binet Comprehension | 0.51 | –0.06 | 0.84 | 0.27 |
| Peabody Picture Vocabulary Test | 0.84 | –0.05 | 0.44 | 0.08 |
| Test of Early Language Development | 0.83 | –0.24 | 0.26 | 0.33 |
| Expressive One-Word Picture Vocabulary Test | 0.88 | –0.10 | 0.36 | 0.13 |
| Stanford–Binet Pattern Analysis | 0.09 | –0.21 | 0.08 | 0.74 |
| Stanford–Binet Copying | 0.55 | –0.39 | 0.30 | 0.45 |
| Stanford–Binet Quantitative | 0.48 | –0.56 | 0.33 | 0.67 |
| Hiskey–Nebraska Picture ID | 0.24 | 0.36 | –0.28 | 0.43 |
| Hiskey–Nebraska Visual Attention | 0.04 | 0.08 | 0.27 | 0.61 |
| Stanford–Binet Memory for Sentences | 0.64 | –0.04 | 0.73 | 0.16 |
| McCarthy Verbal Memory II | 0.63 | –0.43 | 0.29 | –0.27 |
| Annett Pegboard—right hand | –0.06 | 0.73 | –0.43 | –0.09 |
| Annett Pegboard—left hand | –0.12 | 0.80 | 0.17 | –0.03 |
| Seguin Formboard time | –0.20 | 0.80 | –0.07 | –0.16 |

HAD SAMPLE

The factor analysis for the HAD children (N=51) also has four factors (Table 7.10). Loading highly on the first factor, in order of magnitude, are the EOWPVT, PPVT, TELD, S-B Memory for Sentences, McCarthy Verbal Memory II, and, to a smaller extent, S-B Copying and Comprehension. Except for Copying, this first factor seems to be a verbal one, but loading most highly are verbal functions related to lexical/semantic functions and verbal memory.

TABLE 7.11
**Factor structure for the LAD group**

| Task | Factor 1 | Factor 2 | Factor 3 | Factor 4 |
|---|---|---|---|---|
| Stanford–Binet Vocabulary | 0.88 | 0.53 | 0.25 | 0.31 |
| Stanford–Binet Comprehension | 0.87 | 0.48 | −0.21 | 0.26 |
| Peabody Picture Vocabulary Test | 0.49 | 0.87 | −0.18 | 0.28 |
| Test of Early Language Development | 0.42 | 0.78 | −0.06 | 0.60 |
| Expressive One-Word Picture Vocabulary Test | 0.57 | 0.80 | 0.25 | 0.48 |
| Stanford–Binet Pattern Analysis | 0.82 | 0.26 | 0.36 | 0.53 |
| Stanford–Binet Copying | 0.84 | 0.34 | 0.33 | 0.54 |
| Stanford–Binet Quantitative | 0.81 | 0.41 | −0.26 | 0.52 |
| Hiskey–Nebraska Picture ID | 0.41 | 0.18 | −0.35 | 0.87 |
| Hiskey–Nebraska Visual Attention | 0.53 | 0.46 | −0.30 | 0.91 |
| Stanford–Binet Memory for Sentences | 0.83 | 0.61 | −0.31 | 0.46 |
| McCarthy Verbal Memory II | 0.27 | 0.75 | 0.04 | 0.07 |
| Annett Pegboard—right hand | −0.26 | 0.01 | 0.94 | 0.35 |
| Annett Pegboard—left hand | −0.27 | −0.09 | 0.93 | −0.29 |
| Seguin Formboard time | −0.39 | −0.19 | 0.81 | −0.28 |

On Factor 2 are found the three measures of motor speed. S-B Vocabulary, Comprehension and Memory for Sentences load on Factor 3, which thus seems to represent verbal tasks requiring formulation of verbal output.

Factor 4 has loadings from S-B Quantitative and Pattern Analysis, and H-N Visual Attention, and to a lesser extent S-B Copying and H-N Picture Identification, representing visuospatial and constructional skills and visual attention.

LAD SAMPLE

The factor analysis for the LAD children (N=125) also resolves four factors (Table 7.11). Factor 1, accounting for the most variance, includes, in order of magnitude, S-B Vocabulary, Comprehension, Copying, Memory for Sentences, Pattern Analysis and Quantitative. Factor 2 has high loadings for PPVT, EOWPVT, TELD, McCarthy Verbal Memory II and S-B Memory for Sentences. Factor 3 has high loadings for the three motor speed tests. Factor 4 has high loadings for H-N Visual Attention and Picture Identification. Thus, Factor 3 represents motor speed, Factor 2 represents lexical/semantic functions and verbal memory, Factor 4 represents visual attention, and Factor 1, although more difficult to interpret, seems to contain both language and visual tests that have a high demand for formulating verbal output or a problem solving strategy.

NALIQ SAMPLE

The factor analysis for the NALIQ group (N=110) resolves three factors (Table 7.12). On the first factor are found S-B Comprehension and Vocabulary, TELD, EOWPVT, S-B Memory for Sentences, PPVT, McCarthy Verbal Memory II, and, to a lesser extent, S-B Copying and Pattern Analysis. This factor clearly has high loadings for all language variables.

**TABLE 7.12**
**Factor structure for the NALIQ group**

| Task | Factor 1 | Factor 2 | Factor 3 |
|---|---|---|---|
| Stanford–Binet Vocabulary | 0.84 | 0.63 | –0.12 |
| Stanford–Binet Comprehension | 0.85 | 0.58 | –0.28 |
| Peabody Picture Vocabulary Test | 0.79 | 0.37 | –0.25 |
| Test of Early Language Development | 0.83 | 0.29 | –0.22 |
| Expressive One-Word Picture Vocabulary Test | 0.83 | 0.49 | –0.28 |
| Stanford–Binet Pattern Analysis | 0.59 | 0.83 | –0.29 |
| Stanford–Binet Copying | 0.69 | 0.78 | –0.17 |
| Stanford–Binet Quantitative | 0.19 | 0.81 | –0.04 |
| Hiskey–Nebraska Picture ID | 0.51 | 0.58 | –0.31 |
| Hiskey–Nebraska Visual Attention | 0.44 | 0.80 | –0.41 |
| Stanford–Binet Memory for Sentences | 0.80 | 0.60 | –0.27 |
| McCarthy Verbal Memory II | 0.77 | 0.24 | –0.03 |
| Annett Pegboard—right hand | –0.98 | –0.24 | 0.95 |
| Annett Pegboard—left hand | –0.21 | –0.22 | 0.94 |
| Seguin Formboard time | –0.41 | –0.67 | 0.63 |

Factor 2 contains high loadings for S-B Pattern Analysis and Quantitative, H-N Visual Attention, S-B Copying, and to a lesser extent S-B Vocabulary and Comprehension, and H-N Picture Identification. Although there is some representation for language measures on this factor, as there is for visuospatial tasks on Factor 1, Factor 2 represents visuospatial and visual attention skills. Factor 3 contains the three measures of motor speed.

COMPARISON AND INTERPRETATION OF THE FACTOR STRUCTURES FOR THE FOUR GROUPS
The factor structures for all four groups share certain features: each has a factor for motor speed, and the quantitative skill loads with visuospatial skill for each group. Each group has at least one factor for language and one for visuospatial skills. The NALIQ group has the simplest structure, with three factors for motor speed, visuospatial skills and language. The HAD group has a similar structure, except that the language factor breaks into a factor for lexical/semantic functions and verbal memory and a factor for formulated output. The DLD group has a structure similar to the NALIQ group, except that the visual factor breaks into a factor for attention to visual detail and a factor for visuospatial problem solving. The factor structure for the LAD group is similar to that of the NALIQ children, except that all cognitive tests with problem solving or formulation —demands that, presumably, are dependent on fluid, as opposed to crystallized visual and verbal intelligence—form a separate factor, leaving mainly simpler tests loading on the visual and verbal factors.

These analyses may suggest that the DLD children have a severity-of-language deficit that explains most of the variance across all language functions, that the HAD children experience difficulty in verbal formulation and problem solving that may be relatively independent of language functions and that does not extend to the visual

148

domain, and that the LAD children have deficits in formulation and problem solving that pervade both visual and language domains.

## Discussion

The neuropsychological and language data revealed substantial similarities and differences between the HAD and DLD children, and between the NALIQ and LAD children. Language profiles of the DLD children as a group were relatively flat. Previous literature had suggested discrepancies in the relative level of development of various aspects of language in DLD children (Aram and Nation 1975). In particular, studies have suggested deficits (either delay or deviance) in phonology (Leonard 1988, Tallal 1988), and delayed development of morphology and syntax, and discrepant development between the two (Johnston and Kamhi 1984). Some delay in DLD children is also apparent in lexical and relational semantic development (Johnston *et al.* 1981, Johnston 1988) and in pragmatic functions (Shatz *et al.* 1980, Leonard *et al.* 1982, Rowan *et al.* 1983), although most studies conclude that DLD children's lexical/semantic and pragmatic development is spared, relative to language-age-matched normal children. The relatively flat profile of mean language scores for the DLD children in the present study (depicted in Fig. 7.1) is confirmed by the factor analysis, which finds one primary language factor for the DLD group. This finding may be due in part to the use of composite scores (such as the TELD and S-B Verbal Reasoning) and multifactorial tests (such as S-B Absurdities), as well as to the inclusion of the total, heterogenous DLD sample. We expect individual differences and uneven profiles may appear when subgroup analyses using the complete set of language variables are performed.

HAD children, as a group, showed more uneven profiles, with strengths in written language and in naming, and notable deficits in comprehension, verbal reasoning, formulated output of connected speech, and rapid word retrieval within categories. The LAD children were severely impaired, relative to the NALIQ children, on all language measures. Few studies have examined language profiles in either DLD or verbal AD children, although many studies over the past 30 years have documented deficits in specific aspects of language (Menyuk 1978). Unlike DLD children whose phonology and syntax are regularly affected, phonological development may be somewhat delayed but otherwise normal in many verbal autistic children (Tager-Flusberg 1981, Paul 1987). Studies by Waterhouse and Fein (1982) and Tager-Flusberg (1989) found normal sequential emergence of grammatical forms, but restricted variety of usage; syntax was generally normal for language age in autism (Tager-Flusberg 1981, 1985, 1989; Waterhouse and Fein 1982; Swisher and Demetras 1985; Paul 1987). In contrast, a variety of abnormalities in semantic usage, including unevenness in the development of the receptive and expressive lexicons, reliance on syntactic rather than semantic content for comprehension, and a limited vocabulary within word classes have been reported (Simmons and Baltaxe 1975, Prior and Hall 1979, Tager-Flusberg 1981, Waterhouse and Fein 1982, Lord 1985, Paul *et al.* 1988). Some studies, however, have shown an overlap in the kinds of language deficits exhibited by DLD and AD children (Allen 1989, Tuchman *et al.* 1991a, Allen and Rapin 1992). Pragmatic functions are particularly

149

impaired, including poor conversational skills and inadequate use of language to request or share information (Shapiro *et al.* 1972, Baltaxe 1977, Fay and Schuler 1980, Hurtig *et al.* 1982, Paul and Cohen 1984*a*, Tager-Flusberg 1989). The findings in our study are consistent with this body of literature, especially in the finding that expressive vocabulary is superior to receptive vocabulary (see Waterhouse and Fein 1982). Our findings put a slightly different slant on autistic children's language by emphasizing that it suffers dramatically when there is a demand for self-organized verbal output. This is consistent with the results of Minshew *et al.* (1992) and Minshew and Goldstein (1993) who found high-functioning autistic individuals most deficient on tasks involving complex language comprehension, verbal reasoning and semantic organization of verbal memory.

Direct comparison of DLD and HAD children showed the HAD children to be superior on early acquisition of written language but more impaired on all measures of comprehension and all measures requiring formulated verbal output, on functional use of receptive skills, and on rapid word retrieval. Few recent studies have compared language in DLD and autism directly (see Bartak *et al.* 1975; Bartolucci *et al.* 1976; Cantwell *et al.* 1978, 1989). Data from our study are consistent with prior research, suggesting relative DLD deficiency in phonological and syntactic abilities, and relative AD deficiency in semantic and pragmatic skills. These data differ in that they highlight AD children's difficulty with comprehension and self-organized output, rather than identifying deficiency within the domain of syntax or semantics *per se*.

On visuospatial and quantitative tasks, the HAD and DLD children had scores within the normal range on all measures, while the scores of LAD and NALIQ children were rather evenly depressed. This is consistent with the few studies examining visuospatial abilities in DLD children (Stark *et al.* 1983). The measures employed in the current study would not be expected to identify the deficiency in processing rapid visual information in DLD children reported by Tallal and Stark (1981). In the literature on autism, as well, high-functioning autistic children have been shown to have relatively preserved visual–perceptual and visuospatial abilities (Prior 1979, Lincoln *et al.* 1988, Smalley and Asarnow 1990) and to process pictures in terms of semantic rather than structural content (Pring and Hermelin 1993).

We found visual memory to be impaired in both high-functioning groups, more severely in the HAD than in the DLD group. Verbal memory was more impaired than visual memory in both of these groups, but the DLD children made good use of semantic structure, showing their worst deficits on meaningless material (digits), while the HAD children had the opposite pattern, with their worst deficits on the most highly semantically structured material (stories). Both lower-functioning groups were impaired on all memory tasks, the LAD children showing a more severe impairment on the verbal memory tasks than on the visual memory tasks, whereas the NALIQ children showed equal deficits across visual and verbal memory. The factor analytic findings indicated that, at the age of the current sample, memory functions are not generally independent of the domain of the material to be remembered; for all groups, visual memory loaded with visual tests and verbal memory loaded with language tests.

The finding of deficiency in DLD children's visual memory adds to the small but growing body of evidence that their deficits are not restricted to the language domain. There is ample evidence of difficulty with verbal memory in DLD children, including problems with rehearsal (Kirchner and Klatzky 1985), retrieval (Wiig *et al*. 1982) and preservation of sequence (Graham 1980, Wiig and Semel 1980), but other studies point to difficulty with memory for visual material, as the material becomes complex or lengthy (Wyke and Asso 1979). Note that the visual memory test with the lowest scores was a meaningless visual sequence that is analogous to digit span; perhaps if visual memory had been tested with more meaningful non-arbitrary sequences, the children would have shown the same improvement they showed in the verbal domain when meaning of the items to be remembered increased.

The question of memory in high-functioning autism is under-studied and results are contradictory. Although all studies document verbal deficits, some find that the highest-functioning autistic children can use meaning to aid recall (Fyffe and Prior 1978), but others find this ability to be deficient (Hermelin and O'Connor 1970, 1975; Waterhouse and Fein 1982; Minshew and Goldstein 1993). Tager-Flusberg (1991) found that autistic children do not tend to use intrinsic semantic organization spontaneously, but, like normal children, can use semantic cues to aid retrieval; this raises the possibility that verbal material is not encoded aberrantly, but that semantic organization is not activated spontaneously by the child during retrieval. Interpretation of findings in visual memory tasks is not yet clear; Ameli *et al*. (1988) described poor memory for meaningless visual material, but Fama *et al*. (1992) and Barth *et al*. (1995) reported normal visual memory in high-functioning autism. Given the small number of studies and the variability in subject selection criteria, ages, levels of function, and methods and stimuli for testing memory, these contradictions are not surprising. The current study does suggest the presence of visual memory deficiencies in HAD children, but the complex questions of autistic memory remain to be resolved.

The HAD children, as a group, showed a profile of skills on motor tasks similar to that of the DLD group, but they were worse across-the-board than the DLD children. Both groups showed a small but significant motor impairment, relative to norms, that was greater in the right hand. Both autistic groups, relative to their comparison groups, showed some deficits in praxis. The finding of deficits in motor speed and praxis in the HAD children is consistent with previous reports of motor planning deficits summarized by Huebner (1992). The NALIQ children showed bilateral motor difficulties not attributable to their lower MA alone. Factor analyses for all groups showed a clear and distinct motor factor that was largely independent of cognitive skills. Even for the total sample, where only two factors appeared, one represented all cognitive skills, and one represented motor skill. The motor asymmetry, with both DLD and HAD children showing greater impairment in the right hand, is provocative in terms of lateralized impairment, but must be viewed cautiously, because examination of the group means reveals that these differences are statistical and rather subtle, and may be of little clinical significance in any given case. The neurologists did not find right/left differences in either gross or fine motor skill, but previous research has shown that pegboard tests may be more sensitive for detecting mild motor deficits in children than the clinical neurological examination (Rapin *et al.* 1966).

Previous factor analyses of intellectual abilities, as measured by WISC-R subtests, in high-functioning autism suggested a factor for verbal skills and a factor for visuomotor skills, similar to the factor structure for normal children (Lincoln *et al.* 1988). The current study, using more varied measures and examining the factor structure with diagnostic groups, yielded more refined information. Factor analyses of the cognitive battery for each group showed at least one factor for language, one for visuospatial and quantitative function, and one for motor speed. The HAD group's language factor split into two, one primarily representing lexical semantic verbal memory functions, and one representing formulated output and verbal reasoning. The DLD children's visuospatial factor split into two, with one factor representing visuospatial problem solving, and one representing attention to visual detail. The LAD children's language and visuospatial factors split into three: one representing visual and language problem solving, one representing simpler language functions, and one representing attention to visual detail. Thus, the exploratory factor analyses support the traditional distinction between motor, visual and language processing in all groups, but do not support the separation of verbal memory from other verbal functions, or the separation of visual memory from other visual functions, at least at the developmental levels tested. Factor analyses of the cognitive battery administered to the children at school age may support these further distinctions in a set of hierarchically arranged factors. The current factor solutions, if valid, support the notion that the DLD children, as a group, may have a single underlying verbal factor influencing the severity of their language disorder, while the HAD children have separable deficits of more strictly linguistic lexical/semantic and verbal memory functions and of more conceptual and formulated language. As just pointed out, the finding of a single large language factor in DLD does not preclude the existence of weaker or less prevalent dissociable language deficits in subgroups of DLD children.

The Vineland—the parent report instrument presented in this chapter—is quite consistent with formally tested functions, in both communication/language and motor skills. There were a few exceptions, for example parents reported that their children's receptive language was superior to their expressive skills, an impression that data from the formal tests did not support. Nonetheless, the overall consistency across domains of measurement supports the reliability and validity of both the formal test measures and the parent reports.

## Clinical implications

Neuropsychological findings have at least two kinds of clinical utility. First, finding that a child shows a specific pattern of strengths and weaknesses may tend to confirm or refute a diagnosis under consideration. Although the diagnosis of autism rests primarily on behavioral manifestations, a child may manifest a cognitive pattern typical or atypical for that disorder. In contrast, the DLD children, as a group, showed no distinctive pattern on the tests used within the language domain, although there was some indication that they may have had mild deficits in the development of the functional use of expressive language, and that written language deficits may emerge in the early school years. Uneven abilities did appear, however, in the overall relationship of verbal, nonverbal, memory and motor functions. Second, the strengths and weaknesses of children in any diagnostic group may lead to specific recommendations, especially in educational practices.

The most noteworthy aspect of the group language profiles was the difficulty the high-functioning autistic children had with verbal fluency and with comprehension measures, and their relative sparing of written language and confrontation naming. Although analysis of individual differences is not presented here, clinical experience confirms the validity of these findings; autistic children with large discrepancies in favor of expressive over receptive vocabulary (as measured by formal testing) are common in clinical practice, as are autistic children with sparing of written over oral language, including the extreme case of hyperlexia. Such sparing of written language and confrontation naming in the face of severe deficits in meaningful communication are often taken by the diagnostician as a sign of high-functioning autism, and thus tend to constitute 'bad' diagnostic news, rather than the sign of spared intelligence that parents often hope that it represents. The extent to which the sparing of written language can lead to a channel for truly meaningful communication awaits follow-up studies. The HAD children were also found to be especially deficient on tasks requiring the child to formulate and produce connected speech, such as explaining the meanings of words or absurdities. This is also confirmed by clinical practice, where autistic children are often observed to find it very difficult to put their knowledge into an organized, fluent and accurate verbal output.

Diagnosis of the severely affected LAD child is, unfortunately, often clearer than the diagnosis of the HAD child. Current results do suggest that even for these difficult-to-test children, superiority in nonverbal over verbal scores and marked superiority of confrontation naming over receptive vocabulary may be more consistent with LAD than with NALIQ and may thus support a diagnosis of AD.

In analysis of spontaneous discourse, HAD children initiated as many utterances to the adults as did the DLD children, but they responded less to the adults' initiations and made more meaning and pragmatic errors, while the LAD children were severely impaired on almost all measures. Echolalia marked the utterances of the LAD children, but did not differentiate the HAD from DLD children. These findings also serve to quantify somewhat the clinical impression of abnormal interaction with HAD children. The current findings are, however, probably an underestimate of these abnormalities, since they did not involve observation of peer interactions, and since the adults in the interaction, in an effort to maximize language, tended to follow the children's conversational lead rather than try to keep them focused on topics of the adult's choosing. In clinical evaluation, it is important both to gauge the child's pragmatic competence in situations that maximize that competence, on topics of interest to the child, and to stress pragmatic skills by trying to get the child to address topics of more conventional interest introduced by the adult. Assessment of the child in these situations will identify types of inadequacies (topic shifting, personal distance, inadequate eye contact, failure to respond, restricted and perseverative usages, etc.) that can be addressed in language therapy.

Verbal memory tests can also help to differentiate cognitive patterns typical of either DLD or HAD. Memory deficits that are ameliorated by an increase of semantic organization are more characteristic of DLD children, while memory deficits that are essentially unaided by the semantic content are more characteristic of HAD children. The HAD children seem not to focus their attention automatically on the meaning of verbal input, as do normal and even DLD children. They may therefore benefit from training that focuses them on the meaning of what is said, such as visualizing or drawing scenes of short verbal passages, or restating the most essential elements of these passages.

Motor testing indicated that both HAD and DLD children had motor deficits, especially in gross motor abilities, that were more consistent with their language deficits than with their NVIQ. LAD children had functional motor deficits consistent with their cognitive impairment, and NALIQ children tended to have motor deficits even greater than their cognitive disability. While these were not optimally detailed motor examinations, results strongly suggest the value of a detailed motor examination in children with language disorders, autism or mental retardation who might benefit from the provision of occupational therapy targeted to the mitigation of the functional consequences of specific motor deficits.

Results of factor analyses must be regarded as preliminary, since they resulted from exploratory analyses and have not been replicated. If confirmed, they might suggest that clinical evaluations of the abilities of DLD children include a separate estimate of children's visuospatial abilities and their accurate attention to visual detail, whereas clinical evaluations of HAD children focus on lexical abilities as distinct from ability to formulate verbal output.

In terms of educational practice, an important cautionary note for teachers and parents is not to overestimate an autistic child's language ability from high scores or obvious strengths on naming or reading. A child with a tested comprehension ability of 3 years, but naming skill equivalent to that of a 6-year-old and reading decoding skill equivalent to that of a 9-year-old still has very limited comprehension, and must be given verbal input carefully tailored in content and structure to his true comprehension level.

# 8
# BEHAVIOR SCALES

*L. Waterhouse and D.A. Allen*

Documenting children's behavioral development is best done by formal observation coupled with structured assessment (Lord *et al*. 1994). However, for behaviors which are expressed only within narrow developmental windows or infrequently in the child's repertoire, reasonable time constraints in testing preclude efforts to document them. When interview raters forget instances of behavior, and consequently fail to endorse interview items, the child's behavioral repertoire will be reported as more limited than it is. When interviewers are over- or under-inclusive in generalizing across instances, they may characterize the pattern of the child's behavioral expression inaccurately. Finally, because interviewers or raters may have a constrained range of experience of child development, their judgment of qualitative features of behavior may reflect idiosyncratic or training biases of interpretation based on these constraints (Stone and Rosenbaum 1988). Despite these limitations, carefully obtained interview and rating data are an important adjunct to data obtained through testing and structured observation.

There were many important developmental behaviors of children in this study that we could not observe or assess in a structured fashion. To document these behaviors, we used behavior interview and clinical rating scales and asked parents and teachers about their observational experience with the children. We also asked child psychiatrists to fill out two rating scales on each child they interviewed.

Interview and rating instruments have significant limitations. First, they require that interviewers or raters recall specific instances of the child's behavior. Second, they require them to generalize about these events. Third, they may require raters to judge qualitative features of behavior. These three processes potentially yield three types of problems in validity.

## Method

We employed three interview measures: the Wing Autistic Disorders Interview Checklist (WADIC—Appendix 1); the Vineland Adaptive Behavior Scales—Interview Edition (Sparrow *et al*. 1984)*; and the Wing Schedule of Handicaps, Behaviour and Skills (HBS—Appendix 5). In addition to these measures, we employed a clinical rating scale, the Social Abnormalities Scales I and II (Appendix 2). These instruments and the administration procedures used have been described in detail in Chapter 4.

---

*In most cases the mother filled out the WADIC and was interviewed with the Vineland, but in a few cases it was the child's teacher who provided the information.

**TABLE 8.1**
**Autistic behaviors endorsed by parents on the WADIC, by group***

| Area of problem | DLD (N=201) % | HAD (N=51) % | LAD (N=125) % | NALIQ (N=110) % |
|---|---|---|---|---|
| A. Social Interaction | | | | |
| Non-verbal communication | 9 | 90 | 86 | 17 |
| Joint attention | 14 | 98 | 96 | 34 |
| Greeting | 11 | 80 | 93 | 20 |
| Comfort seeking | 6 | 63 | 64 | 15 |
| Giving comfort | 6 | 80 | 77 | 18 |
| Imitation | 6 | 84 | 90 | 22 |
| Friends | 8 | 90 | 86 | 21 |
| Pretend play | 11 | 88 | 86 | 25 |
| Social rule use | 8 | 61 | 74 | 21 |
| B. Communication | | | | |
| Pragmatics | 8 | 84 | 91 | 26 |
| Comprehension | 19 | 84 | 87 | 34 |
| Speech mechanics | 19 | 84 | 50 | 24 |
| Prosody | 15 | 63 | 37 | 15 |
| Abstract language | 13 | 90 | 70 | 29 |
| C. Activity | | | | |
| Motor stereotypies | 7 | 61 | 81 | 23 |
| Sensory motor behaviors | 4 | 22 | 56 | 20 |
| Object perseverations | 10 | 61 | 64 | 15 |
| Maintaining sameness | 1 | 16 | 20 | 4 |
| Routines fixed | 3 | 39 | 26 | 5 |
| Perseverative interests | 9 | 51 | 18 | 10 |
| Empty life | 0 | 31 | 28 | 4 |

*All four-way group differences significant at $p < 0.05$.

## Findings

Tables 8.1–8.12 present findings provided by the five behavior scales and contrast the views of parents, psychiatrists and teachers of the children.

*Parents' views*

WING AUTISTIC DISORDERS INTERVIEW CHECKLIST

Table 8.1 presents the comparative frequency of behaviors endorsed by parents on the WADIC. All 21 items across the three domains—impaired social interaction, impaired communication, and impaired activities—discriminated the four study groups significantly. The total number of checks across all groups fell into a bimodal distribution, with most of the children in both autistic groups (HAD and LAD) being highly deficient and far fewer children in the two non-autistic groups (DLD, NALIQ) being deficient. This finding suggests that the distinction of autistic *vs* non-autistic is not an arbitrary cut in some larger continuum of DLD, NALIQ, HAD and LAD. The WADIC thus is a questionnaire that separates two groups, autistic from non-autistic.

A substantial majority (61–98 per cent) of both HAD and LAD children were reported to have impairment in each of the nine skills in the Social domain, *viz.* (A1) nonverbal interaction; (A2) social play; (A3) greeting behavior; (A4) comfort seeking behavior; (A5) giving comfort; (A6) imitation; (A7) making friends; (A8) pretend play; and (A9) social rule use. The most consistent abnormalities noted in both groups were in the areas of nonverbal communication, joint attention and social play, imitation and peer relationships.

Likewise, a majority (63–90 per cent) of HAD children were impaired in the five items of the Communication domain: (B1) pragmatics; (B2) comprehension; (B3) speech mechanisms; (B4) prosody; and (B5) symbolizing skills in language. A majority of LAD children were stated to have impairment in pragmatics, comprehension and symbolizing skills in language. The low percentage of deficits in prosody (37 per cent) and poor speech articulation reflects the large number of nonverbal or minimally verbal LAD children (see Table 6.9, p. 112).

A majority of both the HAD and LAD children were reported to experience two areas of dysfunction in their activities: (C1) motor stereotypies; and (C2) perseveration with objects. The HAD and LAD groups differed in that high rates of sensorimotor abnormalities were reported for the LAD but not the HAD children, while high rates of obsessive or perseverative interests were reported for the HAD but not the LAD children. Surprisingly, one behavior often identified as diagnostic of autism—insistence on maintenance of sameness in the environment—was reported for very few HAD (16 per cent) or LAD (20 per cent) children. It may be that this behavior appears later in the course of development.

In contrast to the findings for HAD and LAD children, the parents of the DLD and NALIQ children endorsed no more than a small percentage of items across the WADIC. The range for DLD is 0–19 per cent, and that for NALIQ is 4–34 per cent.

Parents of DLD children reported that between 6 and 14 per cent of their children experienced problems in the Social domain. The highest level (14 per cent) of endorsement of dysfunction appeared for item (A2), social play. In the Communication domain it is somewhat surprising that, for each of the five items listed, parents of fewer than 20 per cent of the DLD children reported impairment. This low level of endorsement may be attributable to the fact that the intent of the checklist is the identification of children with autistic behaviors and not those with non-autistic language disorders. Since the parents or caretakers of all the DLD children in the study had identified them as having moderate to severe language disorders, they may have interpreted the WADIC Communication items as identifying more severe communicative impairments than their children's, or may have endorsed one but not other aspects of language dysfunction.

Few parents of children in the DLD group reported impairments in interests and motor behaviors. None reported their child to have a life without interests, but 10 per cent reported that their child had perseverative or repeated behaviors with unusual objects, and 7 per cent reported motor stereotypies. This is in contrast to parents of the three other study groups. 23 per cent of NALIQ children's parents reported them to have motor stereotypies, as did 61 per cent of parents of HAD children and 81 per cent of parents of LAD children.

## TABLE 8.2
**Vineland Adaptive Behavior Scales interview form administered to mothers of subjects: standard scores for four domains and composite score***

| | DLD | | HAD | | LAD | | NALIQ | |
|---|---|---|---|---|---|---|---|---|
| | Mean | (SD) | Mean | (SD) | Mean | (SD) | Mean | (SD) |
| Communication domain | 78.90 | (12.15) (N=197) | 79.70 | (20.39) (N=50) | 52.70 | (13.32) (N=125) | 63.29 | (12.16) (N=103) |
| Daily Living domain | 84.85 | (14.62) (N=197) | 69.76 | (14.95) (N=50) | 51.49 | (15.95) (N=125) | 64.39 | (14.75) (N=103) |
| Socialization domain | 85.12 | (13.11) (N=197) | 69.04 | (12.28) (N=50) | 55.84 | (9.36) (N=125) | 68.90 | (11.59) (N=103) |
| Motor Skills domain | 84.62 | (17.11) (N=190) | 79.14 | (15.40) (N=37) | 58.85 | (14.08) (N=87) | 62.13 | (13.33) (N=84) |
| Composite score | 78.97 | (12.82) (N=197) | 68.52 | (13.75) (N=50) | 49.37 | (11.03) (N=125) | 59.41 | (10.40) (N=103) |

*All four-way group differences significant at $p<0.05$.

## TABLE 8.3
**Vineland Adaptive Behavior Scales interview form administered to mothers of subjects: ratio scores for subdomains of the Communication domain***

| | DLD (N=197) | | HAD (N=50) | | LAD (N=125) | | NALIQ (N=103) | |
|---|---|---|---|---|---|---|---|---|
| | Mean | (SD) | Mean | (SD) | Mean | (SD) | Mean | (SD) |
| Receptive skills | 83.85 | (24.83) | 72.60 | (33.34) | 35.82 | (22.01) | 61.80 | (26.11) |
| Expressive skills | 68.46 | (18.55) | 64.74 | (28.16) | 31.50 | (18.91) | 46.91 | (19.00) |
| Written skills | 68.48 | (33.95) | 91.20 | (41.31) | 45.21 | (25.76) | 48.60 | (22.73) |

*All four-way group differences significant at $p<0.05$.

## TABLE 8.4
**Vineland Adaptive Behavior Scale interview form administered to mothers of subjects: ratio scores for subdomains of the Daily Living domain***

| | DLD (N=197) | | HAD (N=50) | | LAD (N=125) | | NALIQ (N=103) | |
|---|---|---|---|---|---|---|---|---|
| | Mean | (SD) | Mean | (SD) | Mean | (SD) | Mean | (SD) |
| Personal skills | 104.01 | (19.06) | 68.46 | (18.79) | 47.08 | (16.59) | 60.43 | (18.87) |
| Domestic skills | 100.41 | (20.47) | 68.90 | (22.08) | 46.21 | (19.67) | 61.74 | (21.72) |
| Community skills | 79.17 | (22.22) | 59.90 | (24.73) | 33.74 | (17.96) | 53.18 | (24.49) |

*All four-way group differences significant at $p<0.05$.

158

Parents of NALIQ study subjects did endorse social impairments as characteristic of their children, but on no item did more than a third of them identify their children as impaired. 15 per cent endorsed the item 'failure to seek comfort', and 34 per cent endorsed 'impairment to social play' for their children.

In summary, most of the features of behavior included in the Social and Communication domains typified a majority of both HAD and LAD children. Their parents also reported that a majority of them had motor stereotypies and object perseveration. In contrast, a majority of the parents of the DLD and NALIQ subjects did not identify their children as having these developmental problems. It may seem surprising that many parents of DLD children failed to characterize them as having difficulty in communication, but this may be due to the fact that DLD children did not have the kinds of language impairments typical of autistic children described in the WADIC. More than half of these parents apparently did not see salient language impairment in their DLD children, even though those children had been identified by clinicians as having language disorders.

VINELAND ADAPTIVE BEHAVIOR SCALES (ABS)

Tables 8.2–8.5 present data from the Vineland ABS. These scales were administered in interview form to parents of all study children in all study groups. All inter-group comparisons were significant at the p≤0.01 level.

Table 8.2 presents the standard scores and standard deviations for the four domains of the Vineland ABS and the composite score for all four domains. The pattern of standard scores and the composite score is as follows: DLD>HAD>NALIQ>LAD. [There was only one exception to this: in the Communication domain, the HAD children had a mean standard score (79.70) almost equal to that of the DLD children (78.90), explainable due to the relative HAD weakness in receptive and expressive skills but relative strength in written skills (see below).] Composite scores of the four study groups were quite evenly distributed along a developmental continuum: the mean standard score of DLD children was close to 80 (78.97), compared to a standard score of 100 for normal peers of their chronological age; the mean score of HAD children was nearly 70 (68.52), that of NALIQ children was just under 60 (59.41) and that of LAD children just under 50 (49.37). The NALIQ children had slightly more advanced development in interpersonal skills than the HAD children, despite their lower intellectual level.

Group comparisons of raw scores within subdomains generally showed the same pattern (DLD>HAD>NALIQ>LAD). However, there were some variations in this picture. HAD children were reported to have better writing skill than DLD children (Table 8.3). NALIQ children were reported to have slightly more advanced development in interpersonal skills than HAD children (NALIQ = 53.09, HAD = 49.10), even though HAD children had higher NVIQs than NALIQ children (Table 8.4). The highest rates of endorsement for the DLD children occurred on language comprehension and the production of intelligible and syntactically correct speech, whereas the LAD children were most frequently reported to express poor joint attention and social play, impaired language comprehension, symbolic function and pretend play, and inappropriate pragmatic use of language.

159

**TABLE 8.5**
**Study subjects raw scores on the Vineland Maladaptive Behaviors Scales areas I and II**
**administered to mothers of subjects in interview***

|  | DLD | | HAD | | LAD | | NALIQ | |
|---|---|---|---|---|---|---|---|---|
|  | Mean | (SD) | Mean | (SD) | Mean | (SD) | Mean | (SD) |
| I: Maladaptive behaviors | 9.21 | (5.79) (N=38) | 11.67 | (7.43) (N=33) | 15.22 | (7.42) (N=82) | 9.63 | (6.82) (N=49) |
| II: Maladaptive thought processes | 0.74 | (1.36) (N=34) | 3.38 | (3.33) (N=32) | 4.66 | (3.35) (N=74) | 1.20 | (1.71) (N=44) |

*All four-way group differences significant at p<0.05.

Mean raw scores for the Motor subdomain, presented in Table 7.7 (p. 142) and discussed in Chapter 7, again rank the children in the same way: DLD>HAD>NALIQ>LAD. This report corresponds in broad outline with the findings of the neurological examination for fine motor and gross motor skills (Table 6.3, p. 103). In accordance with parents' reports, the cognitively disadvantaged LAD and NALIQ children generally performed less well than DLD and HAD children on gross and, especially, fine motor tasks, with the LAD group inferior to all groups.

Many parents reported themselves unable to remember times of gross motor milestones for their children other than age of walking (see Tables 5.14 and 5.15, pp. 77–78). As can be seen in Table 5.14, age of walking was delayed in the LAD and NALIQ groups but not in the DLD and HAD groups. Parental report on developmental history of the child is thus in line with parental report on the Vineland, where parents of LAD and NALIQ children reported less maturity of gross and fine motor development than did parents of HAD and DLD children.

On the Vineland ABS Maladaptive Scales I and II, both HAD and LAD groups had significantly higher scores than those of the DLD and NALIQ groups; NALIQ children had slightly higher scores than DLD children (Table 8.5). Overall, psychiatrists endorsed many more items on Scale I, which describes developmentally abnormal behaviors, than on Scale II, which asks about aberrant thought processes.

Comparing the reports of parents of AD children on the Vineland ABS, which focuses on the acquisition of normal behavioral skills, with their reports on the WADIC, which focuses on aberrant behaviors, revealed interesting group differences. Although parents of HAD subjects reported their children to be more advanced in the four Vineland ABS domains than did parents of LAD children, both sets of parents reported social and communication abnormalities on the WADIC which on most items were roughly comparable.

In summary, parents of DLD children reported fewer problems on the WADIC than did parents of children in all three other study groups. Compared to parents of NALIQ, LAD and HAD children, parents of DLD children reported the highest developmental levels for their children on the Vineland ABS. Parents of NALIQ subjects identified their children (on the Vineland ABS) as developmentally more advanced than did parents of LAD children. Moreover, parents of NALIQ children endorsed relatively few specific abnormalities for their children on either the Vineland ABS Maladaptive Scales or the WADIC.

*Psychiatrists' views*

SOCIAL ABNORMALITIES SCALES I AND II

Psychiatrists, who evaluated only children who obtained two or more checks in Area A or at least one in each of Areas A, B and C of the WADIC, completed the Social Abnormalities Scales I and II (Tables 8.6 and 8.7) immediately after observing and interviewing each child in a standard psychiatric clinical evaluation session. Each of the 21 items discriminated the four study groups (DLD, HAD, LAD, NALIQ); all chi squared comparisons are at the p≤0.01 level. The strongest discrimination is between the autistic/non-autistic groups. The psychiatrists endorsed very few social abnormalities in either the DLD or NALIQ groups (see below). In the aggregate, more LAD than HAD children were reported to exhibit social abnormalities, but there were exceptions. There was essentially no difference between the LAD and HAD groups on 'excessive fears', 'unusual preoccupations', 'echolalic', and 'overstimulated in social contexts', and a marginal difference on 'clingy/dependent'. They differed most on 'in a shell', 'unaware of social rules', 'lacks empathy', 'doesn't discriminate strangers' and 'obsessive rituals'. Highest endorsement rates for the HAD children were on 'cannot hold a conversation', 'unmotivated emotional outbursts', 'aberrant eye contact', 'lacks empathy' and 'unusual preoccupations'.

The psychiatrists evaluated the subsample of DLD and NALIQ children who had received two or more checks in area A or at least one each in areas A, B and C of the WADIC at initial sample screening as less impaired than did their parents. Ratings by psychiatrists for DLD children ranged from zero (for nine of 21 items), to 16 per cent (for the item 'cannot hold a conversation'). Note that in the DLD subsample the psychiatrists rated included only 37 children, which is less than 20 per cent of the total sample of 201 DLD children. Because the psychiatrists determined that these 37 children did not express symptoms or behaviors characteristic of autism, the children remained in the DLD sample for the study.

Child psychiatrists also rated the subset of 42 NALIQ children (40 per cent of the sample of 110 children) described in Tables 8.6 and 8.7 because they had sufficient numbers of items endorsed by their parents in the initial WADIC screening. As with the DLD subsample they evaluated, psychiatrists rated these 42 NALIQ children as having few autistic symptoms or behaviors. They were not diagnosed as autistic and remained in the NALIQ sample.

There were six of the 21 items on the Social Abnormalities Scales I and II that psychiatrists endorsed in none of the NALIQ children. These were: (i) ignores people; (ii) withdraws from touch; (iii) prefers to be alone; (iv) socializes with mother only; (v) distant while talking; and (vi) has obsessive rituals. On the other hand, they reported that 26 per cent of NALIQ children 'cannot hold a conversation', 12 per cent 'seem unaware of social rules', and 10 per cent 'are clingy and dependent.' In general, psychiatrists

TABLE 8.6
**Psychiatrists' endorsements of abnormalities on the Social
Abnormalities Scale I\***

|  | DLD (N=37) % | HAD (N=50) % | LAD (N=121) % | NALIQ (N=42) % |
|---|---|---|---|---|
| 1. 'In a shell' | 0 | 26 | 69 | 2 |
| 2. Ignores people | 0 | 8 | 43 | 0 |
| 3. Withdraws from touch | 3 | 10 | 29 | 0 |
| 4. Prefers to be alone | 0 | 16 | 44 | 0 |
| 5. Uses others for needs | 3 | 11 | 41 | 2 |
| 6. Aberrant eye contact | 0 | 44 | 68 | 2 |
| 7. Lacks empathy | 5 | 43 | 78 | 5 |
| 8. Never initiates interaction | 8 | 34 | 69 | 5 |
| 9. Doesn't discriminate strangers | 8 | 6 | 40 | 5 |
| 10. Sociable with mother only | 0 | 23 | 52 | 0 |
| 11. Unmotivated emotional outbursts | 10 | 46 | 65 | 9 |

\*All four-way group differences significant at p<0.05.

**TABLE 8.7**
**Psychiatrists' endorsements of abnormalities on the Social
Abnormalities Scale II\***

|  | DLD (N=37) % | HAD (N=50) % | LAD (N=121) % | NALIQ (N=42) % |
|---|---|---|---|---|
| 1. Excessive fears | 0 | 19 | 20 | 5 |
| 2. Unaware of social rules | 3 | 31 | 70 | 12 |
| 3. Unusual preoccupations | 8 | 40 | 47 | 5 |
| 4. No social modesty | 0 | 9 | 29 | 8 |
| 5. Clingy/dependent | 3 | 23 | 35 | 10 |
| 6. Echolalic | 0 | 31 | 31 | 5 |
| 7. Distant while talking | 0 | 30 | 58 | 0 |
| 8. Overstimulated in social contexts | 6 | 29 | 31 | 3 |
| 9. Cannot hold conversation | 16 | 53 | 79 | 26 |
| 10. Obsessive rituals | 3 | 26 | 60 | 0 |

\*All four-way group differences significant at p<0.05.

reported that only a few NALIQ children expressed any of the other abnormalities
indexed by the Social Abnormalities Scales.

In summary, psychiatrists evaluated 42 NALIQ and 37 DLD children whose parents
endorsed more than two items in Area A or at least one in each of Areas A, B and C of
the WADIC. Psychiatrists did not find these children to have a range of social abnormalities that was sufficient to identify them as autistic. In order to increase the reliability of
this finding, videotapes of a clinical play session of these children were viewed by a

second child psychiatrist who evaluated them blind to the child's diagnosis. There was 100 per cent agreement between first and second child psychiatrists. In general, psychiatrists reported a lower prevalence of specific social and communication dysfunctions for DLD and NALIQ children than did their parents. The psychiatrists also identified fewer social abnormalities and aberrant behaviors in the HAD and LAD groups than did the parents of those children. Even though the 21 items of the WADIC and the 21 items of the Social Abnormalities Scales I and II cannot be paired for content, the two sets of terms contain comparable information. Thus we conclude that there were distinct differences in assessment of abnormalities when the ratings of parents and psychiatrists are compared.

It is worth bringing out the parallel between the study neurologists and psychiatrists, both of which had a higher threshold for behavioral abnormalities than parents. There are at least three possible reasons for this. The first has to do with sampling: psychiatrists (and neurologists) spent only 30–60 minutes in the process of psychiatric (neurological) evaluation; therefore, their experience of the child was narrow. Second, because parents have a social and emotional relationship with their child, it is likely that parents feel the lack of normal interaction and the presence of bizarre and disruptive behaviors more keenly than would a physician. A possible third reason why parents saw their children as more impaired than did child psychiatrists and neurologists is the difference between parents and physicians in their background bases of comparison. Child psychiatrists and neurologists see a great variety of children—including severely mentally retarded and emotionally and neurologically disabled children. This range of clinical experience is likely to be far wider than the experience of most parents or caretakers. The effect of clinical experience may be to place a given child's behavior in a wider context of impairment, and thus reduce the judgment of severity of symptom expression. Nevertheless, as parents have access to such a rich sample of the child's behaviors, physicians are well advised to give more weight for diagnosis to parental reports than to the necessarily restricted observations they can make in their offices.

*Teachers' view*
WING SCHEDULE OF HANDICAPS, BEHAVIOURS AND SKILLS
Tables 8.8–8.12 outline responses of the children's teachers to the HBS. In large part, these data confirm the picture created by the reports of parents and the rating of the child psychiatrists.

There were some surprising findings, however. Teachers reported that 50 per cent of HAD children and 68 per cent of LAD children had age appropriate intonation patterns (Table 8.8). These teacher endorsements are different from those of parents to a slightly different but related item on the WADIC (Table 8.1). On the WADIC, 63 per cent of parents of HAD children reported that their children had impaired intonation patterns, while only 37 per cent of LAD parents reported such problems for their children. This teacher report also differed from the neurologists' perceptions: according to the neurologists, two thirds of verbal children in both autistic groups had aberrant prosody (Table 6.9, p. 112). It may be that the wording of the specific question in the two instruments

163

**TABLE 8.8**

**Handicaps, Behaviour and Skills Schedule: teacher judgments of study subjects' language development (percentage judged to have age-normal skills)***

| Item (#) | DLD (N=174) % | HAD (N=50) % | LAD (N=121) % | NALIQ (N=104) % |
|---|---|---|---|---|
| Comprehension (7a) | 73 | 35 | 9 | 32 |
| Grammar (8a) | 63 | 44 | 14 | 35 |
| Question formation (8b) | 74 | 52 | 18 | 54 |
| Intonation patterns (11g) | 96 | 50 | 68 | 90 |
| Articulation (8c) | 25 | 55 | 19 | 26 |

*All four-way group differences significant at p<0.05.

**TABLE 8.9**

**Handicaps, Behaviour and Skills Schedule: teacher judgments of study subjects' social development (percentage judged to have age-normal skills)***

| Item (#) | DLD (N=174) % | HAD (N=50) % | LAD (N=121) % | NALIQ (N=104) % |
|---|---|---|---|---|
| Display of affection (20a) | 95 | 80 | 88 | 89 |
| Friendships (20b) | 98 | 67 | 39 | 86 |
| Social play (21a) | 98 | 80 | 55 | 89 |
| Self-recognition (15k) | 98 | 100 | 66 | 90 |
| General sociability (22a) | 93 | 54 | 28 | 86 |

*All four-way group differences significant at p<0.05.

led parents and teachers to base their ratings or judgments on different experiences or different aspects of children's expressive language.

It was interesting to find that teachers judged 88 per cent of LAD children to be affectionate (Table 8.9), even though they judged only half of the HAD children and one quarter of the LAD children to be sociable. Unfortunately, because this question was not asked in the same manner on any other rating or interview instrument, we could not directly compare data on this item with data collected on other instruments.

Teachers reported that more DLD and NALIQ children showed normal communication skills than did HAD and LAD children (Table 8.10). In particular, they saw more NALIQ children as normal in a variety of communication skills than HAD children. Teachers (Table 8.11), as did neurologists (Table 6.10, p. 114), reported a fairly high frequency of echolalia in both the HAD and LAD groups (delayed echolalia—teachers: HAD = 51 per cent and LAD = 41 per cent; neurologists: HAD = 36 per cent, LAD = 53 per cent). Teachers also reported pronoun reversal (HAD = 39 per cent, LAD = 37 per cent), a feature of autistic speech neurologists failed to report. In contrast to their statements about autistic children, teachers reported delayed echolalia in only 3 per cent of

**TABLE 8.10**

**Handicaps, Behaviour and Skills Schedule: teacher judgments of study subjects' nonverbal communication (percentage judged to have age-normal skills)***

| Item (#) | DLD (N=174) % | HAD (N=50) % | LAD (N=121) % | NALIQ (N=104) % |
|---|---|---|---|---|
| Symbolic gestures (13b) | 84 | 30 | 14 | 54 |
| Facial expression (13c) | 79 | 32 | 27 | 53 |
| Eye contact (19a) | 89 | 26 | 17 | 67 |
| Communication initiation (14b) | 93 | 66 | 32 | 80 |
| Story-telling (14c) | 94 | 58 | 27 | 80 |

*All four-way group differences significant at $p < 0.05$.

**TABLE 8.11**

**Handicaps, Behaviour and Skills Schedule: teacher judgments of study subjects' abnormal communication (percentage judged to have abnormal communication)***

| Item (#) | DLD (N=174) % | HAD (N=50) % | LAD (N=121) % | NALIQ (N=104) % |
|---|---|---|---|---|
| Immediate echolalia (11a) | 2 | 39 | 33 | 11 |
| Delayed echolalia (11b) | 3 | 51 | 38 | 6 |
| Pronoun reversal (11c) | 5 | 39 | 37 | 8 |

*All four-way group differences significant at $p < 0.05$.

**TABLE 8.12**

**Handicaps, Behaviour and Skills Schedule: teacher judgments of study subjects' abnormal behaviors (percentage judged to express abnormal behaviors)***

| Item (#) | DLD (N=174) % | HAD (N=50) % | LAD (N=121) % | NALIQ (N=104) % |
|---|---|---|---|---|
| Distress at sounds (23a) | 9 | 28 | 45 | 23 |
| Obsessed with sounds (23b) | 2 | 10 | 34 | 5 |
| Attracted to lights (24a) | 2 | 10 | 34 | 5 |
| Obsessive interest in spinning objects (24b) | 4 | 26 | 50 | 9 |
| Spinning self (26c) | 5 | 18 | 29 | 3 |
| Self-injurious behavior (25g) | 2 | 6 | 22 | 7 |
| Resistant to change (27a) | 17 | 68 | 65 | 22 |

*All four-way group differences significant at $p < 0.05$.

DLD and 6 per cent of NALIQ children (neurologists: DLD = 9 per cent, NALIQ = 26 per cent) and pronoun reversal in only 5 per cent of DLD and 8 per cent of NALIQ children (neurologists: 0 per cent for both groups).

Teachers stated that more HAD and LAD than non-autistic children were unusually sensitive to features of the environment, or unusually interested in objects and sounds (Table 8.12). They also identified a majority of HAD and LAD children as resistant to change (HAD = 68 per cent; LAD = 65 per cent). Teachers reported a higher level of self-injurious behavior for LAD children (22 per cent) than for any other study group (HAD = 6 per cent; DLD = 2 per cent; NALIQ = 7 per cent).

In summary, teachers' descriptions of children's behaviors, as witnessed in the classroom, supported the picture of abnormal and normal developmental behaviors reported by parents and child psychiatrists on our other interview and rating scales.

## Discussion

Taken together, the findings from the three behavioral instruments (WADIC, HBS, Vineland) and the clinical rating scale (Social Abnormalities Scales I and II) yielded a picture of severe social and behavioral abnormality and developmental delay for the LAD sample, and a relative absence of abnormal social and motor behaviors in the DLD sample. Moreover, the DLD sample approached normal levels of adaptive skill development. The HAD sample was reported by parents and teachers and described by psychiatrists as exhibiting severe social and emotional abnormalities. The NALIQ sample was seen as significantly developmentally delayed, but with fewer of the social, emotional or motor abnormalities of the LAD and HAD children. The observed differences between our AD and NALIQ samples parallel the findings of previous studies that have described greater social impairment in autistic than in mentally retarded children (DeMyer *et al.* 1972, Wing and Gould 1979, Freeman *et al.* 1981).

Our observation of a wide range of social and communication impairments in autism is consonant with most studies of the behavioral characteristics of high- and low-functioning autistic individuals (Rutter 1974; Bartak and Rutter 1976; Wing and Gould 1979; Lord 1985; Prior and Werry 1986; Waterhouse *et al.* 1987; Bryson *et al.* 1988; Rutter and Schopler 1988; Wing 1988; Braverman *et al.* 1989; Gillberg 1990, 1992; Frith 1991; Tsai 1992). Variant patterns of social development, yet with some similarities of language impairment, in autistic and language disordered children, are also consonant with the findings of previous studies comparing those two clinical groups (Bartak *et al.* 1975, 1977; Cohen *et al.* 1976; Cantwell *et al.* 1978; Rutter 1979; Udwin and Yule 1983; Paul and Cohen 1984*b*; Tuchman *et al.* 1991*a*; Allen and Rapin 1992).

We did not find much evidence for symptomatology suggesting psychopathology in the DLD sample (Beitchman *et al.* 1986*a*). Mayes *et al.* (1993) found, in a study of 40 DSM III-R autistic children, 40 PDD-NOS (less classically autistic) children and 40 children with DLDs, that impaired conversational skill was the only point of similarity between PDD-NOS and the DLD children, whereas indices of social deficit, such as withdrawal and the absence of friendships, clearly differentiated these two groups. Our study confirms a clear differentiation between DLD and HAD children.

In the present study we found 11 children among the 201 classified as having DLD who had some autistic features. These features were largely limited to aspects of impaired social communication. The psychiatrists found that these 11 children did not meet diagnostic criteria for DSM III-R Autistic Disorder, nor did they show enough autistic-like features or have social deficits severe enough to place them in the PDD-NOS group. Thus, while essentially all autistic subjects in the present study evidenced some form of language disorder, the children with DLD generally did not express the social impairments associated with autism.

The neurologists and psychiatrists based their diagnostic endorsements on their review of background information and on a clinical interview with the child. The neurologists and psychiatrists endorsed fewer social abnormalities in the autistic children than did the parents and teachers. Thus they had a higher threshold for endorsing social deviance: the one-to-one interaction with an adult in a relatively structured office visit provides an impoverished environment for evaluating sociability, compared to a home or classroom situation. This is why physicians put so much emphasis on historical data, which, as was shown in Chapter 5, supply reliable and highly discriminating diagnostic information, provided the questions probe aspects of behavior covered by autistic questionnaires.

In general, teachers' ratings of the children on the HBS conformed to results from parent's responses to the Vineland interview and the WADIC. A few noteworthy results were that teachers judged 88 per cent of LAD children to be affectionate, they reported a high frequency of echolalia and pronoun reversal in both autistic groups in marked contrast to the non-autistic groups, and they reported many more autistic children (about 66 per cent) as resistant to change than were endorsed on a comparable item on the DSM III-R. Ratings confirmed the sizable superiority of DLD over HAD children in language comprehension and prosody, and the superiority of the HAD children in articulation. Teachers also stressed the special communicative deficits of both autistic groups in use of symbolic gestures, facial expression and eye contact.

These findings raise two questions: (1) what gives rise to the differences in ratings of the same child by different informants?; and (2) how can we summarize behavior patterns for DLD, HAD, LAD and NALIQ children using information from multiple informants?

*Source of discrepancy in ratings*
The most elemental source of discrepancy in the behavioral ratings considered here is that each rater used a different instrument. Different wording of the same question on the four instruments most likely contributed to the differential responses. However, even with identically worded items or the use of a single instrument by the different informants, there are additional sources of variation. Dihoff *et al.* (1993) have argued that ordinal (continuous) diagnostic criteria promote higher levels of diagnostic agreement among professionals than nominal (dichotomous) criteria. The Social Abnormality Scales I and II are nominal. The WADIC is a categorical nominal scale with ordinal developmental item exemplars. The Vineland ABS is developmentally ordinal within

specific nominal domains. The HBS contains nominal items, some of which are coded by developmentally ordinal sub-items and others by general severity (also ordinal).

It may be more difficult to find inter-rater agreement for ordinal symptom severity than for ordinal scales based on development because severity may be indexed quantitatively by the presence of a greater or lesser number of instances of a behavior, qualitatively by an intensity range, or quasi-categorically by shifts in the form of expression of a behavior. In accord with this, Szatmari *et al.* (1994) found that there was good agreement between parents and teachers on the Vineland ABS ordinal developmental scales, but virtually no agreement between parents' and teachers' ratings of PDD children on the Autistic Behavior Checklist (ABC) (Aman and Singh 1986), a nominal scale. Szatmari and colleagues also reported that parental stress was associated with parents endorsing greater numbers of impairments on the ABC.

Pearson and Aman (1994) outlined a further complexity in the relationship between differential ratings, severity and development. They analyzed parent and teacher ratings of developmental maturity and expression of hyperactivity in children with a range of developmental disorders. From regression analysis they concluded that both parents and teachers take mental age into account when rating deviant behaviors in children with developmental disorders. If the same expression of a behavior will be rated with greater severity in children with higher mental ages than in children with lower mental ages, it may be difficult to obtain ratings of the severity of aberrant behaviors in DLD, HAD, LAD and NALIQ children that are independent of mental age.

Yet another factor affecting differential ratings of the same child may arise from differences in expectations of that child. Stone and Rosenbaum (1988) reported that parents and teachers rate children differently because they attend to different behaviors. It may be that parents do see their child's developmental status clearly, as Szatmari's group found, but that parents attend to aberrant behaviors with heightened sensitivity because they are responsible for their child's public and private behavior, and must live with the constant effects that aberrant behaviors have on the family. For example, Arbelle *et al.* (1994) found that preschool autistic children are significantly less compliant with parental prohibitions than mental-age-matched controls. If parents are not effective in controlling the aberrant behaviors of children with developmental disorders, they may rate those behaviors as more severe than if they were able to control them.

In this study we found that physicians had higher thresholds for identifying social abnormalities in autistic children than did parents or teachers, even though parents gave both neurologists and psychiatrists a wealth of developmental history on their children. There may be multiple reasons why physicians see autistic children as less abnormal than do teachers and parents. Neurological and psychiatric interviews may last 30 to 60 minutes, whereas teachers are with the children all week, and parents are responsible for their child's entire life. Abnormalities that a child may express during the relatively brief clinical session may have less emotional impact on the physician, and that, coupled with the physician's wider knowledge of the extent of abnormalities possible in children, may make the threshold for physicians higher.

Children are likely to behave quite differently at school, at home, and in the clinician's office. Stone *et al.* (1994) found evidence that context was a crucial differentiator of behavioral ratings for parents and clinicians. They reported, as we have in this chapter, that neither parents nor professionals saw much insistence on maintenance of sameness in autistic children, and that, as Szatmari *et al.* (1994) noted, parents and professionals saw a different pattern of abnormalities in the same children. An important part of context variation is the people present in each context. For example, Routh *et al.* (1978) found that children's play in a structured experimental session was different in the presence of their mothers. Mothers, teachers and clinicians cannot exclude themselves from interactions with the child.

Parent, teacher and clinician ratings are also subject to the effects of their knowledge of child development, behavioral abnormalities and clinical syndromes. Parents certainly know their children better than any professional could, but parents may have little knowledge of, or experience with developmental disorders. Clinicians or other professionals trained to use different diagnostic systems and working in different settings may also have different thresholds for the recognition and rating of behaviors and skills (Waterhouse *et al.* 1992, Reiss 1994).

If discrepancies in behavioral ratings arise because of (1) the nature of scales used (Dihoff *et al.* 1993); (2) raters' subconscious adjustment of ratings in terms of judged mental age (Pearson and Aman 1994); (3) raters' attentional focus (Stone and Rosenbaum 1988); (4) raters' stress level (Szatmari *et al.* 1994); (5) contextual variation in the child's behavior (Routh *et al.* 1978, Stone *et al.* 1994); and (6) diagnostic training effects (Waterhouse *et al.* 1992, Reiss 1994), how can an accurate, reliable composite picture of developmental disabilities be established?

*Establishing a composite behavior pattern*
A first step would be to have parents, teachers and clinicians use the same rating scale. This has not generally been done, in large part because instruments have been developed for specific groups of raters (*i.e.* for parents, or teachers, or psychologists, or other professionals). A second step would be to insure reliability and coverage of the rating instrument. Researchers have been very concerned with reliability of instruments (Sparrow and Cicchetti 1984, Teal and Wiebe 1986, Aman 1991, DiLalla and Rogers 1994, Lord *et al.* 1994, Sturmey 1994). However, this concern has been limited to the reliability of unitary raters.

Even the use of the same reliable instrument across raters, however, will not address the variation in children's behaviors across contexts. If aberrant behavior X is seen at home, and aberrant behavior Y is seen in the clinician's office, then shouldn't the child's repertoire be considered to include both X and Y? We found differences across informants similar to those described by Stone and Rosenbaum (1988), Stone *et al.* (1994) and Szatmari *et al.* (1994). We suggest that the behavior sets generated by different observers should be additive. Another issue is developmental level. If a child is judged to have a developmental level 6 at school and only 4.5 at home, which (6 or 4.5) should be designated as the child's developmental level? Szatmari and colleagues found an 11 point difference between parents and teachers on the Vineland ABS. We also found differences in global ratings of development across informants. We would suggest that those variant levels be identified by context, because—given that the instrument is reliable—they provide additional information about contextual variation in the child's behavior.

There are no standardized rating instruments that combine information from several informants (Aman 1991). Combining information from several informants would require resolution of the balance of the ecological validity of ratings across contexts, and the reliability of the raters within contexts. Yet the development of such an instrument might go a long way toward achieving better consensus among parents and the diverse professionals and therapists attempting to mitigate their children's developmental problems.

In summary, despite discrepancies, in general terms parents', teachers' and psychiatrists' behavioral ratings of DLD, HAD, LAD and NALIQ children shared a similar picture of developmental immaturity in LAD and NALIQ children, severe social abnormality in HAD and LAD children, and impaired language function in all four groups. Our synthesis of findings on these rating scales is consonant with current understanding of these clinical syndromes (Bishop and Rosenbloom 1987, Reiss 1994, Tonge *et al.* 1994). Only the future development of rating instruments which can blend information from different informants will resolve some of the questions raised by the data from this study.

### Summary and conclusions
Overall, the clinical rating scales and informant report instruments provided a detailed picture of the social and behavioral abnormalities and delays in the diagnostic groups. In general, behaviors in the areas of social interaction and play were the most powerful discriminators of the autistic from the non-autistic children. The LAD children were seen as more impaired in social relations than the HAD children, suggesting an association between severity of cognitive impairment and severity of social impairment within the autistic spectrum. The consistent step-wise progression of developmental and diagnostic group differences (DLD>HAD>NALIQ>LAD) in the behavioral data reported by parents, teachers, psychiatrists and neurologists produced a picture of cognitive deficiency in LAD and NALIQ children, severe social abnormality irrespective of NVIQ in HAD and LAD children, lack of autistic symptoms in DLD and NALIQ children, and impaired language function in all four diagnostic groups. These findings suggest that developmental disorders in preschool children are not on a single continuum. Rather, they point to the possibility of collocations of disruptions in different brain systems responsible for cognition, language and social behaviors. The study provided an opportunity to consider some of the sources of similarities and differences in the way the same child was viewed by separate observers and to make a strong recommendation for the development of common instruments suitable for use by all these observers.

### Clinical implications
The findings from application of the behavior scales in this study suggest that optimally reliable diagnostic decisions would emerge from a consultative process that included

parents, teachers, therapists, and other professionals who evaluated the child (*e.g.* neurologist, psychiatrist, psychologist, speech/language pathologist, etc.). Differences between parents', teacher's and other professionals' perceptions of the child highlighted in this study would almost certainly be minimized if they had available a single instrument to index the child's status. The most discriminating single measure for differentiating the four preschool groups we studied was the WADIC. This brief checklist highlighted a different pattern of functioning between non-autistic (DLD and NALIQ) and autistic (HAD and LAD) groups. It also served to differentiate HAD from LAD, and DLD from NALIQ. Moreover, parents and teachers could use the checklist as easily as the evaluating psychiatrists.

The Vineland ABS also differentiated the four groups, but because the four study groups' variances were evenly stepped, from a relatively high developmental age for DLD, lower to HAD, still lower to NALIQ, down to the very low developmental age of LAD, the Vineland did not aggregate HAD and LAD as an autistic axis separate from DLD and NALIQ in any domain. Thus, although the Vineland has been used to discriminate autism from other contrast groups (Volkmar *et al.* 1993), it did not serve to isolate the autistic spectrum in this study. The Vineland was designed to evaluate any developmentally disabled child's skills against those expected of normal age-matched peers. Because it depends on parental or teacher report rather than test data, the Vineland is valuable for assessing developmental mental age without the influence of test performance limits of children's variable attention and motivation. However, its administration requires training and takes more time than shorter checklists.

The HBS is an interview instrument that combines items concerned with autistic spectrum abnormalities with items from the earlier Vineland Test of Social Maturity. As such it mixes two types of items: (1) items that identify a bimodal distribution of autistic (HAD and LAD together) *vs* non-autistic (DLD and NALIQ) study groups; and (2) items that are developmentally stepped across the four study groups (*i.e.* DLD>HAD>NALIQ>LAD). Although the items on the HBS can be divided and scored as two instruments, we believe separate assessment of developmental age and autistic symptomatology is likely to be an easier clinical practice.

The Social Abnormality Scales I and II were developed specifically to supplement questions about autistic behaviors not included in the WADIC. The scales aggregated the HAD and LAD groups as an autistic axis but did not differentiate DLD from NALIQ.

Because we have found important differences in the way instruments may identify and group children, we would suggest that clinical differential diagnosis and assessment would be best served by employing two instruments: (1) a normative developmental measure, such as the Vineland Adaptive Behavior Scales; and (2) a non-normative inventory of abnormalities that covers both early history and present behavior—which in our study would represent items from the developmental history (as discussed in Chapter 5) and the WADIC. There are a variety of other instruments for assessing autistic symptomatology, including the CARS (Childhood Autism Rating Scale—Schopler *et al.* 1986), the ABC (Aberrant Behavior Checklist—Aman and Singh 1986), the ADI-R (Autism Diagnostic Interview, Revised—Lord *et al.* 1994), and others (Aman 1991).

Because the WADIC was such a strong discriminator of our four study groups we would recommend its clinical use, with the proviso that the instrument be modified to identify not only present but also past behaviors of the child. We would further recommend that the modified (past and present behaviors) WADIC be endorsed by the child's parents, and that the unmodified (present behaviors) WADIC be endorsed by his teacher and physicians.

A well standardized single interview checklist based on a set of questions probing for evidence that the child is on the autistic spectrum would help coordinate judgments about symptoms across parent, physician, teacher and other professionals, and would increase the probability of their arriving at a diagnostic consensus. Because preschool children with communication and social impairments are often difficult to assess adequately in a clinical setting, and because the symptoms that need evaluation are complex, a consultative evaluation process wherein all involved in the consultation generate information on the same instrument from the vantage point of different experiences with the child in different environments may provide greater clarity and sharper diagnostic discrimination, and better consensus. We suggest that developing such an instrument is a goal well worth pursuing.

# 9
# PLAY

*L. Wainwright and D. Fein*

Play can be found in a child's behavioral repertoire almost from birth. Present initially as sensorimotor exploration of the world, any item that provides sensory stimulation, especially visual or auditory stimulation, can interest the baby and encourage engagement of existing cognitive and motor schemes (Piaget 1962). At around age 9 months, infants begin to use toys in a more goal directed way (McCall 1974, Fenson *et al.* 1976). This type of play is often labelled functional and consists of activities that create some desired effect, *e.g.* rolling toys with wheels or stacking cubes. Reciprocal play emerges as the infant pushes objects to another person. These first types of play directly reflect the child's limited capabilities for motor output and social and cognitive expression. They lay the foundation for further development by providing an arena where skills can be tested and applied to items in the world.

Symbolic representation first appears when a child is about 12 months old (Belsky and Most 1981). These representations are simple recreations of familiar events in the child's experience, typically involving grooming (*e.g.* combing one's hair) or eating (*e.g.* sipping from a miniature cup as if something were there). The reproduction of familiar scenarios, generally carried out with another individual, testifies to the social and representational nature of symbolic or pretense play.

Symbolic play continues to develop over the next two to three years, becoming more abstract (Werner and Kaplan 1962), less self-referential (Piaget 1962), and increasing in complexity and duration (McCune-Nicolich 1981, Rubin *et al.* 1983).

During the period of infancy and preschool, play serves as a primary means for children to interact with their environment; it is a natural way for them to explore what is cognitively and socially new. Empirical evidence indicates that the development of a child's play follows a distinct and consistent pattern. Probably due to its representational nature, the development of symbolic play has been strongly correlated with the development of language as well as of cognitive and social skills (Bateson 1955, Piaget 1962, Vygotsky 1978, Bates 1979). McCune-Nicolich and Bruskin (1982) investigated the relationship between symbolic play and language by following a small sample of children over the critical months of development of these functions. They found that increased sequencing of representational play emerged at or before the comparable language sequence. They suggested that 'mechanisms other than uniquely linguistic structures should account for the developments in both domains'. Additionally, symbolic play frequently replicates social interaction. As a result, it is likely to mirror social development and to be more influenced by deficits in social knowledge than other, earlier developing forms of play. Therefore, investigation of children's play skills—and particularly their

**TABLE 9.1**
**Play session toys**

| | | |
|---|---|---|
| Action figure | Doll's house and human figures | Pull-toy |
| Baby doll | Dump truck | Puppets |
| Ball | Duplo blocks | Puzzles |
| Blocks | Gum ball machine | Scissors |
| Books (3) | Jack-in-the-box | Tea set |
| Bubbles | Merry-go-round | Wind-up toy |
| Crayons and markers | Paper | Xylophone |

symbolic play skills—should help to illuminate a variety of conditions resulting in a broad range of developmental delays.

Prior studies reported that the play of NALIQ children is consistent with their mental age (Cunningham *et al.* 1985, Power and Radcliffe 1989), but that the play of DLD, and especially autistic, children, is impaired relative to overall mental age (Riquet *et al.* 1981, Ungerer and Sigman 1981, Terrell *et al.* 1984, Power and Radcliffe 1989). In light of these data, we felt that it was important to investigate the play of the children in our study, in conjunction with other cognitive and neuropsychological measures. We hoped not only to replicate previous findings but also to define play deficits specific to sub-types of developmentally impaired children. Because pretense play requires social knowledge (to produce social imitation) and language skills (to share the content of the pretense with another player), along with enjoyment of social interaction, the course of play development may serve as a prognostic indicator that is equal to or better than language itself. While the ability to speak by age 5 years is frequently mentioned as an important prognostic factor for a child's long term outcome, it may be that adequate symbolic play is equally necessary for continued developmental progress.

## Method

We chose to investigate the children's play using a spontaneous play paradigm. This choice deviates from many previous studies which made use of specific play scenarios likely to suggest particular lines of symbolic play. Tests such as the Symbolic Play Test (Lowe and Costello 1976) utilize toys that strongly elicit symbolic play but provide no information about the activity the child might have chosen spontaneously, inasmuch as each set of toys is placed systematically before the child. Children, especially those experiencing developmental delays, can have qualitatively different responses when activities are structured, as compared to when they are left to pursue their own interests. Our spontaneous play paradigm enabled us to quantify the presence of sensorimotor, functional and symbolic play and to determine each child's preferred activity.

## Subjects

Four hundred and thirty-four videotapes of play sessions were available for analysis. 53 children were not included in the play analysis due to scheduling difficulties and some stolen videotapes; no child was excluded for reasons of diagnosis or performance. Of the

434 subjects (89 per cent of the 487 children in the study), 182 (91 per cent of 201) belonged to the DLD group, 48 (94 per cent of 51) to the HAD group, 105 (84 per cent of 125) to the LAD group, and 99 (90 per cent of 110) to the NALIQ group. In addition, the same play paradigm was used with a sample of 41 normal children from a day care center. This sample served as a comparison group inasmuch as there are no normative scores for spontaneous play. Although most children had play sessions of equal lengths, a few sessions were curtailed because of random events, mostly scheduling issues; this accounts for small variations in reported sample sizes across analyses.

**Procedure**

Each child's play and spontaneous language were evaluated on the basis of a 25 minute structured play session. The session was carried out either in available space in laboratory facilities or at the child's school or home. The session was video- and audio-recorded for later analysis. A specific set of toys, which covered a broad range of developmental levels, was used and included sensorimotor toys (jack-in-the-box, pull toy, bubbles, nesting cups, musical toy, unbreakable mirror, pieces of yarn), functional/ constructional toys (crayons and markers, blocks, Lego blocks, a gum ball machine, cars and trucks, balls, puzzles, books) and symbolic toys (baby doll, puppets, doll house, telephone, tea set, action figures) (Table 9.1).

The session was divided into three parts. During the first five minutes each child was introduced to the play area, offered a simple snack and invited to play with whatever toys he liked. The examiner and a familiar adult (a parent or teacher) sat to the side of the play area and talked quietly to one another. This provided an opportunity to record the child's choice of toys and style of solitary play. After five minutes, the examiner told the child that the familiar adult was going to leave and would return in a short time. If the child was highly resistant to this idea, the examiner asked the familiar adult to stay but remain uninvolved with the play. Play with the examiner continued for the next 15 minutes. During this time the examiner attempted to elicit the child's highest level of play and language, using the available toys. Whenever possible, the trained examiner followed the child's lead in play. The examiner was instructed to attempt to elicit symbolic play during the latter portion of the 15 minute period if the child had not demonstrated this activity spontaneously. At the end of the 15 minutes, the familiar adult returned and joined in play with the child for a further five minutes. This final period provided a means for comparing the child's play, language and sociability when engaged with familiar *vs* unfamiliar persons.

**Data analysis**

Data were gathered from the videotape records using time sampling. Each sample consisted of one consecutive minute of play divided into three 20-second segments (total nine segments). A trained observer identified the type of play in which the child was engaged, as well as the specific toy(s) used during each 20 second segment. The first sample was taken during the first five minutes when the child was engaged in solitary play with the familiar adult present in the room. Samples 2 and 3 were taken during the

**TABLE 9.2**
**Play categories**

*Passive Sensorimotor Play*
Looking (just looking at toy)
Passive holding (holding toy without looking)
Passive looking (holding and looking at toy)
Mouthing and sniffing (inappropriately)

*Active Sensorimotor Play*
Active manipulation (investigating a toy)
Waving, dropping or banging
Combinatorial play (stacking or nesting toys)

*Functional Play*
Functional
Constructional

*Symbolic Play*
Symbolic inanimate (*e.g.* animating cars, trucks, etc.)
Symbolic animate (*e.g.* animating dolls, puppets, etc.)
Substitution
Imaginary

*No Toy Play*
No toy play
Cannot see child

15 minute play period alone with the examiner: sample 2 after a four minute warm-up period (selected from minutes 5–7), and sample 3 late in the play period (selected from minutes 11–13). Slight variations in this scheme were sometimes necessary due to fluctuation in the length of sessions (*e.g.* the familiar adult returned too soon), but in all cases at least 30 seconds elapsed at the start of the session before any data were collected, and a four full minutes elapsed between the departure of the familiar adult and the second time sample. This insured that each child had a uniform amount of time to adjust to the setting and to being alone with the examiner.

Four scorers shared the coding of the videotapes. Each was pretrained in the use of the coding scheme; inter-rater reliability was established following independent viewing and coding of at least ten play sessions. Values for reliability within each play code ranged from $r = 0.70$ to $r = 0.98$.

Codes for each type of play were pre-established and covered seven types of sensori-motor activities (looking, passively holding but not directly looking, passively looking while holding, inappropriate mouthing or smelling, waving or banging, stacking, actively manipulating), two types of functional play (functional and constructional), and four categories of symbolic play (symbolic inanimate, symbolic animate, substitution, imaginary) (Table 9.2). There were also codes to indicate inability to see the child's activity and to signal entire 20 second segments during which the child did not play with any of the toys (*e.g.* talked but did not play, wandered, stared, ate the snack, etc.). Each play type was also identified as being elicited by the examiner, or being generated by the child alone or in cooperation with the examiner.

We tallied the number of segments in which each specific play code appeared, with the maximum number of any one type of play equalling 9, inasmuch as each child's data consisted of three one-minute samples divided into nine 20-second segments. We also computed a measure of diversity of toys used, based on the number of toys used in each three minute interval.

We converted the frequency scores of the four play categories into percentages of all activities within each sample. This percentage represented the frequency score of a particular category divided by the sum of the frequencies in all four categories. We used a percentage rather than the absolute frequency to take into account variations in the overall activity level of the children. A child might engage in functional play in all nine 20 second segments and yet also engage in each of the other types of play as well; that child would differ from another child who played only functionally and who would thus obtain a score of 100 per cent for functional play. We also generated a value for the percentage of time during which there was no toy play. This was computed by dividing the frequency score for the 'no toy play' category by the activity in all five categories listed in Table 9.2. In addition to the percentage of activity in each category, we analyzed the number of activities that were produced spontaneously as opposed to those elicited by the experimenter.

The original percentage scores and the percentage scores for non-elicited play were compared using analysis of variance to identify group differences. We repeated these analyses covarying with age, SES and NVIQ. Finally, we examined the relationship between symbolic play and various other measures of symbolic ability and global measures of verbal and nonverbal IQ, as well as the number of checks each child received on part A of the WADIC, by computing correlations between each of these variables and the percentage score for the symbolic play category.

## Results

### Type of play

There were significant differences in the type of play produced by children in the four diagnostic groups (Table 9.3) and less marked differences between time samples (Table 9.4). Focusing first on Sample 1 (Table 9.5)—the sample representing the child's solitary play—there were significant differences between groups for the two types of passive and active sensorimotor play. The three groups with normal NVIQs (Normal, DLD, HAD) did not differ from each other, nor did the two low NVIQ groups (LAD, NALIQ). Covarying type of play for age, sex, and NVIQ left only the LAD group with a greater amount of sensorimotor play and abolished differences between the HAD and LAD groups. These results indicate that the increased percentage of sensorimotor play found in the autistic group is accounted for by diagnosis and not solely by NVIQ.

The groups also differed significantly in percentage of functional play in Sample 1. NVIQ as well as diagnostic group contributed to intergroup differences in that the groups with normal NVIQs produced more functional play than the LAD group and only the normal and DLD groups produced more than the NALIQ group. When this analysis was repeated using covariance, differences were no longer significant, although the

177

**TABLE 9.3**
**Type of play (analysis of variance summary)**

|  | Non-covaried ANOVA | Covaried ANOVA[1] |
|---|---|---|
| Sensorimotor Play | Normal=DLD=HAD<br>NALIQ≤LAD<br>DLD<NALIQ | Normal=DLD=NALIQ<br>DLD<HAD (sample 2 only)<br>NALIQ=LAD (passive)<br>NALIQ<LAD (active)<br>HAD=LAD |
| Functional Play | Normal=DLD=HAD<br>NALIQ=LAD<br>DLD>NALIQ | No significant differences |

[1]Covariates: age, nonverbal IQ and socioeconomic status.

**TABLE 9.4**
**Symbolic play (analysis of variance summary)**

|  | Non-covaried ANOVA | Covaried ANOVA[1] |
|---|---|---|
| Sample 2 | Normal=DLD=HAD<br>NALIQ>LAD<br>DLD>NALIQ<br>HAD>LAD | Normal=DLD=HAD<br>NALIQ>LAD<br>DLD=NALIQ<br>HAD=LAD |
| Sample 3 | Normal=DLD>HAD<br>NALIQ>LAD<br>DLD>NALIQ<br>HAD>LAD | Normal=DLD>HAD<br>NALIQ>LAD<br>DLD=NALIQ<br>HAD=LAD |

[1]Covariates: age, nonverbal IQ and socioeconomic status.

difference between the DLD and LAD groups approached significance.

There was no difference among groups in percentage of symbolic play during solitary play. As can be seen in Table 9.5, the percentage of symbolic play was low in all groups during this period.

In Sample 2 (Table 9.6)—the first sample of play with the examiner—the children in the four groups engaged in significantly different types of play. The groups differed in both active and passive categories of sensorimotor play. The Normal, DLD and HAD groups, which did not differ in amount of passive sensorimotor play, engaged in less of it than did the LAD group. The HAD and NALIQ groups, which did not differ, produced less passive play than the normal and DLD groups. When reanalyzed with covariance, the DLD group had less passive play than the HAD group, whereas differences between the HAD and LAD groups and between the DLD and NALIQ groups became non-significant. The two autistic groups engaged in more active sensorimotor play than their NVIQ-matched non-autistic counterparts. These differences were maintained when the data were covaried.

Differences in functional play in sample 2 can be accounted for primarily by NVIQ. Differences between the DLD group and the NALIQ and LAD groups, with the LIQ

178

**TABLE 9.5**
**Play types: sample 1 (percentage of subjects)**

| | Normal (N=39) Mean (SD) | DLD (N=178) Mean (SD) | HAD (N=45) Mean (SD) | LAD (N=99) Mean (SD) | NALIQ (N=98) Mean (SD) | F | p |
|---|---|---|---|---|---|---|---|
| Passive sensorimotor | 19.5 (21.2) | 22.3 (21.9) | 25.5 (20.8) | 35.8 (27.0) | 29.5 (25.1) | 6.44 | 0.0001 |
| Active sensorimotor | 26.4 (20.1) | 30.0 (24.4) | 22.7 (24.0) | 35.4 (28.8) | 24.9 (23.3) | 2.53 | 0.04 |
| Functional | 38.6 (30.8) | 33.0 (28.0) | 31.5 (31.0) | 19.3 (24.1) | 25.3 (27.4) | 5.68 | 0.0002 |
| Symbolic | 5.2 (12.9) | 4.0 (11.1) | 4.9 (13.8) | 2.5 (8.8) | 4.0 (9.7) | 0.67 | ns |

**TABLE 9.6**
**Play types: sample 2 (percentage of subjects)**

| | Normal (N=41) Mean (SD) | DLD (N=178) Mean (SD) | HAD (N=46) Mean (SD) | LAD (N=105) Mean (SD) | NALIQ (N=99) Mean (SD) | F | p |
|---|---|---|---|---|---|---|---|
| Passive sensorimotor | 24.8 (18.3) | 25.6 (17.7) | 30.9 (20.6) | 38.7 (24.5) | 33.8 (22.1) | 7.99 | 0.0001 |
| Active sensorimotor | 15.8 (17.3) | 12.6 (13.0) | 17.9 (14.5) | 27.3 (21.4) | 19.0 (16.6) | 13.55 | 0.0001 |
| Functional | 34.4 (20.8) | 39.6 (24.4) | 32.9 (28.9) | 29.4 (24.6) | 33.4 (24.1) | 3.14 | 0.0145 |
| Symbolic | 25.0 (26.0) | 21.6 (25.3) | 18.3 (24.2) | 3.5 (8.9) | 13.8 (23.0) | 13.21 | 0.0001 |

**TABLE 9.7**
**Play types: sample 3 (percentage of subjects)**

| | Normal (N=41) Mean (SD) | DLD (N=182) Mean (SD) | HAD (N=48) Mean (SD) | LAD (N=98) Mean (SD) | NALIQ (N=99) Mean (SD) | F | p |
|---|---|---|---|---|---|---|---|
| Passive sensorimotor | 23.1 (18.4) | 25.4 (18.8) | 28.1 (16.4) | 36.9 (23.4) | 31.7 (17.8) | 7.08 | 0.0001 |
| Active sensorimotor | 14.7 (16.8) | 13.8 (15.1) | 18.7 (15.8) | 28.1 (21.5) | 19.1 (17.4) | 11.41 | 0.0001 |
| Functional | 36.3 (23.9) | 37.0 (25.7) | 37.6 (27.8) | 27.0 (24.5) | 35.1 (25.3) | 2.76 | 0.0276 |
| Symbolic | 25.9 (25.9) | 23.8 (28.6) | 15.6 (21.0) | 4.8 (11.3) | 14.0 (18.4) | 12.98 | 0.0001 |

groups having less functional play, were no longer significant when the data were covaried for NVIQ. The amount of symbolic play during Sample 2 did not differ among the groups with normal NVIQs, but these groups produced significantly more symbolic play than the LIQ groups (Table 9.6). There was no difference between the amount of symbolic play in the HAD group as compared to the NALIQ group, which, in turn, had significantly more symbolic play than the LAD group. When NVIQ was taken into account through covariance, differences among groups became non-significant with the exception of the comparisons of the normal and DLD groups *vs* the LAD group and of the NALIQ *vs* the LAD group. The LAD group continued to have the least symbolic play. There was no difference between the HAD and LAD groups when NVIQ was covaried.

Data from Sample 3 (Table 9.7) were similar to those from Sample 2 in terms of sensorimotor and functional play. Amounts of passive and active sensorimotor and functional play continued to differ across groups. Again, the amount of passive and active sensorimotor play differed as a function of NVIQ. Differences between DLD and NALIQ groups, as well as those between HAD and LAD groups became non-significant when NVIQ was covaried, which was not the case with differences between the LAD and NALIQ groups which remained significant. LAD children had a greater amount of sensorimotor play of both types than their non-autistic counterparts, whereas this was true only for active sensorimotor play during Sample 2.

The amount of symbolic play during Sample 3 also differed among groups. The major difference was that the two autistic samples engaged in less symbolic play than their NVIQ-matched counterparts. Differences between the normal and LIQ groups but not between autistic and non-autistic groups became non-significant when NVIQ was covaried (summarized in Table 9.4).

Thus, findings on type of play indicate that more sensorimotor and less symbolic play is characteristic of children with lower NVIQ and also of children with autism. Data also indicate that symbolic play tends to increase in DLD children, but to decrease in HAD children, as the session progresses, suggesting a possible warm-up for the DLD children and a loss of interest or motivation for the HAD children.

*Non-elicited play*

The previous analyses were computed using all of the play exhibited by the child, without taking into account the role of the experimenter in eliciting the activity. Similar analyses were carried out using only play spontaneously produced by the child, without suggestion or elicitation from the experimenter. The outcome of these analyses was virtually identical to the findings for total play, which means that no single group required and/or benefitted in a unique way from the interaction with the examiner.

*'No Toy Play'*

We also compared the groups in terms of the percentage of the child's activity which did not include play with toys. During Sample 1, groups had an average of at least 20 per cent of their activities not involving play with the toys. This was accounted for by a variety of behaviors ranging from eating the snack to exploring the room but not the toys, to rocking or hand flapping. During this sample, there was no significant difference among groups in the percentage of time spent doing something other than playing with toys.

During Samples 2 and 3, the amount of time spent in this type of non-play activity was much less, ranging from 1.3 per cent to 7.0 per cent in Sample 2, and 2.6 per cent to 13.4 per cent in Sample 3. There were significant differences among groups within

Samples 2 and 3 (Sample 2: $F = 3.68$, $p<0.0014$; Sample 3: $F = 7.47$, $p<0.0001$). The higher percentage of non-play activity of the HAD group compared to the NALIQ group accounted for group differences in Sample 2. In Sample 3, the LAD group spent significantly more time in non-play activities than the other groups.

*Diversity of play based on toy choice*
The number of toys used by each group during each time sample and throughout the three samples was used as a measure of diversity of choice during play. There was no significant difference among groups for any individual sample. The mean number of toys used during a three minute sample (*i.e.* the three one-minute samples) ranged from 2.48 (SD 1.75) for the HAD group in Sample 1 to 3.63 (SD 1.43) for the normal children in Sample 2. In general, the children used about three toys per three minute sample, irrespective of the portion of the tape analyzed. When the number of different toys used across the three samples was analyzed there was a significant difference among groups ($F = 3.42$, $p<0.009$). The NALIQ group used the greatest variety of toys (mean = 8.15, SD 2.97) and the HAD group used the least (mean = 6.49, SD 2.14).

*Correlations of play with other characteristics*
We computed correlations to investigate possible relationships between the percentage of symbolic play and measures of IQ, language function and social relatedness. We used percentages of symbolic play from Samples 2 and 3 to compute correlations with global measures of verbal and nonverbal IQ. There was no significant correlation between symbolic play and verbal or nonverbal IQ in the normal children or those with DLD. In the NALIQ group, amount of symbolic play and NVIQ were significantly positively correlated in Sample 3 ($r = 0.26$, $p<0.008$) and symbolic play and verbal IQ were significantly positively correlated in both Samples 2 and 3 (Sample 2: $r = 0.27$, $p<0.007$; Sample 3: $r = 0.38$, $p<0.001$).

Symbolic play and IQ were also positively correlated in the autistic groups. The HAD group's play was positively correlated with verbal IQ in both samples (Sample 2: $r = 0.40$, $p<0.0055$; Sample 3: $r = 0.31$, $p<0.036$) and NVIQ in sample 2 ($r = 0.31$, $p<0.036$). There were significant positive correlations in the LAD group between NVIQ (Sample 2: $r = 0.24$, $p<0.01$; Sample 3: $r = 0.22$ $p<0.037$) and verbal IQ (Sample 2: $r = 0.23$, $p<0.016$; Sample 3: $r = 0.24$, $p<0.02$).

The relationship between various language measures and the extent of symbolic play was also determined using correlations (Table 9.8). A child's MLU had a significant positive correlation with the extent of symbolic play in the DLD, LAD and NALIQ groups but not in the normal or HAD children. Note, however, that the correlation in the normal group was very low but that that in the HAD group was approximately equal to that in the other diagnostic groups. The lack of significant findings for the normal group is believed to be related entirely to sample size. When the strength of the correlations for the DLD and HAD groups was compared there was no significant difference between the specific *r* values computed (McNemar 1969). There was a significant relation in the DLD and HAD groups between their level of symbolic play early in the play session and

181

**TABLE 9.8**
**Correlations of language measures with symbolic play: samples 2 and 3**

|  |  | *Normal* | *DLD* | *HAD* | *LAD* | *NALIQ* |
|---|---|---|---|---|---|---|
| MLU | Sample 2 | 0.13 | 0.26** | 0.23[†] | 0.47*** | 0.40*** |
|  | Sample 3 | 0.04 | 0.25** | 0.32[†] | 0.52*** | 0.35*** |
|  | N | 37 | 144 | 33 | 58 | 74 |
| Brown's Stages | Sample 2 | 0.20[†] | 0.27*** | 0.43* | 0.10 | 0.47[†] |
|  | Sample 3 | –0.20[†] | 0.11 | 0.35[†] | 0.02 | –0.02 |
|  | N | 31 | 125 | 29 | 24 | 9 |
| PPVT standard | Sample 2 |  | –0.03 | 0.35* | 0.10 | 0.04 |
|  | Sample 3 |  | 0.10 | 0.25 | 0.14 | 0.04 |
|  | N |  | 176 | 43 | 55 | 82 |
| PPVT raw | Sample 2 |  | 0.11 | 0.35* | 0.29* | 0.13 |
|  | Sample 3 |  | 0.21** | 0.25[†] | 0.39*** | 0.23* |
|  | N |  | 176 | 44 | 61 | 85 |

*p<0.05; **p<0.01; ***p<0.001; [†]*ns* (probably due to sample size).

**TABLE 9.9**
**Correlations of Stanford–Binet scores with symbolic play in Samples 2 and 3**

|  |  | *DLD* | *HAD* |
|---|---|---|---|
| Verbal Reasoning | Sample 2 | 0.05 | 0.21 |
|  | Sample 3 | 0.11 | 0.35* |
|  | N | 171 | 42 |
| Vocabulary | Sample 2 | –0.03 | 0.37* |
|  | Sample 3 | –0.02 | 0.28[†] |
|  | N | 165 | 37 |
| Comprehension | Sample 2 | 0.11 | 0.32* |
|  | Sample 3 | 0.16 | 0.38* |
|  | N | 174 | 36 |
| Absurdities | Sample 2 | 0.03 | 0.03 |
|  | Sample 3 | 0.13 | 0.44* |
|  | N | 150 | 26 |

*p<0.05; [†]*ns* (probably due to small sample size).

Brown's stages of language development (Brown 1973) determined by SALT analysis of their language (see Chapter 7). These correlations were not significant in the LIQ groups, although the NALIQ group had a relatively high correlation. Again, the lack of significant findings in this group for their early play is probably due to the very small sample size. Finally, the standard score on the PPVT was positively correlated with symbolic play for the HAD group. When raw scores were correlated both the HAD and LAD groups had significant relationships for the early play sample and the DLD, LAD and NALIQ groups had significant relationships for the later play sample.

**TABLE 9.10**
**Comparative views of subject's play (percentage with deficiency)**

| Rater | DLD % | HAD % | LAD % | NALIQ % |
|---|---|---|---|---|
| Play session sample (functional or symbolic play) | 41 | 39 | 67 | 53 |
| Neurologist observation (social play) | 17 | 63 | 92 | 48 |
| Parent report (social play) | 21 | 49 | 73 | 40 |
| Teacher report (social play) | 36 | 67 | 84 | 58 |
| Teacher report (play with representational toys) | 1 | 8 | 52 | 13 |

We examined the relationship between S-B verbal scores and symbolic play for the DLD and HAD groups* (Table 9.9). There were some positive correlations between symbolic play measures and standard scores for Verbal Reasoning, and the Vocabulary, Comprehension and Absurdities subtests during some of the play samples for the HAD group but not the DLD group. Except for Vocabulary and Comprehension, their Verbal Reasoning scores were more likely to be positively correlated with symbolic play late in the play session (Sample 3) than during the first sample with the examiner.

The relationship between symbolic play and a number of social measures was also determined using correlations. First, the number of checks a child received on part A of the WADIC—the portion dealing with the child's sociability—was correlated with play. There was a significant negative correlation between the presence of symbolic play and the number of checks on the WADIC in the LAD group (Sample 2: $r = -0.25$, $p < 0.009$; Sample 3: $r = -0.24$, $p < 0.014$) but not in other groups. When the total number of checks on the WADIC was correlated with play the only significant finding was again in the LAD group; they had a negative correlation between total checks and symbolic play in Sample 2 of the play session ($r = -0.20$; $p < 0.037$).

Finally we compared the quantitative data derived from Sample 2 of the formal play session (first play period with the examiner—Tables 9.4 and 9.6) with the neurologists' impressions of the children's play and with parents' and teachers' responses to questions regarding play. Table 9.10 indicates that the four types of observers were in fair agreement regarding the relative prevalence of children with deficits among the four groups, even though the data they provided were not entirely comparable: the data from the play session represent lack of either functional or symbolic play during a one minute sample with the examiner; the neurologists played briefly with the children and rated the quality of their symbolic play (see Table 6.7, p. 109); data from the parents represent their endorsement of lack of play or manipulative play only (Table 5.24, p. 90); data from the teachers refer to lack of social play and of imaginative play with representational toys.

*The numbers of individuals in the LAD and NALIQ groups who were fully testable with verbal subtests of the Stanford–Binet were so small as to make it impractical to perform these analyses. The normal children were not tested with the S-B.

Table 9.10 shows that, in general, the two autistic groups were viewed as inferior to the non-autistic groups and the play of the DLD group was the best and that of the LAD group the worst among the four groups. Agreement regarding social play was closer than observations of functional or symbolic play with toys and reports from teachers on play with representational toys. The teachers, who had extensive contact with the children, reported that virtually all of them, except for the large majority of those in the LAD group, played with representational toys even though the percentage who did so during the one minute sample of the play session was lower.

**Discussion**
The existing literature suggests that the development of play is linked to the acquisition of cognitive and social skills as well as language. This is especially true of symbolic play because of its representational nature and the time period during which it emerges as an essential component of play. Therefore, the discussion of the findings in our study will focus on differences among the groups in their ability to play symbolically. Note, however, that because the play measures represent percentages of total activity, significant increases in symbolic play necessarily meant decreases in other play categories.

The data indicate that the relative amount of symbolic play depends on at least three factors. First, symbolic play depends on the availability of a partner in play. This is demonstrated by its noticeable absence during the first sample of the play session, when the children played alone. Even the normal children exhibited very little pretense play under these circumstances. Our findings suggest that symbolic play is a more social form of play than either sensorimotor or functional play. This has important implications for the populations represented in this study. The impaired social skills of autistic children automatically put them at a disadvantage for the development of this form of play.

Another possibility to account for the virtual absence of symbolic play during the period of solitary play may be that children were reluctant to play in this manner in a very new setting. If this were true, one would expect to see an increase in symbolic play from Sample 2 to Sample 3, when the child should have become increasingly comfortable. Our data do not show such an increase for the normal children and therefore do not provide support for this explanation. Still another possibility is that an observer is likely to have difficulty identifying symbolic play when a child is alone because of the absence of the language and gestures a child might use to identify the substance of the pretense to another player.

Secondly, the data indicate that symbolic play is related to a child's IQ, as shown by the several cases where differences between the NALIQ and the cognitively normal control and DLD groups became non-significant when data were covaried for IQ. Consistent with our findings using a spontaneous and unstructured paradigm, several investigators (*e.g.* Cunningham *et al.* 1985, Power and Radcliffe 1989) assessed play using the standardized scenarios of the Symbolic Play Test (Lowe and Costello 1976). Their findings indicate that children with developmental delays who have even cognitive profiles (comparable to our NALIQ group) show overall delays in the development of symbolic play, and that their level of play is consistent with their mental age. In this cognitively subnormal population, immature play parallels cognitive level, suggesting that mental impairment affects the rate but not the sequence of development of symbolic play. The same was true of differences between the HAD and LAD groups which disappeared following covariation. IQ influences the content of play across developmental categories inasmuch as covariation of IQ abolished intergroup differences for sensorimotor and functional as well as symbolic play. This conclusion is also supported by the significant correlations between measures of IQ and symbolic play in the LIQ groups as well as the HAD group.

Finally, diagnosis accounted for some group differences in symbolic play. Previous studies have found severe impairment of symbolic play in autism (Riquet *et al.* 1981, Ungerer and Sigman 1981, Mundy *et al.* 1987). In free play situations investigators found that in AD subjects both the frequency of play and its developmental level were well below those in non-autistic subjects matched on mental age (Riquet *et al.* 1981). In situations in which an examiner modelled symbolic play, the AD children's play level rose over their free play abilities, but it continued to be below that of mental-age-matched comparison groups. Furthermore, the AD subjects' functional level of play was correlated with receptive language ability, while symbolic play was correlated with both receptive and expressive language ability (Mundy *et al.* 1987). The present study reports somewhat different findings. Although the LAD group stood out by the sparseness of their symbolic play, the HAD group demonstrated relatively strong symbolic play in Sample 2 when they produced as much symbolic play as the other two normal NVIQ groups. This finding demonstrates that they had symbolic schemes available for use. However, by the third sample, when a child had been playing with the examiner for seven to ten minutes, the amount of symbolic play declined in the HAD group to the point where it resulted in a significant difference between that group and the DLD and normal groups. The HAD group's decline in symbolic play (a decline also seen in the LAD group) must be compared to the other two groups' maintenance or slight increase in play of this type during Sample 3. It seems, therefore, that although the higher functioning autistic children could produce symbolic play they seemed unable or unwilling to sustain it for very long. This observation is consonant with the work of Lewis and Boucher (1988) who found that high-functioning autistic children can produce symbolic play but need to be coaxed through elicitation, showing that symbolic play does not seem to be their preferred mode of play.

The emergence of increasingly complex symbolic play may also be delayed in children with DLDs, although to a lesser extent than their language (Terrell *et al.* 1984, Power and Radcliffe 1989). Terrell and her colleagues found that scores on the Symbolic Play Test were significantly below the normative data for their sample's chronological age. However, when compared with a group of language-matched children (younger children with equivalent language ages), the DLD group played in a more symbolically mature way, indicating that, although their symbolic play function was impaired, it was not as impaired as the symbolic function that mediates language. These findings suggest that in DLD, delays in the development of play may result from some disturbance in general representational functioning or in the normal coordination of language and other representational systems during development. Contrary to some of these earlier studies, however, we did not find significant differences in play between the DLD group and age-matched control children. This may be due to our paradigm which enabled the children to choose their own materials, and which presented a great range of toys from which to choose. This paradigm may have highlighted their representational abilities because they were able to choose areas of strength upon which to build scenarios. It is also possible that spontaneous play allowed them to rely on gesture and action more than would have been the case in a more formalized testing situation, thereby masking their developmental weakness. Finally, in other studies data generally were collected from the time a child began to play. Our long period of warm-up at the start of the period of play with an adult (four minutes) may have allowed the children to feel more comfortable and therefore to engage in higher levels of play by the time the data were collected.

Other potential differences among diagnostic groups failed to reach significance. We had expected that we would find differences between the frequencies of play elicited by the examiner and non-elicited play. This unexpected result may be accounted for by our play paradigm. Examiners were trained to allow each child as much freedom to direct their play as possible, therefore they were not inclined to elicit play directly. The data support this, with relatively small amounts of elicited play. Also, play was attributed to the child if, once the topic or toy was introduced, the child maintained interest without further prompting. The group that prompted the most eliciting behavior on the part of the examiners was the LAD group. However, this group was also the least responsive to the experimenters and thus it was relatively impervious to the examiner's influence. Since the child's and not the examiner's behavior was being recorded, the child's behavior continued to be identified as a spontaneous choice because the attempted elicitation was ignored.

The 'no toy play' measure warrants a few comments. Its presence, which 'competed' with play, was noticeably higher in Sample 1, where it accounted for 20 per cent or more of the children's activity, than in the other two samples. This was true for all groups. This finding probably reflects the effects of both a new situation and the absence of a partner for play. Significant differences during play with the examiner were related to higher levels of non-playing activity in the autistic groups. This may reflect these children's temporary disengagement from interaction (and therefore play) with another person, and/or their inability to sustain play themes throughout the 15 minute period.

There was a relationship between some of the language measures and symbolic play. The strongest of these was MLU, supporting the assumption that ability to represent longer strings of ideas verbally should be related to representing symbolic acts in play. There does seem to be a point at which length of utterance is great enough that it no longer relates to symbolic ability, as seen in the absence of this correlation in the normal children. It is also noteworthy that the HAD group's S-B Language scores were correlated with symbolic play measures, with the strongest correlations being in areas that require the individual to express ideas about social convention (Comprehension subtest) and unusual or humorous events (Absurdities). These correlations were strongest in the later sample of play when the HAD group was exhibiting a decline in symbolic play.

This suggests that for this group of children the ability to use language to convey information about social aspects of life is related to their ability to act out those social aspects in a sustained manner in their play. It is important to keep in mind, however, that these correlations, though significant, were still low and so account for a small amount of variance in these variables.

Finally, some of the findings of the relationship between the children's symbolic play and their parents' and teachers' and the neurologists' impressions of their overall social functioning described in Chapters 6 and 8 need to be highlighted. Like the language measures, these correlations were low despite their statistical significance, therefore it is important to recognize that many other factors also account for variability in these measures. There was a negative correlation in the LAD group between symbolic play and the WADIC which measured the degree of their social impairment: increasing social impairment was associated with a decline in the amount of symbolic play. We also found significant correlations between various dimensions of social responsiveness measured by the Vineland and play. One finding of note was that correlations which existed between social abilities and play in DLD children were significant only during the first period of play with the examiner—the period in which the children would be less familiar with the situation and examiner. The children's play was unrelated to these measures as they remained in the play situation for longer periods of time. This supports our conclusion that the lack of significant play findings for the DLD group is, in large part, related to our paradigm of extended play.

The HAD group, on the other hand, again had significant correlations which appeared in the later sample when, as a group, their symbolic play was declining. This indicates that while their ability to play symbolically may not be predicted, based on their overall language or social ability, their ability to sustain that form of play can be predicted, to some extent, by these measures.

The quality of symbolic activity was not measured in these analyses. Ongoing work is examining the play of the clinical groups and the normal children for complexity and other qualitative features, and this work may reveal more about group differences.

The data, taken as a whole, support the hypothesis that symbolic play is a representational function dependent not only on general cognition but also on social functioning. The autistic groups' impairment indicates a two part process to symbolic representation in play. Those children who are lower functioning have limited use of symbolic play as shown by their low percentage of symbolic play throughout these analyses. The higher-functioning autistic children seem to develop, or perhaps can be taught, symbolic play, but they cannot or will not sustain the play for regular use. Therefore, the absence of symbolic play can serve as a diagnostic criterion in cognitively subnormal children suspected of falling on the autistic spectrum. With higher-functioning children, it is not so much the presence of symbolic play but the ability to sustain and elaborate symbolic representation that seems to be diagnostically significant.

It continues to be important to consider the role of language comprehension and expression in the development of play as a whole and, in particular, of symbolic play. The absence of differences in symbolic play between the normal and DLD groups would suggest that language variation may not play a major role in symbolic play, at least in children with mental ages above 3 years.

## Summary of findings

All groups showed very little symbolic play during their solitary play time. During play with the examiner, the autistic groups showed more active and passive sensorimotor activity than the other groups. Percentages of time spent in functional play were equivalent among the groups when NVIQ was covaried. In the first interactive segment sampled, the LAD children showed very low rates of symbolic play, which continued to be significantly different from the other groups' even when IQ was covaried. The HAD children had a rate of symbolic play that was not higher than that of the LAD children when IQ was covaried. The HAD children were lowest in symbolic play among the normal NVIQ groups, but the comparison did not reach significance. In the later interactive segment, the DLD children were again equivalent to the normal children in rates of symbolic play, but the HAD children were significantly lower. The LAD children also showed lower rates of symbolic play than the NALIQ children. Differences between normal and low IQ groups disappeared when IQ was covaried, but the autistic children remained lower in rates of symbolic play than their non-autistic comparison groups.

There was no group difference in rates of elicited *vs* non-elicited play. Non-play activity tended to be higher in the autistic children during interactive, but not solitary segments. Across the three one-minute segments, the NALIQ children used the greatest diversity of toys, and HAD children the least.

There was no significant correlation between symbolic play and IQ for the DLD and normal children. The NALIQ and both AD groups of children did show modest but significant correlations between symbolic play and both verbal and nonverbal IQ. The LAD, but not the HAD children had modest but significant negative correlations between symbolic play and number of checks on the autistic diagnostic checklist. The fact that IQ did not correlate significantly with symbolic play within the normal and DLD groups, but did for the AD and NALIQ children, combined with the fact that many group differences in symbolic play between high- and low-functioning children disappeared with covariation of IQ, suggests that IQ is indeed related to symbolic play, but not when it is within the normal range.

Diagnosis also contributed to differences in symbolic play. The LAD children had very sparse symbolic play in all segments. The HAD children had relatively strong symbolic play in the first interactive segment, but it declined by the second interactive segment, compared to the play of the non-autistic groups, which remained level or increased over time. This suggests that although the HAD children have the competence to engage in symbolic play schemes, they lack the sustained motivation to do so. Contrary to results from some other studies in the literature, the DLD children did not differ from normal children in symbolic play.

## Clinical implications

Typically, observation of spontaneous play with representational toys is not part of a routine pediatric, neurological or neuropsychological evaluation. Speech and language pathologists are more likely to engage children in play, but it is generally for the purpose of evaluating the child's conversational abilities and the richness of his vocabulary and syntactic competence, rather than for examining the quality of the play. Psychiatrists use symbolic play extensively, with the goal, in most cases, of using it as a tool for understanding and treating the child's emotional state.

What the study demonstrates is that attention to how the child plays and what toys he selects often provides extremely useful information, even though it does not, alone, yield a reliable differential diagnosis among the common causes of preschool developmental impairment. Lack of symbolic play or repetitive manipulation should alert the clinician to the possibility that the child is autistic as well as communicatively and/or cognitively impaired. The study shows that poorly developed language alone is not a sufficient explanation for deficient play and that cognitive impairment, if less than severe, often does not either. The study also shows that looking at what the child does with the toys on his own is not nearly as informative as attempting to engage him in interactive representational play. Furthermore, the increasing differentiation between DLD and HAD children as the play session progressed suggests that an inability to sustain symbolic play with the examiner, rather than an inability to engage in symbolic activity, may be more clinically relevant to high-functioning autism. Restricted diversity of toy choices and increased periods of non-toy-play may also be consistent with a diagnosis of autism. We speculate that early symbolic play may turn out to be as potent a predictor of outcome as the presence of early communicative language, but this remains to be evaluated in a follow-up study. This study suggests that symbolic play is such an efficient and potentially enlightening addition to the mental status assessment of young children as to recommend that it be widely used by all the clinicians concerned with the evaluation of developmentally impaired preschool children.

# 10
# CLASSIFICATION ISSUES

*I. Rapin, D.A. Allen, D.M. Aram, M.A. Dunn, D. Fein, R. Morris and L. Waterhouse**

> "The much maligned science of taxonomy, the ordering and classification of organisms, takes a culturally imposed backseat to the more interventionist and generalizing work style of experimentation and quantification. But taxonomy should be viewed as one of the most fundamental, and most noble, of scientific pursuits—for what can be more basic than parsing nature's rich and confusing complexity? Our categories, moreover, record our modes of thought, and taxonomy therefore teaches us as much about our mental functioning as about nature's variety." (Gould 1994)

As stated in the above epigraph and discussed in Chapter 1, classification, an inductive, descriptive, observational approach to science, is often regarded as inferior to and less exciting than deductive, hypothesis-driven, top-down science. Yet until one has surveyed the territory one cannot draw maps. Several decades have been devoted to the description of the developmental disorders of brain function in children, with the tacit assumption that dyslexia, developmental language disorder, other learning disabilities, attention deficit disorders, motor ineptness, tone deafness, mental retardation without autism, and autistic disorders are discrete entities. Much of the research to date has concentrated on one or another of them, often studied mainly from the point of view of the one discipline most concerned with the diagnosis or habilitation of the children with that particular disorder.

Anyone who works with these children has been frustrated at times by the fuzzy boundaries of the developmental disorders, yet issues of classification have only recently come to the forefront of research (*e.g.* Stanovich 1991, Shaywitz *et al.* 1992). A major goal of this project, described in Chapters 4–9, was to compare groups of preschool children with developmental disorders of verbal and/or nonverbal communication selected according to criteria widely accepted by researchers and clinicians. The project enabled us to examine some of these criteria more critically, using a new empirical approach to classification developed by R.R. Golden (see footnote 2, p. xii).

## Levels of classification
### Level I
Studies concerned with the differential diagnosis of the developmental disorders considered in this monograph (DLD, AD, NALIQ) and with the boundaries between these disorders and normalcy are referred to in Chapter 1 as Level I research. Behavioral classification at Level I is of great importance to the educational administrators who

*I. Rapin assumed major responsibility for this chapter; other participating investigators are listed alphabetically.

must provide remediation for developmentally disabled children. Not only must they decide whether a child's needs will best be met in a class for the mentally retarded, the neurologically impaired, the language disordered or the autistic, they must first decide whether that child's deficits are severe enough to mandate remediation. Thus Level I is concerned with identification of developmental disorders and their base rates in the total population of children, as well as with differential diagnosis among major developmental disorders.

The matter of the etiology (biological or environmental cause) of the developmental disorders is also largely, but not exclusively, a Level I issue. These classification issues have enormous political and fiscal importance, as well as impacting on training programs for professionals who will evaluate and educate the children, not to mention the often overwhelming impact on families of a diagnosis of developmental disability in a child.

Many affected children have prototypic disorders that pose no particular problem for classification, but it is common for a child to have deficits that qualify for more than one disorder, for example, language disorder and autism. Does this mean that the child has two disorders, or that there is an overlap between two separable disorders, or that one causes the other? Cross-disciplinary studies to attempt to resolve some of these dilemmas are relatively recent, as are studies concerned with the relationships between what are generally considered distinct developmental disorders such as, for example, dyslexia and attention disorders, dyslexia and language disorders.

*Level II*

At Level II the concern is not identification of disabled children but gaining a detailed understanding of the specific behavioral and cognitive deficiencies responsible for individual children's developmental disabilities; it is also trying to identify the dysfunctional systems in the brain responsible for the deficits in these tightly defined subgroups. In order to advance this second goal, classification at Level II seeks to determine whether there are subtypes within disorders identified at Level I. Like Level I, Level II has an impact on those concerned with habilitation because of the need to identify specific cognitive and other behavioral deficiencies that might be remediated with an effective educational approach targeted at particular cognitive deficiencies.

The other major importance of Level II classification is gaining an understanding of the neuropathophysiology of the developmental disorders. At present, their classification is based entirely on behavioral criteria, consisting of attempts to define and quantify the children's most salient symptoms. However, advancing genetic, neuroscientific, neuropsychological, neurophysiological and neuroimaging technologies are now making it possible to investigate the neurological basis of the developmental disorders whose neurophysiological and neuropathological basis was, until recently, virtually entirely conjectural. These biological studies are predicated on the availability of tight, valid behavioral classifications because, in order for neuroscientists to elucidate the burning questions of the neuropathophysiology of particular behaviorally defined deficits and their genetic or acquired etiology, they need to study 'pure' cases, groups of prototypic children with disorders tightly defined at the behavioral level, so as to minimize the noise that falsely diagnosed cases would introduce into biologic studies.

### Classification at Level I: identifying major developmental disorders and setting boundaries between them

*Traditional classification of DLD based on discrepancies among quantitative test scores*
As discussed in Chapter 2, identification of children with DLDs is based on a combination of inclusionary and exclusionary criteria. DLD is widely considered a well defined entity on the basis of some saliently deficient aspect of children's language development (inclusionary criterion). Chapter 2 reviews some of the problems associated with the use of exclusionary criteria to diagnose DLD, such as hearing loss, known brain lesions, defined genetic or malformation syndromes, mental retardation, autistic behaviors and environmental deprivation. The boundaries of these exclusionary criteria are not crisp, and defining a disorder largely on the basis of negative criteria says very little or nothing about its characteristics. Chapter 2 then goes on to discuss studies of DLD that used discrepancies between some psychometric test(s) of language skills and chronological age, mental age or NVIQ for diagnosis, as opposed to qualitative clinical criteria used by experienced clinicians and educators sensitive to deficiencies or deviance in children's conversational language.

Criteria for the identification of children with DLD vary a great deal, both among clinicians and among researchers. Standardized psychometric discrepancy criteria, which are often used for the purpose of defining research samples and children who are entitled to special education, tend to be more restrictive and perhaps less sensitive to language impairment than is clinical judgment based on a child's language performance in naturalistic contexts. We summarize briefly here two Level I studies conducted as part of our effort at classification, studies aimed at increasing congruence between a clinical diagnosis of DLD and diagnosis by standardized criteria.

• *Use of discrepancy criteria for a diagnosis of DLD* (Aram *et al.* 1993). The purpose of this study was to evaluate the reliability, coverage and usefulness of both clinical and research definitions of DLD children. Subjects in the study were the 252 children whom clinicians referred to the present study as language impaired. All met the exclusionary criteria intended to eliminate hearing deficits, bilingualism, mental retardation, autism, and major neurological or orofacial abnormalities as causal factors for the language impairment.

Initially, a series of formulas for establishing discrepancies between nonverbal and language abilities was applied, using the Visual/Abstract Reasoning domain of the Stanford–Binet and the Test of Early Language Development (TELD). These various discrepancy criteria included: a discrepancy ≥1 SD between these two tests; a discrepancy of the standard error of means ≥7 points, or using an individualized residual regression score; a disparity between mental age and language age derived from these two tests greater than or equal to 12, 18 or 24 months; a discrepancy between chronological age and language age greater than or equal to 12 months; and finally an absolute TELD cut-off score <85 (Table 10.1). Even the best of these psychometrically defined formulas

**TABLE 10.1**
**Alternative discrepancy criteria for capturing children as developmentally language disordered using S-B and TELD scores: number and percentage of 252 subjects[1]**

| Criterion | N | % |
|---|---|---|
| S-B–TELD discrepancy (≥1 SD —15 points) | 149 | 59.1 |
| S-B–TELD standard error of means ≥7 points | 167 | 66.3 |
| S-B NVIQ–TELD residual regression | 44 | 17.5 |
| Mental age–language age | | |
| ≥12 months | 136 | 54.0 |
| ≥18 months | 72 | 28.6 |
| ≥24 months | 18 | 17.1 |
| Chronologic–language age ≥12 mo | 124 | 49.2 |
| TELD Score <85 | 130 | 51.6 |

[1]S-B = Stanford–Binet; TELD = Test of Early Language Development.

identified only two-thirds of the clinically defined population of DLD children.

After reviewing alternative nonverbal and language measures we concluded that using either an S-B–TELD discrepancy ≥1 SD or a mean length of utterance (MLU) standard age score <85 was the most inclusive discrepancy criterion for capturing children among those identified clinically as DLD; yet even this formula failed to identify 20 per cent of the clinically defined population. These results demonstrated the significant mismatch between clinical and research definitions of DLD and led to a second study summarized below.

• *The use of spontaneous language measures in identifying children with specific language impairment: an attempt to reconcile clinical and research incongruence* (Dunn *et al.* 1996). The investigators examined (1) differences in performance on the standardized tests described in Chapter 4 and in spontaneous language in groups of children clinically diagnosed as language disordered who were or were not identified as DLD through the standard discrepancy criteria used to select the DLD group described in this monograph, and (2) the utility of objective measures of MLU, syntax, semantics and pragmatics derived from a spontaneous language sample as criteria for discriminating clinically identified preschool children from normally developing preschool children.

Preschool children diagnosed as DLD according to psychometric discrepancy criteria were in general significantly more impaired in performance on all standardized tests of language and in MLU than were clinically identified children who did not meet these criteria. However, spontaneous language data indicated that children clinically identified as DLD produced a significantly higher percentage of errors in spontaneous speech than normal controls, whether they met psychometric discrepancy criteria or not. These data are consistent with the notion that preschool children clinically identified as specifically language impaired who are not classified as DLD by standard psychometric criteria do have language deficits, but in aspects of language that are poorly assessed by standardized language tests. On average they speak in phrases of normal length but have predominantly expressive language impairment involving more errors in syntax, semantics and pragmatics than expected for age.

Logistic regression analysis indicated that a combination of MLUs, percentage of structural errors, and chronological age constituted the optimal subset of variables for predicting a clinical diagnosis of DLD. This criterion discriminated clinically diagnosed DLD preschool children from normally developing controls and captured a higher percentage of the clinically identified DLD children than did even the best psychometric discrepancy criteria. It classified 96.5 per cent of the clinically diagnosed DLD children as DLD (high sensitivity), but only 48.8 per cent of the control children as normal (poor specificity).

Sensitivity and specificity provide only part of the information required to judge the utility of various measures for classifying preschool children as DLD. Another important component is base rate (*i.e.* the frequency with which specific language impairment is seen in the population of interest). The base rate for DLD in this study was 83 per cent. Base rate information is taken into account by examining positive and negative predictive values, which were 90.2 per cent and 74.0 per cent respectively. This positive predictive value implies that a clinician using these variables to identify DLD would have a hit rate of 90.2 per cent and a false positive hit rate of 9.8 per cent. The negative predictive value implies that a correct classification of not-DLD would be made 74 per cent of the time when no diagnosis is indicated.

Longitudinal follow-up to determine outcome in preschool children meeting standardized psychometric discrepancy criteria and those meeting only spontaneous language criteria will be important for confirming the prognostic significance of DLD diagnosis based on different criteria.

### Traditional classification of autistic disorders on the basis of standardized behavioral inventories

Autism is in many ways the most complex of the developmental disorders of brain function. The American Psychiatric Association uses the umbrella term Pervasive Developmental Disorder (PDD) to cover the entire range of its severity. The term PDD is felicitous because it indicates that disorders on the autism spectrum are not limited to deficits in traditional neuropsychological functions such as sensorimotor abilities, cognition, memory, attention and language, but that they involve other dimensions of human function such as sociability, insight, verbal and nonverbal language use, affect, play, range of interests and choice of activities, and aberrant behaviors. Because there are no standardized tests that quantitate these defining deficits of PDD, diagnosis cannot rest on discrepancy criteria between psychometric tests of particular cognitive/language functions, as is the case for DLD. Instead, current progress toward increasing specificity in making a diagnosis of AD uses a polythetic approach. Diagnosis rests on the number and distribution of aberrant behaviors parents or professional observers endorse from any one of a validated series of descriptors of autistic characteristics. With this approach, no single behavioral abnormality is necessary or sufficient to the diagnosis, which requires a defined minimum number of checks within defined categories.

Chapter 3 pointed out that, despite considerable progress in the definition of what constitutes the autistic spectrum, its borders remain fuzzy. There is fuzziness between the autistic spectrum and mental retardation, DLDs (especially those which affect reception), and childhood-onset schizophrenia. Chapter 3 also stressed the vastly heterogeneous etiologies of autism (Gillberg and Coleman 1992), and the fact that DSM IV and ICD-10 exclude from the diagnosis of AD children with autistic behaviors secondary to defined etiologies such as fragile X syndrome, congenital rubella and a host of others, but they include Rett syndrome, a probably specific biological disorder. DSM IV and ICD-10 include as a separate subgroup of PDD the behaviorally defined group of non-retarded, mildly affected children with adequate expressive language at the levels of phonology and syntax who currently go under the diagnosis of Asperger syndrome, even though there is no unanimity on whether or not Asperger syndrome represents a behaviorally or etiologically specific subgroup among PDD children (Frith 1991).

This section summarizes two studies we carried out concerned with the classification of autism. The first investigates the consequences, in terms of the number of children captured, of applying a series of DSM and ICD algorithms to the 194 children referred to the study as being on the autistic spectrum. The second study compares the 176 children captured by the DSM III-R criteria for AD—the criterion used to select children for the study described in this monograph—with the 18 children who did not meet these criteria but who were studied nonetheless in order to test the validity of these criteria. Following this, we summarize the preliminary results of a novel statistical approach to classification developed by R.R. Golden, the regression-mixture taxometric method; this was used for the identification of children on the autistic spectrum and to discriminate them from the non-autistic DLD and LIQ children, comparing the number of children captured in the autism taxon with those captured with DSM and ICD criteria.

• *Comparison of DSM and ICD criteria for making a diagnosis of autism* (Waterhouse *et al.* 1996). As described in Chapters 4 and 8, all children among those referred to the study who were found to be socially impaired on the basis of the WADIC criteria were interviewed by a child psychiatrist who gave them a DSM III and a DSM III-R diagnosis; the psychiatrist also completed the Social Abnormalities Scales I and II. Then, using items taken from the formal psychiatric evaluation and from parent interview data (WADIC, Vineland ABS, Vineland Maladaptive Scales, Family Questionnaire, HBS), we identified Autistic Disorder according to the criteria of DSM IV and Childhood Autism according to the criteria of ICD-10*.

Psychiatrists diagnosed 98 children as having DSM III Early Infantile Autism or Autism Residual State, 176 children as having DSM III-R Autistic Disorder, and 18 children as having DSM III-R PDD-NOS (Table 10.2). The DSM IV algorithm yielded 115 cases of Autistic Disorder, and the ICD-10 algorithm 125 cases of Childhood Autism.

*Both these classification systems were published after completion of the study.

**TABLE 10.2**
**Scores for nonverbal IQ (NVIQ) and Vineland Adaptive Behavior Scales (ABS)
composite for 176 children diagnosed with DSM and ICD systems**

| Groups | Test | DSM III | DSM III-R | DSM IV | ICD-10 |
|---|---|---|---|---|---|
| AD + Autistic Residual | NVIQ | 49 (N=112) | 62 (N=176) | 58 (N=115) | 59 (N=125) |
| Non-autistic PDD (remainder) | NVIQ | 78 (N=82) | 73 (N=18) | 71 (N=79) | 73 (N=69) |
| AD + Autistic Residual | ABS | 48 (N=112) | 55 (N=176) | 54 (N=115) | 53 (N=125) |
| Non-autistic PDD | ABS | 64 (N=82) | 67 (N=18) | 60 (N=79) | 62 (N=69) |

Non-autistic PDD corresponds to PDD not otherwise specified or PDD-NOS of DSM
III-R, and to other categories on the autistic spectrum in DSM III (see Table 10.3).

Despite these sharp differences in sample coverage, all four diagnostic systems—
DSM III, DSM III-R, DSM IV and ICD-10—generated samples of positively diagnosed
autistic cases with nearly identical patterns of impairment on key diagnostic features.
More than 90 per cent of the children in each of the four defined autistic groups expressed marked social withdrawal, inadequate imitation, impaired reciprocal play, inappropriate social greetings, poor eye contact and deficient non-verbal communication.
The NVIQ of those diagnosed as autistic by DSM III, the most stringent diagnostic
system, was on average about 10 points lower than the NVIQ of those diagnosed by the
three other algorithms (Table 10.2). On the Vineland ABS, their mean composite standard scores were congruent with their NVIQ and were three or more standard deviations
below the mean for normal children of their age. The scores on the Vineland ABS of
DSM III-R PDD-NOS children were about one standard deviation higher but still more
than two standard deviations below expected means.

In general, then, we have found the functioning of the four overlapping samples of
children with AD identified by the four systems to be similar in social impairment, IQ
and level of developmental maturity even though each system captured a vastly different
number of children among those referred to the study. There were substantial differences
between subgroups of PDD children captured by the four diagnostic systems; these subgroups will be discussed later when we consider Level II subtype classification issues.

• *Comparison of children who met DSM III-R criteria for AD with those diagnosed as
PDD-NOS.* Of the 194 children clinically identified as being on the autistic spectrum,
176 fulfilled DSM III-R criteria for the diagnosis of Autistic Disorder, while 18 failed to
meet full autism criteria and were designated as PDD-NOS. In this study, we compared
the AD subjects with the PDD-NOS subjects in order to determine the amount of overlap
and/or differentiation of these two groups.

As discussed in Chapter 4, the AD population was compared to two non-autistic
contrast groups on the basis of NVIQ: (1) a group of DLD children who, by definition,

had NVIQs ≥80, and (2) a group of NALIQ children with NVIQs <80. In order to match the contrast groups, the AD population was divided into HAD (NVIQ ≥80) and LAD (NVIQ <80) subsamples to match the contrast groups. For the purposes of this study, the PDD-NOS group was divided along these same NVIQ lines so as to make direct comparisons with the contrast groups, rather than treating AD and PDD-NOS as a single diagnostic group, irrespective of IQ.

Of the 18 children diagnosed as PDD-NOS, nine had NVIQ ≥80 and nine had NVIQ <80. The overall patterns on most key variables for both groups were as follows. The NVIQ ≥80 PDD-NOS group had scores that were higher than those of the HAD group but lower than those of the DLD contrast group. Likewise, the NVIQ <80 PDD-NOS group had scores that were higher than the those of the LAD group but lower than those of the contrast NALIQ group. The same patterns were found with Vineland Composite and subdomain scores, Peabody Picture Vocabulary Test scores and S-B Verbal Reasoning scores.

While all of the 18 children who failed to meet AD criteria by DSM III-R met PDD-NOS criteria according to psychiatric evaluation, their DSM III diagnoses were almost identical. In the NVIQ ≥80 group seven children were diagnosed with Atypical PDD; in the NVIQ <80 group six were. In the NVIQ ≥80 group one child was diagnosed with Childhood Onset PDD; in the NVIQ <80 group three were. In the NVIQ ≥80 group one child was diagnosed with questionable Schizophrenia in Childhood. The Social Abnormalities scores were not significantly different in the HAD and LAD comparison groups.

This study suggests that NVIQ is an important factor in studying AD and PDD-NOS subjects. It also suggests that when this intelligence factor is considered, there is not a significant difference between those children who are diagnosed as autistic and those who are diagnosed with PDD-NOS.

*The regression-mixture taxometric method: a new approach to differential classification of AD* vs *non-AD subjects*
The regression-mixture approach to classification is described in more detail by Golden and Mayer (1995). Briefly, a regression-mixture analysis attempts to detect the existence of a quasi-dichotomous entity underlying a behavioral syndrome. This is accomplished through the use of available 'fallible' neurobehavioral indicators (test scores or scales), singly or in combination. The choice of indicators is informed by accepted diagnostic criteria and by clinical criteria for hypothesized groups or subgroups.

The following sequence of tests was performed (until failure) for each clinically conjectured autism and language disorder syndrome. (1) Logistic regression and regression classification trees were used to develop and identify those indicators (test scores or scales comprising items assessing related behaviors)—taken singly and in combination—that best predicted clinical diagnosis. (2) Next, these indicators were used to attempt taxometric detection of a latent taxon or subtaxon (conjectured 'natural' group or subgroup), employing consistency requirements across methods and indicators. (3) If a taxon was detected, then, for each individual child, the probability of being a member of the taxon was estimated and used for classification. (4) Estimates of taxon base rate, misclassification rates, indicator validities and other latent parameters (and associations with diagnosis and other classification systems, measurements and ratings) were used to learn more about the nature of the detected taxon. What is described in this chapter is a preliminary application of this method to the children in the study; more detailed aspects will be dealt with in future papers.

The goal of the analysis was to determine whether AD is taxonomic and whether there are subtaxa within AD and DLD, that is, whether there are strong statistical indications that there is a conjectural quasi-dichotomous abnormality whose presence or absence underlies the manifest behavioral symptoms of these children. Future goals are (1) to develop objective empirical methods for preschool classification of AD and DLD; (2) to develop a valid neurobehavioral nosology of these disorders and their major subtypes, as discussed later; (3) to identify those 'dimensions' (language, non-verbal intelligence, autistic behavior, etc.) within the autism taxon and its complement that are most powerful for defining the taxon and that can be used as strong indicators for creating this nosology. Other future goals will be to identify preschool predictors of school-age functioning and extend the preschool nosology to school-age children.

IDENTIFICATION OF THE AD TAXON

From the several hundred available preschool tests, ratings and measurements, we identified those that had shown promising discriminate validities for each of the clinical diagnoses (present *vs* absent) of AD and DLD (Table 10.3). Each was considered as a multifactorial (hence, fallible) indicator—but hopefully with discriminant validity—for major latent autism and language taxa. We developed four autism indicator scales (AutNeu—items from the mental status part of the neurological examination and Vine-land Socialization domain; AutPsy—WADIC and its subscales; AutPar—parent questionnaire regarding autistic behaviors; AutTch—Wing Teacher questionnaire) as follows. (1) Items having face validity (to clinicians) for diagnosis of autism and some evidence of statistical validity were selected. (2) Items with a common format were combined (using unweighted sums) to form one or more subscales. (3) These subscales, sex and SES were used as predictors in logistic regression prediction of diagnosis. (Age was not included as a predictor, as the DLD sample was younger than the other two samples.) (4) The weighted composite in logit form (*i.e.* predicted probability of positive diagnosis by logistic regression) was used as a candidate indicator.

The results of the preliminary taxometric analyses provide strong corroboration for the existence of a 'latent' autism 'taxon', dichotomously distinct from DLD and NALIQ. Using the total sample of 556 children, the four autism indicator scales we developed (AutNeu, AutPsy, AutTch, AutPar) each had sensitivities between 0.75 and 0.85 and specificities between 0.85 and 0.95 for a clinical diagnosis of autism. In Figure 10.1, we show the results of regression-mixture analysis of an average composite of the four rating scales (composite rating logit) as a function of a second logit of NVIQ (adjusted for sex and SES). Note that: (1) there is about a 10 per cent overlap between the ellipses representing the latent autism taxon and its complement, indicating that there are children whose membership is indeterminate; (2) there are a few children whose clinical classi-

198

TABLE 10.3
**Selected preschool candidate indicators of latent autism taxa and complement, autism and DLD subtaxa and complements**

| Preschool test/scale | Name | Taxa/subtaxa detected[1] | Test performance to detect DLD clinical subtypes[2] |
|---|---|---|---|
| Neurological examination mental status scale | AutNeu | Autism taxon + subtaxa | |
| History: Parent questionnaire autism scale | AutPar | Autism taxon + subtaxa | |
| WADIC autism scale | AutPsy | Autism taxon + subtaxa | |
| Wing Teacher Questionnaire autism scale | AutTch | Autism taxon + subtaxa | |
| Peabody Picture Vocabulary | Peabody | Aut subtaxa Lang subtaxa | DLD subtypes (2<3, 4<5,6) |
| Bayley/S-B non-verbal IQ | BSB NVIQ | Aut subtaxa DLD subtaxa | DLD subtypes (1<2, 3<4) |
| S-B Verbal Reasoning | SBVrRea | DLD subtaxa | Receptive language |
| Vineland Communication | ViLang | Aut subtaxa DLD subtaxa | Receptive language, DLD subtypes (1<2) |
| Vineland Daily Living | ViDLvg | Aut subtaxa | DLD subtypes (1<2) |
| Vineland Sociability | ViSoc | Aut subtaxa | DLD subtypes (1<2) |
| One-Word Picture Vocabulary Test | OneWord | Aut subtaxa DLD subtaxa | DLD subtypes (2,6<3,4,5) |
| Syntax: mean length of utterances | MLU | DLD subtaxa | DLD subtypes (2,6<3,4,5) |
| Phonetic Articulation Test | PhonArt | DLD subtaxa | DLD subtypes (3,4>1,5,6) |
| Cycle—Receptive Language | CycleR | DLD subtaxa | Receptive language |
| Spontaneous play | Play | Aut taxon Aut subtaxa | |
| Social Abnormality Scales | SocAbn | Aut subtaxa | |

[1]S-B = Stanford–Binet; Aut = autism; Lang = language.
[2]Clinical language subtypes: the numbers refer to the clinical subtypes proposed by Rapin and Allen (1983, 1988) and briefly described in Appendix 4.1 (pp. 55–57): 1 = verbal auditory agnosia; 2 = mixed receptive/expressive phonological/syntactic deficit; 3 = lexical syntactic deficit; 4 = semantic–pragmatic deficit; 5 = phonologic production deficit; 6 = verbal dyspraxia. Symbols < and > denote significant differences in medians.

fication is almost certainly erroneous (*i.e.* black circles and white diamonds); and (3) there are some outliers and individuals with stippled shading whose classification is ambiguous.

Table 10.4 presents the data in tabular form, comparing taxometric assignments with the clinical diagnoses of autism/non-autism mentioned above. The table indicates that 63 of the 556 study children had a greater than 50 per cent chance of belonging to a taxometric class (autistic/non-autistic) inconsistent with their assigned diagnosis (see also Figs. 10.2–10.5 below). The autism taxon extends the boundaries of the clinical dia-

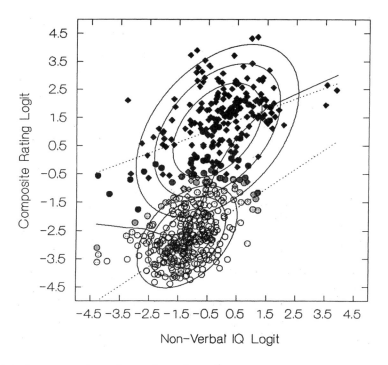

**Fig. 10.1.** Autism taxon and complement for total sample.

Result of regression-mixture analysis of an average composite [Composite Rating Logit (logit = predicated probability of positive diagnosis by logistic regression)] of the four indicator rating scales (AutNeur, AutPsy, AutPar, AutTch—see Table 10.3) as a function of a second logit of nonverbal IQ (Stanford–Binet NVIQ adjusted for sex and SES). Individual children in the clinically defined autistic group [HAD, LAD, plus the 5 per cent who did not meet AD criteria (PDD-NOS)] are depicted as diamonds, children in the clinically defined non-autistic group (NALIQ, DLD, plus the 20 per cent who did not meet DLD criteria) are depicted as circles. Shading indicates the probability that a child belongs in the Autism taxon (black = 1.0, clear = 0.0). The concentric ellipses show probabilities of 0.9 (inner ellipse), 0.75 (middle ellipse), and 0.5 (outer ellipse) that individuals belong to the latent autism taxon (upper ellipses) or its complement (lower ellipses). The solid line shows the strongly sigmoidal smoothed regression line for the entire sample, which indicates possible taxonicity. The dotted lines are the individual regression lines for the taxon and its complement.

gnoses to include 17 of the DLD and 34 of the NALIQ children. Figure 10.1 shows that these individuals are mostly in the area of high taxonomic overlap. When the autistic status of 15 of 18 children diagnosed as PDD-NOS was clarified by using the estimated individual probabilities of being in the autism taxon (see below), along with further clinical assessment, 12 were unambiguously reclassified as autistic, three as not autistic, and three were indeterminate. Finally, we note from Figure 10.1 that, like clinical diagnosis, the autism taxon base rate as a function of non-verbal intelligence is very high for low IQ scores and decreases monotonically to nearly zero for high IQ scores—a

TABLE 10.4

**TABLE 10.4**
**Taxometric classification *vs* preschool clinical diagnosis**

| Taxometric classification | Preschool clinical diagnosis | | | |
|---|---|---|---|---|
| | *HAD + 9 PDD-NOS* | *LAD + 9 PDD-NOS* | *DLD + 51 no DLD criteria* | *NALIQ* |
| Autistic (AD) (N=232) | 53 | 128 | 17 | 34 |
| Non-AD (N=313) | 8 | 4 | 233 | 68 |
| Missing (N=11) | 0 | 1 | 2 | 8 |
| Total (N=556) | 61 | 133 | 252 | 110 |

The taxometric regression-mixture analysis was carried out on 545 children (total sample of 556 minus 11 with missing data). The probability cut-off for assignment to the AD taxon was set at 50%. This table includes the 18 children diagnosed as PDD-NOS by the psychiatrists (not as DSM III-R Autistic Disorder)—the nine with NVIQ ≥80 with the HAD group plus the nine with NVIQ <80 with the LAD sample; similarly, the 51 children who did not meet DLD criteria for inclusion in the DLD group (see Chapter 4) are included with the DLD group. (Differences in number within clinically defined categories result from the reclassification of five children with clerical errors identified unmistakeably by taxometrics. Recalculation of key variables indicated that correction produces negligible change in results.)

direct contradiction of the DSM III-R instruction that a diagnosis of autism requires that autism symptomatology be out of proportion with mental age.

As indicated in Chapter 4, various statistical consistency tests were applied to the taxa and subtaxa. With regard to the autism taxon, classification was consistent (but not perfect) across sources of clinical data: each of (a) behavioral ratings by the neurologist or (b) psychiatrist, (c) parental interviews (WADIC, history form), and (d) teacher questionnaires (HBS) can be used to classify children as autistic or not. Taxometric analyses indicate that, with respect to the autism taxon, the sensitivity of each is 0.8–0.9 and the specificity of each is 0.9 or higher. However, we note that differences in types of information obtained across sources makes finer comparisons difficult.

CLASSIFICATION OF INDIVIDUAL CHILDREN

The regression-mixture analyses just described enabled the taxometric classification of individuals, as shown in Figure 10.1. It also yielded a profile based on data from different raters (neurologist, psychiatrist, teacher, parent) for each individual child indicating the probability of being a member, or not, of the autism taxon (Figs. 10.2–10.5). Each of the figures shows in different shadings, for individual children in one of the four clinically diagnosed groups, the taxometric probability of him belonging in the Autism taxon. Each small profile represents one child. Each of the four diagnostic scales (AutNeu, AutPsy, AutTch, AutPar) used for taxometric classification is represented on the abscissa of each child's profile, and for each scale, elevation along the ordinate marks the probability that the child is autistic. A profile that has the shape of a tall black rectangle represents a child who has a 100 per cent probability, on each scale, of being autistic, whereas a flat line represents a zero probability. Note that, with a few excep-

# DLD GROUP

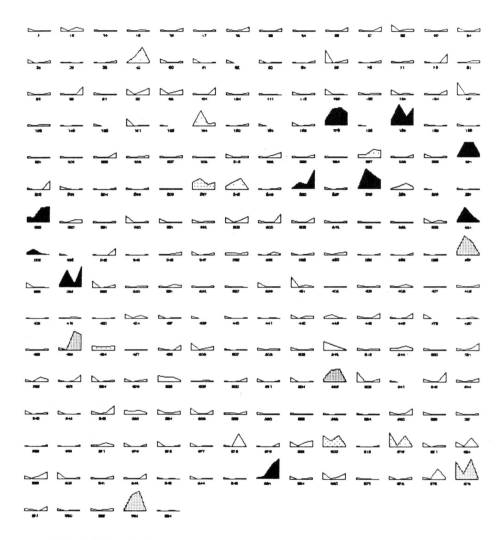

**Fig. 10.2.** Probability of individual children in the DLD group being members (or not) of the Autism taxon.

Each small diagram represents a child. (Beneath these diagrams, but illegible here, a code number identifies the individual child.) Each of the four rating-scales (AutNeur, AutPsy, AutTch, AutPar—see Table 10.3) used for regression-mixture classification is represented on the abscissa of each child's profile, and for each scale, elevation along the ordinate marks the probability that the child is autistic. Shading indicates the overall probability of the child being in the Autism taxon (black = 1.0, clear = 0.0). A profile that has the shape of a tall black rectangle represents a child who has 100 per cent probability on each scale of being autistic, whereas a flat line denotes a probability of zero.

# HAD GROUP

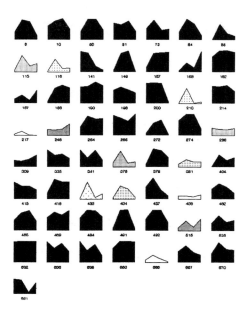

**Fig. 10.3.** Probability of individual children in the HAD group being members (or not) of the Autism taxon. (See Fig. 10.2 for explanation of diagrams.)

tions, children clinically diagnosed as DLD have a low probability of being classified with the regression-mixture method in the autism taxon, and that the reverse is true of children with a clinical diagnosis of LAD. Taxometrics classifies a significant minority of NALIQ children in the autism taxon; HAD children have more irregular profiles than LAD children, indicating somewhat less severe and more variable behavioral assessments, but nonetheless most are classified in the autism taxon.

Discordances between clinical diagnosis and taxometric classification may be due to disagreement among clinicians as to diagnosis, to the unreliability of preschool measures, or to errors either in clinical diagnosis or in measurement. Follow-up studies may help resolve some of these issues. One must not forget, however, that there are individuals with genuinely ambiguous group membership and that any measure has a (hopefully) small but irreducible error rate.

In summary, the overall disagreement between original clinical classification and the regression-mixture taxometric identification was 10 per cent, but taxometrics was very efficient at picking up children who were not prototypic of their diagnostic class. The contribution of taxometrics is the provision of an objective method for classification that supplies probabilities about group membership. Finally, taxa are not groups defined by

# LAD GROUP

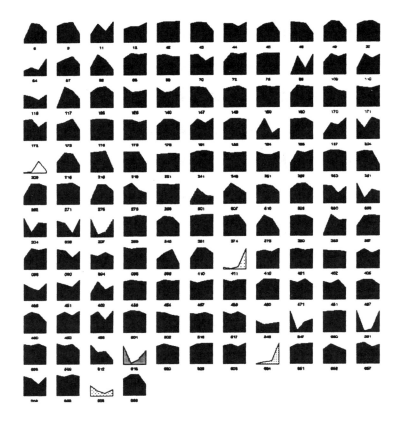

**Fig. 10.4.** Probability of individual children in the LAD group being members (or not) of the Autism taxon. (See Fig. 10.2 for explanation of diagrams.)

arbitrary criteria; they have a high probability of identifying membership in dichotomous groups that may share an underlying biological characteristic.

## Classification at Level II: identifying major subtypes in DLD and AD
*Subtyping in DLD*
Subtyping of DLD has a long history. Myklebust (1954), Morley (1957, 1965, 1972) and de Ajuriaguerra *et al.* (1976) were among early investigators who pointed out that DLD is not a homogeneous disability and that there are children who have predominantly expressive disorders, whereas in others both reception and expression are deficient. As long ago as 1930, Worster-Drought and Allen described children whose comprehension was so profoundly impaired that they were essentially word-deaf and, therefore, virtually

# NALIQ GROUP

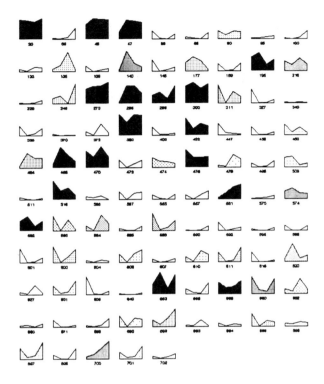

**Fig. 10.5.** Probability of individual children in the NALIQ group being members (or not) of the Autism taxon. (See Fig. 10.2 for explanation of diagrams.)

nonverbal because deficient comprehension precludes the acquisition of expressive language; this syndrome is now generally referred to as verbal auditory agnosia (VAA). Aram and Nation (1975) subtyped DLD children into six syndromes on the basis of their comprehension, production and repetition at the phonological, syntactic and semantic language levels. The clinical classification proposed by Rapin and Allen (1983) was based on the characteristics of preschool children's spontaneous language at these same linguistic levels. They proposed three major groupings, each with two subgroups: (1) children with comprehension deficits at the level of phonology and therefore also with severe expressive deficits were classified as having either VAA if comprehension (and therefore expression) was very severely compromised, or mixed receptive/expressive (phonological–syntactic) deficit if comprehension was superior to expression; (2) those with vastly better comprehension than expression (or normal comprehension) were classified as having either verbal dyspraxia if expressive language was minimal, or

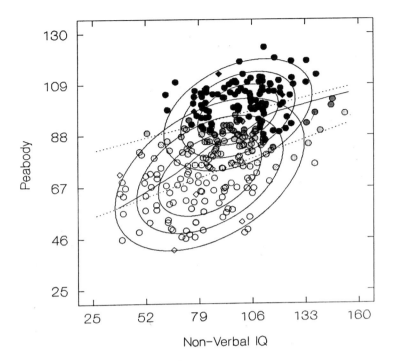

**Fig. 10.6.** Language Subtaxa A and B within the weighted Autism complement sample.

Result of regression-mixture analysis of scores on the Peabody and Stanford–Binet NVIQ. Individual children in the Autism complement (non-autistic groups) are depicted as diamonds if they were clinically diagnosed as belonging to the original autism group (AD plus PDD-NOS) and as circles if they were clinically diagnosed as belonging in the non-autistic group (NALIQ, DLD, plus the 20 per cent who did not meet DLD criteria). Shading indicates the probability that a child belongs in the A (Expressive) Language subtaxon (black = 1.0, clear = 0.0). The concentric ellipses show probabilities of 0.9 (inner ellipse), 0.75 (middle ellipse), and 0.5 (outer ellipse) that individuals belong to Language subtaxon A (receptive) (upper ellipses) or its complement, Language subtaxon B (receptive/ expressive) (lower ellipses). The solid line shows the sigmoidal smoothed regression line for the entire sample, which indicates possible taxonicity. The dotted lines are the individual regression lines for the subtaxon and its complement.

speech programming deficit if they spoke much more but did so unintelligibly; (3) children with adequate phonology and syntax but with word retrieval deficits and comprehension deficits at the level of the sentence were classified as having semantic–pragmatic deficit if they were verbose, or lexical–syntactic deficit if expressive speech was sparse and phonology and syntax immature.

RECEPTIVE *VS* EXPRESSIVE SUBTAXA

Using the sample of children classified as belonging in the Autism complement (*i.e.* those not in the Autism taxon, comprising both DLD and NALIQ children), a regression-

TABLE 10.5
Taxometric classification *vs* original preschool clinical diagnosis

| Taxometric classification | Clinical classification | | | |
|---|---|---|---|---|
| | DLD + 51 no DLD criteria | HAD + 9 PDD-NOS | LAD + 9 PDD-NOS | NALIQ |
| Language A (N=176) | 159 | 4 | 1 | 12 |
| Language B (N=137) | 74 | 4 | 3 | 56 |
| Autism A (N=115) | 17 | 49 | 30 | 19 |
| Autism B (N=117) | 0 | 4 | 98 | 15 |
| Missing (N=11) | 2 | 0 | 1 | 8 |
| Total (N=556) | 252 | 61 | 133 | 110 |

The regression-mixture taxometric analysis includes the total sample of 556 children (minus the 11 with missing data). The 51 children who did not meet DLD criteria for inclusion in the DLD group (see Chapter 4) are shown with the DLD group. Among the 18 children who were diagnosed as PDD-NOS by the psychiatrists (not as DSM III-R autistic disorder), the nine with NVIQ ≥80 are shown with the HAD group, the nine with NVIQ <80 are shown with the LAD group. The numbers in each of the columns show how children were classified by the regression-mixture taxometric analysis compared to their original clinical assignments.

mixture analysis was carried out as described above. From the many preschool tests, ratings and test scores, those that had promising discriminate validity for a diagnosis of DLD and the clinical subtypes proposed by Rapin and Allen (1983, 1988) and Allen (1988, 1989)—*i.e.* the Peabody and other tests of receptive language listed in Table 10.3—were identified and made into scales. Using these scales and adjusting for sex and SES, an attempt was made to subtype the children; it provided evidence for one subtaxon with a higher IQ and predominantly expressive language deficits (Language A) and another subtaxon (its complement) with a lower IQ and receptive (and expressive) deficits (Language B). In Figure 10.6, we show the results of the regression-mixture detection of Language subtaxa A and B on the basis of the Peabody and NVIQ. The area of overlap between the ellipses is greater and the regression curve less sigmoidal than for the detection of the Autism taxon depicted in Figure 10.1; in other words, the evidence for taxonicity of expressive *vs* receptive/expressive DLD subtaxa is less strong. Twice as many of the children in the clinically diagnosed DLD group (159 *vs* 74) were classified in Language A as in Language B (Table 10.5). Interestingly, among the NALIQ children, 12 were classified in Language A and 56 in Language B.

• *Subtaxon of DLD with impaired phonology.* Factor analysis of the language test scores depicted in Table 7.9 (p. 146) indicated that the tests with strongest loading on the language factor were S-B Vocabulary and Memory for Sentences, the Peabody, the TELD and the EOWPVT. The Phonetic Articulation Test (PAT), which loaded on a separate factor, was used for taxometrics to attempt to detect a phonologically impaired DLD subtaxon. Using the sample consisting of those classified as belonging to the non-autistic complement and the PAT scores for the production of labial consonants (Lips) *vs* lingual consonants (Tongue), the smoothed regression curve had the sigmoidal shape suggesting

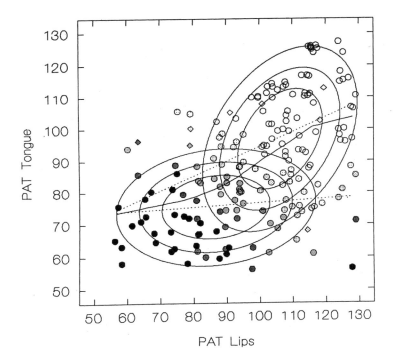

**Fig. 10.7.** Attempt to detect a phonologically impaired DLD subtaxon using the Phonetic Articulation Test (PAT) within the weighted Autism complement sample.

Result of regression-mixture analysis of scores on the PAT for the production of labial consonants (Lips) and lingual consonants (Tongue). Individual children in the Autism complement (non-autistic groups) are depicted as diamonds if they were clinically diagnosed as belonging to the original autism group (AD plus PDD-NOS) and as circles if they were clinically diagnosed as belonging in the non-autistic group (NALIQ, DLD, plus the 20 per cent who did not meet DLD criteria). Shading indicates the probability that a child belongs to the subtaxon with impaired phonology (black = 1.0, clear = 0.0). The concentric ellipses show probabilities of 0.9 (inner ellipse), 0.75 (middle ellipse), and 0.5 (outer ellipse) that individuals belong to the latent phonologically impaired subtaxon (lower ellipses) or its complement (upper ellipses). The solid line shows the sigmoidal smoothed regression line for the entire sample, which indicates possible taxonicity. The dotted lines are the individual regression lines for the subtaxon and its complement.

dichotomous taxonicity and the existence of two overlapping groups of children (Fig. 10.7). The black circles correspond to children who have a high probability of belonging to the subtaxon with impaired phonology, and the more numerous children with clear symbols, those belonging to its complement. The proportion of children with agreement between membership in an expressive phonological subtaxon and clinical rating of intelligibility according to the score in the neurological examination was 0.80.

An attempt to detect subtaxa that might correspond to the six Rapin and Allen clinically conjectured subtypes of DLD failed (see Table 10.3). There was a suggestion that

**TABLE 10.6**

Distribution of 194 children originally referred to the study as clinically autistic across diagnoses in each of the DSM and ICD classification systems and of those (N=232) among the original sample of 556 taxometrically classified as belonging to the autism taxon and subtaxa[1]

| DSM III | | DSM III-R | | DSM IV | | ICD-10 | | Subtaxa | |
|---|---|---|---|---|---|---|---|---|---|
| Early Inf Aut | 111 | AD | 176 | AD | 112 | Childh Aut | 123 | ADB | 117 |
| COPDD | 9 | PDD-NOS | 18 | PDD-NOS | 26 | Atyp Aut | 3 | ADA | 115 |
| Atyp PDD | 21 | | | Other PDD | 35 | Other PDD | 45 | | |
| Childh Schizo | 33 | | | | | Overact Dis | 5 | | |
| No Dx | 20 | No Dx | 0 | No Dx | 21 | No Dx | 18 | | |
| Total | 194 | | 194 | | 194 | | 194 | | 232 |

[1]The 194 children include those referred to the study as clinically autistic; the group comprises the 176 children with DSM III-R autistic disorder plus the 18 diagnosed as PDD-NOS not included in the analyses described in other chapters of the monograph. The group of 232 children refers to those among the 545 (556 minus 11 with missing data) which the regression-mixture analysis assigned to the autism taxon and subsequently divided into autism subtaxa A and B.

COPDD = childhood onset pervasive developmental disorder; Atyp PDD = atypical pervasive developmental disorder; Childh Schizo = childhood onset schizophrenia; No Dx = no diagnosis; PDD-NOS = pervasive developmental disorder not otherwise specified; Overact Dis = overactive disorder; ADB = autism B subtaxon (lower functioning); ADA = autism A subtaxon (higher functioning).

Language A might be a subtaxon, corresponding to the lexical syntactic and semantic pragmatic syndromes, distinct from its complement because phonology is typically spared in these children, who score better on the PAT. There are a number of reasons that may account for failure to detect more of the clinically identified groups, but it may be that the clinically conjectured language disorder subgroups are in fact non-taxonic. It may also be that there were too few indicators that discriminated subgroups. Further studies are needed to examine this question.

*Subtyping in autism*

There is a debate in the literature on whether autism is a unique behavioral syndrome with a wide range of severity or whether there are subtypes in autism that point to potentially separable underlying brain dysfunctions. There is no debate regarding the fact that autism is heterogeneous at the etiologic level (for reviews, see Gillberg 1992, Gillberg and Coleman 1992). For the purpose of prognostication, several writers (*e.g.* Rutter 1979, Rutter and Garmezy 1983, Cohen *et al.*1987, Lord and Venter 1992, Tsai 1992) have proposed dividing the children either on the basis of whether they have acquired expressive speech by the age of 5 years, or on the basis of an IQ >70. Verbal autistic persons with an IQ >70 are regularly referred to as 'high-functioning'.

As discussed in Chapters 3 and 8, both DSM and ICD classifications partition the children on the PDD (autistic) spectrum into several subtypes, based not on IQ but on the number of abnormal behaviors endorsed by parents or observers. Table 10.6 shows the number of children among the 194 in the clinically diagnosed PDD sample (51 HAD, 125 LAD, 18 PDD-NOS) captured by each system. It shows that the number of children

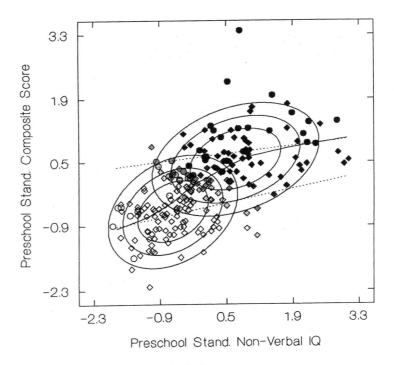

**Fig. 10.8.** Autism subtaxa (A and B) within the Autism taxon.

Result of regression-mixture analysis, using as indicators a composite of scores chosen on the basis of clinical criteria and the Stanford–Binet NVIQ standard scores. Individual children in the Autism complement are depicted as diamonds if they were clinically diagnosed as belonging to the original autism group (AD plus PDD-NOS) and as circles if they were clinically diagnosed as belonging in the non-autistic group (NALIQ, DLD, plus the 20 per cent who did not meet DLD criteria). Shading indicates the probability that a child belongs to the higher functioning Aut A subtaxon (black = 1.0, clear = 0.0). The concentric ellipses show probabilities of 0.9 (inner ellipse), 0.75 (middle ellipse), and 0.5 (outer ellipse) that individuals belong to the higher-functioning Aut A subtaxon (upper ellipses) or its complement, the lower-functioning Aut B subtaxon (lower ellipses). The solid line shows the sigmoidal smoothed regression line for the entire sample, which indicates possible taxonicity. The dotted lines are the individual regression lines for the subtaxon and its complement.

**TABLE 10.7**
**Estimates of taxonomic class base rates and misclassification rates**

| Taxonomic class | N | Sample[1] | N | Base rate | Misclass. rate |
|---|---|---|---|---|---|
| Autism | 232 | Total | 545 | 0.434 | 0.051 |
| Autism A | 115 | } Autism | 232 | 0.490 | 0.133 |
| Autism B | 117 | | | 0.510 | 0.133 |
| NonAutism | 313 | Total | 545 | 0.566 | 0.051 |
| Language A | 176 | } NonAutism | 313 | 0.528 | 0.161 |
| Language B | 137 | | | 0.472 | 0.161 |

[1]'Sample' refers to the sample used for each taxometric analysis. Total sample excludes 11 with missing data.

who were not diagnosed in each of the systems was comparable. As stated earlier, those diagnosed non-autistic PDD by the DSM and ICD algorithms had mean NVIQ scores 10–15 points higher than those diagnosed AD (Table 10.3). The mean Vineland ABS scaled scores of the PDD-NOS group were also higher than those of the AD groups, confirming that these children were less severely impaired in everyday life, as one might have anticipated because they had fewer checks on the DSM and ICD scales.

Using the sample of children classified as belonging in the Autism taxon, a regression-mixture analysis was carried out. Indicators were chosen on the basis of clinical criteria. The analysis produced evidence of two subtaxa corresponding to a higher functioning (Autism A) and lower functioning (Autism B) group (Fig. 10.8). Table 10.5 shows the correspondence with clinical diagnoses. The correspondence between HAD and Autism A is stronger than that between LAD and Autism B. Autism A lowers the HAD-defining NVIQ cut-off score of 80 (which, recall, was selected for the sole purpose of comparing HAD with DLD children, who by definition had an NVIQ cut-off of 80) to an optimal cut-off score of about 65.

Finally, the taxonomic class base rate and probability of misclassification in the Autism taxon, and in the Autism and Language subtaxa, are shown in Table 10.7. Note that the misclassification rate is lowest for the Autism taxon *vs* its complement (Non-Autism) and is 10 per cent overall, whereas it reaches 30 per cent for the subtaxa.

**Summary**

This chapter has summarized progress made toward developing a valid classification of preschool children with inadequate communication skills. We have shown that, depending on what cut-off scores are used when using psychometric discrepancy scores for DLD and on the number of items endorsed on an autism questionnaire, one will capture a markedly different number of disabled children. We have also shown that clinically referred children not captured by diagnostic criteria widely used by investigators and clinicians do not differ markedly from those who are captured, although they tend to be somewhat less severely affected.

In the case of DLD, spontaneous language criteria alone capture more of the children identified by clinicians than combined test and spontaneous language discrepancies. A spontaneous language criterion that included MLU, percentage of structural errors and chronological age had a higher sensitivity for a diagnosis of DLD in preschool children than any one of the psychometric discrepancies. It is important to consider both sensitivity and specificity in making a diagnosis. As is well known, the greater diagnostic specificity that follows moving one's cut-off score toward the more stringent end of a scale results in less sensitive detection, and the decision of where to make diagnostic cuts is a matter of cost-effectiveness, given the base rate of the condition of interest (the lower the base rate, the more expensive are the false positive diagnoses incurred in the attempt to avoid missing a rare affected individual). It is also a matter of one's goals: to try to determine the neurological basis of particular disorders one wants tightly defined groups with as specific as possible a diagnosis so as to avoid introducing random noise into the system.

Regression-mixture analysis as summarized in this chapter supported the hypothesis that autism is taxonic, that is, it provided strong statistical evidence for an underlying 'fundamental' quasi-dichotomous brain abnormality responsible for the behaviorally defined syndrome. Taxometrics also provided strong evidence for two subtaxa in autism and somewhat less strong evidence for receptive and expressive subtaxa in DLD. Taxometrics did not find that DLD was taxonic with respect to NALIQ (no language criterion was applied to NALIQ children, who were chosen on the basis of their NVIQ—in fact, it is likely that some of these children were language disordered as well as cognitively impaired); it provided only weak evidence for further subtaxa in DLD. Logistic regression predictors of diagnosis yielded individual profiles for each child, indicating her probability of belonging in the Autism taxon. These profiles provided the opportunity to detect children who were potentially misclassified into clinical groups because of measurement or clerical errors, or for other reasons. Validation of taxometric diagnoses must await longitudinal follow-up of children classified at preschool age and their study with independent neurological measures such as brain morphometry, functional neuroimaging or neurophysiological evoked activity during the performance of relevant cognitive tasks.

**Clinical implications**

In looking at the many problems inherent in classifying children with developmental disorders of higher cerebral function, our study has highlighted the inherent arbitrariness of diagnoses for defining what are often looked upon as clear-cut entities, diagnoses that are based on cut-off scores on standardized neuropsychological/language tests as well as on clinical criteria; it indicated that sources of disagreement between clinicians and researchers may in some cases be due to the fact that standardized instruments do not assess behavioral features to which clinicians are sensitive (this was the case for children referred to this study by clinicians as DLD). The cost of diagnostic criteria with high sensitivity is overdiagnosis, and that cost escalates in the case of conditions with a low base rate within the population.

The regression-mixture taxometric method has provided strong statistical evidence supporting the existence of a fundamental underlying quasi-dichotomous basis for autism, and provided no evidence indicating that autism is a more severe variant of language disorder or mental retardation. There was only about a 10 per cent overlap among the 556 children in the study partitioned into the autism taxon *vs* its non-autistic complement (the DLD and NALIQ children). It also provided empirical evidence for at least two subtaxa in autism. These subtaxa have much in common with the widely accepted 'high-functioning' and 'low-functioning' autism groups described in the literature. The taxometric analysis also provided preliminary empirical evidence for the existence of at least two latent subtaxa in DLD, expressive and receptive/expressive, again supporting previous work. The analysis did not support the taxonicity of six proposed subtypes of DLD defined on the basis of clinical assessment of receptive and expressive language.

A strength of the regression-mixture taxometric approach is that it does not depend on a particular set of indicators, so that measures used by neuropsychologists, neurologists, and speech/language pathologists, as well as questionnaire data from parents and teachers, yield convergent results. The concordance of this empirical classification with clinical classification validates clinical diagnosis and provides a strong incentive to iteratively refine both clinical criteria and diagnostic indicators until a 95 per cent concordance between the clinical and empirical classifications is achieved. This level of concordance will optimize future research aimed at identifying the genetic, pathological, pathophysiological and neuropsychological bases of these developmental disorders.

The basic result of the regression-mixture method is that the three sets of indicators found most effective for separating autism from non-autism were the classic autistic behavioral items used as a function of NVIQ. To identify subtaxa within the Autism taxon, one uses NVIQ as a function of the autistic behaviors. Finally, to identify the receptive subtaxon within the DLD group (or the autistic complement), one uses the language measures as a function of NVIQ.

Rather than the finding of a continuous distribution of scores, the identification of autism and DLD subtaxa within autism and its complement has major research and practical implications, because these groups were not defined by an arbitrary cut along some continuous variable, and therefore they may have an as yet undefined biological validity. The support for taxonicity provides a strong incentive for attempting to define the dichotomous biological factors underlying the taxa and subtaxa. Obviously, stability of the taxa and subtaxa as the children reach school age must be determined, because stability would provide further evidence for their validity and biological basis.

A major asset of the logistic regression method is that it provides statistical evidence for determining the probability that an individual child does or does not belong to a taxon or subtaxon, using simple scaled psychometric criteria. This type of evidence is valuable because it flags children with equivocal diagnoses and picks out those with possibly erroneous diagnostic assignments. Provided the taxa and subtaxa turn out to be stable in later childhood, being able to define the probability that a preschool child belongs to one or another subgroup will be valuable for parents asking for prognostic information, which has been notoriously difficult to supply at preschool age. It will also be valuable for educators planning a particular child's habilitation.

Despite the further work required to confirm the preliminary results of the regression-mixture method applied to data from this cohort of communicatively disabled children, the results illustrate the potential contribution of this novel empirical approach to classification, a contribution that may prove useful for validating clinical classifications. It may also prove useful by providing investigators of the neurological basis of these disorders with more tightly defined groups, which will enhance the probability of arriving at meaningful brain–behavior correlations.

### ACKNOWLEDGEMENT

The investigators express their gratitude to Dr Robert R. Golden for generously discussing and making available the preliminary results of analyses of the data from this cohort using his regression-mixture method and for reviewing a preliminary draft of Chapter 10. Responsibility for preparation of this chapter is entirely that of the authors, not of Dr Golden.

# 11
# OVERVIEW AND CONCLUSIONS

*D. Fein, D.A. Allen, D.M. Aram, M.A. Dunn, R. Morris, I. Rapin and L. Waterhouse\**

**Goals and scope of the project**

This monograph has presented the results of a study characterizing the social composition (Chapter 4), developmental, medical and family history (Chapter 5), neurological status (Chapter 6), language and cognitive development (Chapter 7), behavioral development and abnormalities (Chapter 8), and play skills (Chapter 9) of three clinical populations of preschool children: 201 clinically diagnosed as DLD; 176 diagnosed (by DSM III-R criteria) as AD; and 110 diagnosed as NALIQ (NVIQ <80). These groups of young children with inadequate communication skills were formed according to widely accepted consistently applied criteria and were studied uniformly. The study describes and contrasts the findings in these groups.

We undertook this project with the goal of attempting to generate an improved classification system for early developmental disorders affecting communication and sociability. We reviewed some bases for classification (Chapter 1) and compared a wide variety of classification systems for DLD (Chapters 2 and 10) and four diagnostic systems for the identification of autism (Chapters 3 and 10). Our aim was to delineate operationally defined entities that would be reliable, valid and clinically useful, and have good coverage for the affected children. A key element of this was the preservation of the clinical essence of the major entities under study—AD, DLD and NALIQ—and the identification of reliable indicators to differentiate the disorders. Another goal of the project was to define meaningful subgroups of these major disorders, through both statistical exploration of results, and attempted validation of clinically derived subgroups. To this end, the monograph presents the results of an innovative quasi-dichotomous taxometric method for separating AD from non-AD children and for detecting subgroups among children with AD and DLD (Chapter 10). In this chapter, use of the term 'taxonomic' denotes results of these specific empirical analyses.

**Classification issues**

Young children with developmental disorders affecting communication represent a challenge for both clinicians and researchers. These children have many overlapping behaviors and symptoms. Standardized evaluation is difficult because of the dearth of sensitive and valid assessment instruments for preschool children, and the lack of a widely accepted and validated classification system with which to communicate about the children, predict their development, or group them for research purposes.

*D. Fein assumed major responsibility for this chapter; other participating investigators are listed alphabetically.

The criteria used to form the groups—DLD, NALIQ and AD [the latter arbitrarily divided at an NVIQ cut-off of 80 into high AD (HAD) and low AD (LAD) groups, as described in detail in Chapters 2, 3, 4 and 10]—conform quite well to established clinical and research practice. They overlap to a considerable degree with the empirically derived taxa described in Chapter 10, except that the NVIQ that best discriminates the (higher functioning) Autism A subtaxon from the (lower functioning) Autism B subtaxon is 65, close to the Full Scale IQ of 70 widely used in the literature to separate high- and low-functioning autism groups (Rutter and Garmezy 1983, Cohen *et al.* 1987, Sheslow and Adams 1990, Lord and Venter 1992, Tsai 1992).

The results presented in this monograph represent the first step toward developing a valid and objective classification system for developmental disorders. The first goal of the project was to create definitions of the major entities under study which would preserve the essence of the disorders as clinically conceived, but which would meet rigorous classification standards. The success of the classification depends in part on its achievement of (i) validity, (ii) coverage, and (iii) homogeneity within groups.

*Validity*
Characterization of the four groups was generally in good agreement with previous literature. Results reported here clearly show clinically meaningful and statistically significant differences between children in the four groups. These results, on this large sample of children, provide clear information regarding the best attributes for differentiating such children at preschool age, using the current classification system. Thus, the results suggest good descriptive validity. This type of validity, necessary though it is, is of limited use; predictive validity is of more interest and importance to both clinicians and researchers, but requires a longitudinal design. Of equal validating importance is a classification system's conformity to external bio-behavioral attributes such as brain morphology, electrophysiological responses and neurological findings. How well such a system correlates with developmental outcome and biological attributes may influence its usefulness for devising a specific intervention. Future external validation and longitudinal follow-up studies are required to explore these aspects of validity.

*Coverage*
Coverage of the system for the preschool children referred for communication deficits seems good: 88 per cent of the clinically referred children were diagnosable by the algorithms used. Of the children who were not diagnosable by these procedures, the majority had been referred as language disordered, suggesting that children referred as possibly on the autistic spectrum were better covered by the diagnostic criteria used. Characteristics of children referred as either language disordered or autistic who were not diagnosable by the criteria used for the study are summarized in Chapter 10.

A degree of diagnostic overlap was indicated by the number of children referred for one diagnosis but classified by study criteria into another group, and by reassignment of children from one diagnostic group to another by taxometric analysis. Examination of both these sets of data indicate that few autistic children were reclassified, but that a substantial number of children diagnosed NALIQ were better regarded as autistic; there was little movement in or out of the DLD category, but a substantial number of clinically referred DLD children did not meet the more rigorous inclusionary criteria. Thus, analyses suggest that the clinical and empirical diagnoses of autism are in good correspondence, but that the differentiation between autism and cognitive deficit may be more difficult. In contrast, DLD is more distinct from autism and cognitive deficit, but the clinical and empirical definitions are not in very good agreement.

*Homogeneity*

Even though clear operational criteria were used to group children, it is apparent from the data reported in this monograph that the groups represent very broad and heterogeneous groups and, furthermore, that considerable overlap exists between groups. Social and communication difficulties exist in the DLD and NALIQ groups, language disorders in the NALIQ and AD children, and retardation in the AD children. Ranges and standard deviations on many variables also attest to the heterogeneity within groups. This problem was addressed in two ways. First, alternative systems for classifying children into DLD and AD groups were explored; in general their coverage was less than the systems adopted for forming the groups. Each of these alternative systems differed in its coverage and homogeneity. In the absence of biological 'gold standards' for classification, the system one selects depends on the goals of one's classification (*e.g.* the goal of finding all cases increases the probability of making some false positive diagnoses; the goal of assembling highly homogeneous groups increases the probability of missing some affected children). As is well known, the relative costs of over-inclusion (false positives) *vs* missing cases (false negatives) depends in large part on the base rate of the condition being considered: the rarer it is, the greater the cost of detecting all cases and of spurious identifications.

The second method for addressing heterogeneity within major groups was to seek evidence for the existence of subtypes within the taxometrically defined AD and DLD groups. Evidence for two subtaxa of autism, Autism A and B, was relatively strong, whereas evidence for Expressive and Receptive/Expressive DLD subtaxa was less strong. Stronger taxometric evidence for these and, perhaps, other subtaxa would have required a larger number of subjects.

Another important finding was the generally good consistency of results from different domains of assessment and different types of assessment (formal testing, clinician ratings, informant checklists, time-sampled behavior ratings). For example, poor language comprehension and pragmatics, together with impaired sociability, served best to differentiate the HAD from the DLD children on neuropsychological testing, on psychiatrists' ratings, on neurologists' ratings, and on several parent and teacher reports. Several important exceptions to this consistency across domains and sources of data should be noted: many more teachers than parents described autistic children as resistant to change in routines, an important finding to explore because it may reflect different behavior in different settings, and because this is one of the DSM III-R behavioral criteria for autism. Neurologists described subnormal cognitive skills in only about two thirds of the children found to be deficient on formal measures of intelligence. One reason might have been that intellectual level may be hard to assess accurately in one session of behavioral observation, especially when the physician is also rating many other aspects of the child's functioning; another equally plausible reason was that children may not perform to potential on formal testing; a third reason might relate to the choice of a high cut-off for this study (NVIQ <80), which is higher than the IQ level of 70 usually considered to define the upper level of mental retardation. In most cases, and dependent on the skill of the tester and the experience of the neurologist, the first explanation is probably more valid, and the clinical implication is that formal testing should be performed whenever level of intellectual functioning is in doubt. Another inconsistency was that the child neurologists and psychiatrists endorsed fewer behavioral abnormalities than parent and teacher informants. This result held across all groups; the physician's differential sensitivity was as great as the parent reporters, but their threshold for endorsing an abnormality was higher. Parental report of current and past autistic behaviors showed a bimodal distribution (autistic/non-autistic); this may indicate that such behavioral report data may be stronger indicators of a diagnosis of autism than observations by neurologists and psychiatrists in a single interview of the child.

**Limitations of the study**

Conclusions from the project are constrained by several limitations. A most important one is the lack of a large normal control group for non-standardized measures. Normal children were studied to provide comparisons for the language and play data, but it was not possible to administer the entire battery to a large group of normally developing children. We relied on published norms for standardized tests, an acceptable compromise. We were able to examine differences among the four clinical groups on most variables, but were unable to compare each of the groups to normally developing children, which would have allowed characterization of the profile of development of each group as compared with that seen in normal children.

Another limitation of the study is that it was not designed or executed as an epidemiologic study; therefore estimates of base rates of disorders, required for accurate calculation of diagnostic efficiency, and important in themselves, cannot be made from the data base, nor can estimates of relative rates of disorders in family members be evaluated relative to the general population. Also, the study is not of the universe of preschool children with inadequate communication and social skills because it excluded children with known etiologies, overt brain damage, uncontrolled epilepsy, and hearing and visual losses. Another possible shortcoming of a non-epidemiological study is that the referral-based sample excluded children who had not been brought to the attention of a clinician or who had been judged unimpaired; the children enrolled thus represent an incomplete sample.

A third limitation of the project is that the wide range of functioning of the children necessitated use of some non-overlapping assessment instruments, creating psychometric difficulties for comparing children within and across groups. This issue is discussed in Chapter 4.

Despite these limitations, the project provides data to address the classification issues discussed earlier and helps answer some additional questions regarding differential diagnosis and possible underlying brain deficits and etiologies.

### Best discriminators between autistic and non-autistic groups

There was no single type of assessment or area of function that best differentiated autistic from non-autistic children, but selected groups of items within each area were good discriminators. Family histories were generally not strong discriminators between groups. Although language disorders were highest in families of DLD children, and autism in the siblings of autistic children, there was a suggestion of crossover between groups. A higher proportion of the NALIQ, but not of the LAD, children were from families of lower SES. While acquisition of most language and motor milestones was related to IQ, the autistic children showed more delayed onset of pretend and social play, of achieving toilet training, of asking 'wh–' questions, and of speaking in full sentences than the non-autistic children. Regression in language skills and severely impaired comprehension were much more common in autism, as were sleep disturbances. Neurologically, small heads tended to characterize the NALIQ children and large heads the HAD children.

All behaviors on the autism behavior checklist of the history form strongly differentiated autistic from non-autistic children. The most potent discriminators were nonverbal communication, interactive play and joint attention, peer relationships, pretend play, pragmatic use of language, and motor stereotypies. In the neurological examination, uncooperative behavior, social withdrawal, and flat or depressed affect also characterized many autistic children. On direct observation, the autistic children showed less symbolic play than their comparison groups, with the LAD children showing little symbolic play, the HAD children showing impaired capacity to sustain their symbolic play, and the DLD children needing 'warm-up' time to demonstrate their full symbolic play.

Cognitively, the autistic children as a group had particularly marked deficits on receptive language measures, on functional deployment of their expressive skills, on prosody, prevalence of echolalia and use of scripts, and on formulating connected discourse, but showed spared development of written language, while the DLD children as a group showed relatively even patterns of language skills with relative impairment in written language. Verbal and visual memory was impaired in all groups; the key difference was that the DLD children were able to compensate for deficits if semantic structure was present to organize the information, while the verbal autistic children did as well or better on non-meaningful information.

Motor profiles were generally similar across autistic and non-autistic groups, but the autistic children were more impaired than the DLD children, and showed motor stereotypies not shown by the other groups. The verbal autistic children, however, had better articulation and oromotor skills than the other groups.

### Non-language deficits in the DLD group

Although some investigators have suggested that the deficits presented by language disordered children are specific to language (hence the use of the term 'specific language impairment'), the findings of our study do not support the specificity of this disorder. The DLD group obtained scores >1.5 SD below the mean on the S-B Bead Memory, a test of visual memory. In addition, their performance on several motor tasks evidenced impairment, including borderline overall performance on the composite motor domain of the Vineland, with particular deficits in the gross motor subdomain, and on the Annett Pegboard where right hand performance was >1 SD below average. Thus, while the deficits among the DLD children are most pronounced in areas involving language, impairment is not specific to language alone, but also includes other visual and motor functions.

### Interpretation of differences between the HAD and LAD groups

We divided the AD sample after the fact into HAD and LAD groups by a cut-off at 80 in NVIQ in order to compare DLD with HAD and NALIQ with LAD children. We want to stress again that the division between HAD and LAD does not correspond to the division at IQ 70 used by many investigators in the field to separate high- from low-functioning autistic children, and that it does not correspond either to the recommended cut between Autism A and B discussed in Chapter 10. Although we formed the HAD and LAD groups arbitrarily, we nonetheless found many significant non-cognitive differences between them.

Children in the LAD group were more likely to have seizures, sleep problems, greater delay in developmental milestones and greater severity in autistic symptomatology than those in the HAD group. HAD children were more likely to have large heads than LAD children. LAD children had more apraxia and stereotypies, and poorer representational play than HAD children. About half the LAD children had no speech; no HAD child was mute and some were judged to speak excessively. HAD children showed much better language and cognitive skills than LAD children. While both HAD and LAD children were judged to be severely socially impaired on a variety of variables, LAD children were viewed as more socially impaired than HAD children.

While some portion of the differences between HAD and LAD children may be the result of a general severity factor, the differences cannot be explained entirely by mental age. First, the neuropsychological measures were covaried for IQ and yet some group differences between HAD and LAD remained. Second, data for the developmental histories showed group differences even when the data from the lowest IQ LAD children (IQs ≤50) were excluded.

Current data do not justify reification of HAD and LAD as 'true' subgroups of AD. Our finding of subtaxa within the AD taxon, with overlapping distributions that do not correspond exactly with the HAD and LAD groups, provides empirical evidence for the long-held suspicion of many investigators that there are subgroups within autism. Larger numbers of subjects, as well as longitudinal data, will be required to enable a more detailed analysis of the characteristics of subgroups and, perhaps, the detection of further subtaxa.

### Clues about etiology and localization of brain dysfunction in the four groups

Both HAD and DLD children showed relative deficits in motor skill with the right hand

219

on the Annett Pegboard, possibly suggesting greater left hemisphere involvement. In the LAD group there was a small but disproportionately distributed number of children who had had early encephalitis or meningitis. The NALIQ children showed a higher prevalence than the other groups of preterm birth, small head size, motor delays and abnormalities, and seizures, possibly indicating more diffuse brain involvement, and suggesting that less favorable social/environmental (*e.g.* prenatal) conditions might have played an etiologic role in some cases. The fact that, as a group, the LAD children, who were more retarded than the NALIQ children and shared their high rates of motor impairments and seizures, did not share their low birthweights and lower SES suggests a different set of causes for their cognitive subnormality. The disproportionate number of HAD children with large heads, and the relatively large heads of even the LAD group, suggest a distinctive type of aberrant brain development in autism, rather than a destructive or growth stunting process.

Factors previously cited as possibly contributing to specific syndromes, such as ear infections and perinatal insults, did not differentiate the groups, but the lack of a large normal control group precludes examining the possibility that these factors would be elevated in all of the groups under study. There was no differential prevalence of other psychiatric and medical conditions in the families of children in the four groups; it is possible, however, that links will be found when more homogeneous subgroups of the four major groups are defined. Genetic contributions to DLD and autism were suggested by the differential prevalence of language disorders in the DLD families and autism in the families of autistic children. An epidemiological study with examination of all family members would be required to demonstrate that the prevalences reported in this study are elevated above those in the general population and to determine whether they differentiate among disorders.

## Clinical implications of the project
### Diagnosis
CRITERIA FOR IDENTIFYING DLD

Although many researchers assume that DLDs have a neurological basis, there is as yet no distinctive neurological evidence upon which to base the identification of preschool children as having DLD. Our goal in the present study was to be inclusive but to follow a procedure that would be replicable and that would be consistent with current clinical practice. Therefore we started by using a psychometric discrepancy criterion to identify our DLD cohort, defined as a 15 point discrepancy between verbal and nonverbal standard scores. This criterion captured no more than 60 per cent of the clinically defined sample. Because this criterion yielded inadequate coverage, we added low MLU for age as an additional/alternative criterion to capture our DLD sample.

Both the group of clinically identified DLD children who met the psychometric discrepancy criteria and the group that did not produced a significantly higher percentage of structural and meaning errors in a spontaneous language sample than did normal control children. Therefore, we attempted to develop new diagnostic criteria using data from the spontaneous language sample. An optimal combination of variables that included MLU, percentage of structural errors (percentage of utterances containing a syntactic error), and chronological age identified 96 per cent of the clinically referred children (Dunn *et al.* 1996). Our study shows that MLU and percentage of structural errors provide a more sensitive gauge of syntactic competence across the preschool and early school-age years than psychometric tests of language which address language competence mainly at the single word level. Quantitative measures of syntax in spontaneous language samples seem to provide a more clinically congruent, and perhaps more ecologically valid method for identifying children as DLD than do psychometric data*. Before this more sensitive approach is widely accepted, it will require confirmation through future research.

CRITERIA FOR IDENTIFYING AUTISTIC DISORDERS

Autism is part of a larger set of disorders of sociability, social communication and repetitive behaviors generally referred to as pervasive developmental disorder. For the present study we used DSM III-R criteria for Autistic Disorder to form our sample. DSM III-R was the standard diagnostic instrument at the inception of our study; also, it provided the greatest coverage. Current DSM IV and ICD-10 criteria provide significantly less coverage. Taxometric analysis has suggested that there are two core PDD groups— one a more low-functioning and more severely autistic group whose IQs are likely to be <65 (subtaxon B), and another group with milder symptomatology whose IQs are likely to be ≥65 (subtaxon A). These subtaxa cross diagnostic boundaries of standard psychiatric classification systems. Clinical prototypes of the two subtaxa may be of significant help in understanding the essential nature of the PDD spectrum. The study supports the generally accepted view that both severity of autistic behaviors and NVIQ be used to differentiate children who are likely to be less severely affected from those likely to be more seriously affected.

CONTRIBUTION OF THE HISTORY

Clinicians from many fields are equipped to differentiate autistic children from non-autistic children with language disorders or cognitive impairment, and our study confirms that historical information can be relied upon for making this distinction, provided clinicians are familiar with the symptoms of autism. If they are not, they should use one of several well standardized checklists or questionnaires. These may indicate the presence of an autistic spectrum disorder even if more obvious signs are not readily apparent in the atypical environment of a single office evaluation.

The study illustrates the advantage of using a questionnaire format for eliciting uniform developmental information. A number of standardized questionnaires about early language milestones such as the parent-report MacArthur Communication Development Inventories (Fenson *et al.*1991) and the observational Early Language Milestone Scale (Coplan 1989, Coplan and Gleason 1990) became available after the inception of this

*Although calculating MLU and number of structural errors requires transcribing a spontaneous language sample of no less than 50 (better 100) utterances, and analysis is facilitated by the availability of a specialized computer program, it can be carried out straighforwardly by hand if only these two numbers are of interest.

study. We would recommend that physicians use them in order to sensitize themselves to what is acceptable within the range of early language development and what indicates a potential problem in a young child, so that they can refer the child for a more quantitative assessment. Filling out an identical or congruent questionnaire on each follow-up visit, ideally supplemented with descriptive notes about features it does not cover, provides the longitudinal data required for tracking the evolution of early deficits.

The study confirms the importance of obtaining a detailed family history of disorders of reading and spelling as well as of delayed onset of speech, and of enquiring specifically about other relatives with autistic traits, inadequate socialization skills, severe depressive or manic–depressive illness, and perhaps schizophrenia, if one is interested in pursuing the genetics of these conditions. Again, a standardized format for recording the data is crucial if one's goal is to inform as yet unanswered research questions about the possible relation of early developmental disorders to those of later life.

CONTRIBUTION OF THE MEDICAL/NEUROLOGICAL EVALUATION

Together, the Collaborative Perinatal Project and the present study indicate that the physician plays an important role in evaluating preschool children with developmental disorders of higher cerebral function. The specific contribution of the physician is the focus on potential biological etiologies. Even though there is a small probability of making a specific biological diagnosis in disorders without obvious genetic or physical cause or other detectable evidence of brain dysfunction, the importance of such a finding, when it does occur, may be great. Evaluation of the medical and genetic history and findings on examination of the child guide the physician's choice of potential ancillary tests such as neuroimaging, electrophysiological and newer genetic tests. Such tests are unlikely to alter the prescription for habilitation of the child but they may be essential, in some cases, for excluding a treatable condition, for example hypothyroidism, and for detecting a condition with genetic implications like fragile X syndrome. It will remain the physician's role to interpret the biological implications of the findings, subtle or not, from the aggregate of all the diagnostic investigations so as to provide the parents with the assurance that no biological cause requiring medical intervention, including, perhaps, psychopharmacological medication, has been overlooked.

Even a very detailed medical and classic neurological examination will, however, probably add limited data to the understanding of the child's functioning and needs. When dealing with developmental disorders of brain function, it is the history and the results of age-appropriate standardized psychological and language tests and behavioral questionnaires that are likely to provide the most informative and reliable data for making an accurate diagnosis. Nonetheless, physicians need to learn to pay attention to the various aspects of children's language and to observe their social skills and play—the mental status evaluation in preschool children—because it is this type of observation that will help them decide whether a referral for quantitative behavioral testing is warranted.

CONTRIBUTION OF FORMAL TESTS OF LANGUAGE AND COGNITION

Before considering aspects of the neuropsychological evaluation suggested by the data, we should examine some general issues relevant to neuropsychological evaluation of the populations under consideration.

Individual variation is the rule, not the exception. Examination of standard deviations in the data tables confirms what clinicians observe, namely, that there is tremendous variability among children in levels and profiles of cognitive abilities, even among children who share diagnostic and behavioral features. Therefore, each child must be studied with an open mind and few preconceptions, or important strengths as well as weaknesses will be missed.

In this monograph mean scores for groups of children are presented, with few qualitative observations. Qualitative observations of behavior during testing are extremely important for understanding the child's cognitive style and abilities, and for making recommendations. Of particular importance are children's ability to self-monitor and self-correct, their ability to perform without frequent tangible reinforcers, their motivation and use of specific problem-solving strategies such as verbal rehearsal or self-instructions, or evidence of visual scanning and internal generation of solutions rather than overt trial and error behavior, and expression of pride and mastery. Such behaviors, and even those with some negative connotations such as performance anxiety, will indicate that the child has a general social context in which to view the activity of testing, and has some motivation to succeed and/or to please, and the ability to take an overview of his own behavior; these are important positive prognostic signs for the child's educational success.

Observation of aspects of attention is also crucial. Ability to sustain on-task behavior for reasonable lengths of time is very important for educational success. Materials that trigger loss of attention may suggest or confirm areas that the child finds particularly difficult or aversive. The degree to which task success, interesting materials, or stepped-up tangible reinforcers can boost sustained attention and increase resistance to distraction will be useful information for teachers and parents.

The study indicates that there are some specific findings that the neuropsychological evaluation should include. In general, DLD children had difficulty with some aspects of language testing, but the autistic children had even poorer language skills, especially in the receptive domain. Consonant with much clinical experience, visual cues seemed to facilitate word retrieval, so that confrontation naming was an actual area of strength for the autistic children, contrasted with categorical word retrieval which was very poor. The discrepancy between visual confrontation naming and single word receptive vocabulary (with naming higher) was particularly marked for the high-functioning autistic children, while the DLD children as a group showed no such discrepancy. Another finding that should guide evaluation is that the autistic children had a marked discrepancy between tests of lexical/semantic and rote verbal memory functions, on the one hand, and tests requiring verbal problem solving or self-organized formulated verbal output, on the other, with the latter being especially deficient; these areas, then, should be evaluated separately. As pointed out previously, the autistic child's high confrontation naming ability can easily mislead adults or peers to overestimate the child's language comprehension.

Spontaneous language analysis indicated that DLD children made more discourse errors than normal children, but the autistic children made more errors still. While the DLD and autistic children made equal numbers of syntactic errors in spontaneous language, the autistic children made more semantic and pragmatic errors. Although no standardized measures of these types of errors are in use, the clinician can use the description of these errors in Appendix 4.1 to estimate the degree of deficit the child has in each of these areas. As stated earlier, engaging the children on topics of great interest to them will tend to minimize their pragmatic deficits, while pressing topics of conventional interest will expose more subtle pragmatic deficits; the full range of pragmatic competence should be examined by engaging the child in both ways. Observation of factors in the child's pragmatic style which limit reciprocal interaction (such as inability to maintain a topic, intrusion of perseverative concerns, failure to respond to social initiations, inappropriate or inadequate eye contact, poor social distance, etc.) may help in planning remediation.

Children in all clinical groups showed difficulty with aspects of visual memory, even though visuospatial reasoning was at the average level in the DLD and HAD groups. Therefore, neuropsychological evaluations of DLD children, although they would appropriately focus on language processes, should also examine visual memory abilities. Verbal memory showed different patterns in DLD than in HAD children. The overall degree of deficit was not very different, but the children differed in the type of material that was most difficult for them. The DLD children's performance improved as intrinsic semantic organization increased; they were able to use the meaning of the verbal material spontaneously to encode the information and use the meaning to retrieve more of the information. When material was inherently meaningless, however, as in Digit Span, the autistic children were superior in rote recall. Therefore, examination of verbal and visual memory, using material that varies in degree of intrinsic organization or meaningfulness, will be helpful; the relatively recent Wide Range Assessment of Memory and Learning (Sheslow and Adams 1990) may turn out to be extremely useful in this regard.

The study also suggests that motor testing is important for autistic, NALIQ and DLD children because some children in all groups showed motor deficits. Praxis deficits were found in both autistic groups and in the NALIQ group but not in the DLD group, even though some individual DLD children may have been mildly dyspraxic. Some children in the DLD group had deficits on fine and gross motor testing. Unilateral or asymmetric deficits on quantitative fine motor testing were found for many of the children, and we therefore recommend including a timed pegboard test that evaluates each of the two hands individually.

Although many of the tests were highly intercorrelated within groups, there were certain suggestive dissociations. The DLD children had a factor for visuospatial skills, but a separate factor for attention to visual detail, suggesting that these should be assessed separately. For the autistic children, there was a dissociation between rote memory and simple tests, on the one hand, and complex problem solving and planning tasks on the other. For the LAD children, this distinction cut across both verbal and visuospatial tasks; for the HAD children, this held only for verbal tests. This would suggest that a clinician cannot generalize from an autistic child's single-word or rote memory tests to his general language or cognitive competence; for the LAD group, one cannot generalize from simple visual matching tests to complex visual problem solving.

CONTRIBUTION OF A SYSTEMATIC ASSESSMENT OF BEHAVIOR

The findings from the interviews and scales concerned with behavior suggest that to arrive at optimal diagnostic decisions it is best to use a consultation process that includes parent, teacher and physician (child psychiatrist, child neurologist, or pediatrician with particular interest in developmental disorders). The accumulation of information from three sources using a common instrument or approach followed by discussion yields the most detailed and accurate picture of a child's functioning. The most discriminating single measure for differentiating the four preschool groups we studied was the WADIC. This brief checklist can be used easily by parents or any professional evaluating the child and would provide a brief clear means for coordinating the judgment of parent, physician and teacher or other professional. Because the WADIC in its present form addresses only current behavior, we recommend that parents use a modified version to endorse both past and present behaviors, in order to increase the sensitivity of the diagnosis. This or a similar checklist would seem to be particularly helpful for early preschool determination of the presence of autistic features in the behavior of any clinical population.

CONTRIBUTION OF THE OBSERVATION OF PLAY SKILLS

Observation of play is not a typical component in a routine pediatric, neurological or neuropsychological evaluation. Speech pathologists are more likely to engage children in play, but it is generally for the purpose of evaluating the child's language development and conversational abilities. Psychiatrists use symbolic play with the goal of understanding the child's psychodynamics. However, this study suggests that observation of play with representational toys is an efficient and enlightening addition to the mental status assessment of young children. We therefore recommend that it be widely used by all clinicians concerned with the evaluation of developmentally impaired preschool children, with a focus on children's capacity for advanced representational play, their motivation to sustain such play, and their willingness to incorporate the examiner in their ongoing play.

*Suggestions for intervention based on the neuropsychological profiles*

It is important to state at the outset that research regarding the efficacy of specific remedial approaches is replete with studies that do not disentangle confounding factors. The approaches suggested below have not been proven effective by rigorous studies but are driven by a theoretical perspective based on neuropsychological data.

The major goal for intervention is to find a match between instructional methods and the individual child's learning style as understood through the child's profile of cognitive, linguistic and behavioral strengths and weaknesses revealed by comprehensive neuropsychological investigation. A relatively flat neuropsychological profile, as for example in the NALIQ group, does not provide the specific approaches to remediation afforded by the more irregular profiles of children in the DLD and HAD groups.

There are four basic approaches to remediation: (1) direct intervention ('teach to the deficit'); (2) modification of the environment; (3) teach to the child's strengths; and (4) use strengths to compensate for weaknesses. The general assumption of the neuropsychological model is that there is some degree of neural plasticity in the developing child but that different systems of the brain are not equipotential. In addressing severe impairments it is often necessary to modify the environment or work only toward developing areas of strength. In the very young child direct remediation may be appropriate, but the primary approach with many children involves teaching the child to use strengths to compensate for weaknesses. For example, DLD and HAD children, being the least impaired of the children considered in this study, can benefit from such compensatory strategies.

Clearly, each child has a somewhat different neuropsychological profile that needs to be considered in planning an individualized remedial approach. Within-group variability in groups as broadly defined as those in our study attests to the need for careful consideration of the individual child, yet the group profiles described in this monograph are instructive. We provide here some examples of general approaches to remediation based on these group profiles.

The neuropsychological profile in the DLD group included poor auditory verbal short term memory for material low in meaning, and improvement with increasing meaningfulness of the material; relatively spared visual memory for easily verbally codable material; poor visual sequential memory; and normal nonverbal problem solving. This profile suggests that some teaching methods should be more effective than others. For example, in teaching the young school-aged DLD child sound/letter relationships, learning may be enhanced by embedding the material in a meaningful context. One way would be to embed each letter in the picture of a concrete object beginning with that letter sound (a picture of a snake in the shape of an 'S') and to select pictures from an area of interest to the child. A child who has difficulty with phonemic discrimination or awareness may be helped by employing a mirror to promote the use of the visual cues provided by looking at the face and mouth of the speaker. In teaching DLD children to read words, a word-families approach is helpful because it taxes auditory verbal memory and visual sequential memory much less than sounding out words letter by letter. As words are learned, embedding them in sentences takes advantage of the enhanced memory associated with increasing meaning. Learning to read could be presented as a nonverbal problem solving task using word/picture puzzles or letter/word family puzzles.

The neuropsychological profile in the HAD group included normal nonverbal abilities; poor self-organization of connected speech; poor pragmatics and impaired socialization; inadequate language comprehension; stronger confrontation naming and written language skills than DLD children; better short term auditory verbal memory for non-meaningful material than for meaningful material; relatively spared visual memory; strength in rote learning and good long term memory. In remediating HAD children, it is critical to remember not to judge their language comprehension from their output, because they do not exhibit the more common pattern of better comprehension than expression, at least at the lexical level, typical of most language impaired children. HAD children's prevailing reliance on formulaic expressions can be deceptive inasmuch as they are able to say things that they do not fully comprehend. A concrete, visually based format, for example an adaptation of Pehrsson and Robinson's (1985) Semantic Organizer Approach to Reading and Writing Instruction, may help remediate deficient attention to auditory/verbal meaning and inadequate formulation/organization of discourse. In this approach the child is taught to produce a hierarchically organized semantic network of pictures/written words, where the main topic constitutes the central node, and subtopics and supporting details are branches emanating from that node. In a child with adequate written language skills, written language can be used to enhance auditory verbal comprehension. After some experience with this strategy, the child can be taught to visualize the network to aid in the discussion of a topic. The child is taught a variety of organizational frames/formulas that can be applied in a variety of circumstances.

The autistic children's deficits in behavior and socialization limit their ability to benefit from even a structured teaching situation. The first goal for these children is to foster skills such as sustained attention to task, turn-taking, imitation and self-control. It is usually necessary to address these issues directly in order to provide an environment in which learning can proceed. LAD children tend to have better nonverbal than verbal abilities and they may have adequate rote memories. They tend to learn better in highly routinized/predictable environments and may particularly benefit from individualized highly structured reward-based educational approaches. Higher-functioning verbal autistic children can benefit from working in dyads with children who are less socially impaired in order to learn ways of interacting socially and verbally with their peers.

In our cohort, 6 per cent of DLD, 39 per cent of AD, and 17 per cent of NALIQ subjects were mute or essentially nonverbal (fewer than ten utterances during the entire 25 minute play session). Many of these children appear to have severe deficits in the processing of auditory language. For these children, it is crucial that visual language systems be used in conjunction with oral language in order to provide them with alternatives to the auditory channel alone. Despite normal hearing, these youngsters require some of the techniques that have been successfully utilized with deaf and severely hearing impaired students. Communication boards, picture exchange, computerized programs, sign language and written language can be utilized effectively to supplement oral input.

**Future research**
Ongoing analyses of the database are focusing on the delineation of subgroups within the major clinical entities described here. Repeating some of the analyses described in this monograph on other large groups of children studied with similar or even dissimilar test instruments would strengthen the evidence for subtaxa and the detection of further subgroups. It may well be that additional features, such as genetic links with other disorders or neurological findings, will become significant when larger, more homogeneous

groups are identified and studied. The need to pursue the biological basis of these disorders in homogenous groups of children with tightly defined behavioral characteristics needs no further emphasis here because it is abundantly evident that progress in prevention and pharmacological intervention rests upon biological, not behavioral studies. But in order to increase the probability of making valid brain/behavior correlations it is essential to minimize group variance and thus essential to study groups with rigorously defined behavioral characteristics.

The other major thrust of ongoing research is the longitudinal follow-up of the children at school age and, hopefully, in adolescence. The developmental course of the groups will support or deny the validity of the syndromes defined in the preschool years and will allow clinicians to provide earlier and more accurate prognoses. Such future studies will have both clinical and research importance and will help resolve some of the enigmas that continue to plague our understanding of these complex disorders of early brain development.

# REFERENCES

Adler, S. (1964) *The Non-verbal Child.* Springfield, IL: Charles C. Thomas.

Allen, D.A. (1988) 'Autistic spectrum disorders: clinical presentation in preschool children.' *Journal of Child Neurology,* **3,** S48–S56.

—— (1989) 'Developmental language disorders in preschool children: clinical subtypes and syndromes.' *School Psychology Review,* **18,** 442–451.

—— Rapin, I. (1980) 'Language disorders in preschool children: predictors of outcome—a preliminary report.' *Brain and Development,* **2,** 73–80.

—— —— (1992) 'Autistic children are also dysphasic.' *In:* Naruse, H., Ornitz, E.M. (Eds.) *Neurobiology of Infantile Autism.* Amsterdam: Excerpta Medica, pp. 157–168.

Aman, M.G. (1991) *Assessing Psychopathology and Behavior Problems in Persons with Mental Retardation: a Review of Available Instruments.* Rockville, MD: US Department of Health and Human Sciences.

—— Singh, N.N. (1986) *Aberrant Behavior Checklist: Manual.* Aurora, NY: Slossom Educational.

Ameli, R., Courchesne, E., Lincoln, A.J., Kaufman, A.S., Grillon, C. (1988) 'Visual memory processes in high-functioning individuals with autism.' *Journal of Autism and Developmental Disorders,* **18,** 601–615.

American National Standards Institute (1970) *Specifications for Audiometers. ANSI S3.6–1969.* New York: ANSI.

American Psychiatric Association (1968) *Diagnostic and Statistical Manual of Mental Disorders. 2nd Edn (DSM II).* Washington, DC: APA.

—— (1980) *Diagnostic and Statistical Manual of Mental Disorders. 3rd Edn (DSM III).* Washington, DC: APA.

—— (1987) *Diagnostic and Statistical Manual of Mental Disorders. 3rd Edn—Revised (DSM III-R).* Washington, DC: APA.

American Psychiatric Association (1994) *Diagnostic and Statistical Manual of Mental Disorders. 4th Edn (DSM IV).* Washington, DC: APA.

American Speech–Language–Hearing Association (1983) 'Position paper on social dialects.' *ASHA,* **25** (9), 23–24.

Amiel-Tison, C., Stewart, A. (1989) 'Follow up studies during the first five years of life: a pervasive assessment of neurological function.' *Archives of Disease in Childhood,* **64,** 496–502.

Annegers, J.F., Blakley, S.A., Hauser, W.A., Kurland, L.T. (1990) 'Recurrence of febrile convulsions in a population-based cohort.' *Epilepsy Research,* **5,** 209–216.

Aram, D.M. (1991) 'Comments on specific language impairment as a clinical category.' *Language, Speech, and Hearing Services in Schools,* **22,** 84–87.

—— Nation, J.E. (1975) 'Patterns of language behavior in children with developmental language disorders.' *Journal of Speech and Hearing Research,* **18,** 229–241.

—— Ekelman, B.L., Nation, J.E. (1984) 'Preschoolers with language disorders: 10 years later.' *Journal of Speech and Hearing Research,* **27,** 232–244.

—— Morris, R., Hall, N.E. (1993) 'Clinical and research congruence in identifying children with specific language impairment.' *Journal of Speech and Hearing Research,* **36,** 580–591.

Arbelle, S., Sigman, M.D., Kasari, C. (1994) 'Compliance with parental prohibition in autistic children.' *Journal of Autism and Developmental Disorders,* **24,** 693–702.

Arthur, G. (1952) *The Arthur Adaption of the Leiter International Performance Scale.* Washington, DC: Psychological Service Center Press.

Asarnow, R., Sherman, T., Strandburg, R. (1986) 'The search for the psychobiological substrate of childhood onset schizophrenia.' *Journal of the American Academy of Child Psychiatry,* **25,** 601–614.

Asperger, H. (1944) 'Die "autistischen Psychopathen" im Kindesalter.' *Archiv für Psychiatrie und Nervenkrankheiten,* **117,** 76–136. [*Reprinted in translation in:* Frith, U. (Ed.) (1991) *Autism and Asperger Syndrome.* Cambridge UK: Cambridge University Press, pp. 37–92.]

August, G.J., Stewart, M.A., Tsai, L. (1981) 'The incidence of cognitive disabilities in the siblings of autistic children.' *British Journal of Psychiatry,* **138,** 416–422.

—— Raz, N., Baird, T.D. (1987) 'Fenfluramine response in high and low functioning autistic children.' *Journal of the American Academy of Child and Adolescent Psychiatry*, **26**, 342–346.

Bagley, C., McGeein, V. (1989) 'The taxonomy and course of childhood autism.' *Perceptual and Motor Skills*, **69**, 1264–1266.

Bailey, A., Luthert, P., Bolton, P., LeCouteur, A., Rutter, M., Harding, B. (1993) 'Autism and megalencephaly.' *Lancet*, **341**, 1225–1226. *(Letter.)*

Baker, L., Cantwell, D.P. (1987) 'A prospective psychiatric follow-up of children with speech/language disorders.' *Journal of the American Academy of Child and Adolescent Psychiatry*, **26**, 546–553.

Baltaxe, C.A.M. (1977) 'Pragmatic deficits in the language of autistic adolescents.' *Journal of Pediatric Psychology*, **2**, 176–180.

—— Simmons, J.Q. (1975) 'Language in childhood psychosis: a review.' *Journal of Speech and Hearing Disorders*, **40**, 439–458.

Baron-Cohen, S. (1991) 'Do people with autism understand what causes emotion?' *Child Development*, **62**, 385–395.

Bartak, L., Rutter, M. (1976) 'Differences between mentally retarded and normally intelligent autistic children.' *Journal of Autism and Developmental Disorders*, **6**, 109–120.

—— —— Cox, A. (1975) 'A comparative study of infantile autism and specific developmental receptive language disorder: I. The children.' *British Journal of Psychiatry*, **126**, 127–145.

—— —— —— (1977) 'A comparative study of infantile autism and specific developmental receptive language disorders. III. Discriminant function analysis.' *Journal of Autism and Childhood Schizophrenia*, **7**, 383–396.

Barth, C., Fein, D., Waterhouse, L. (1995) 'Delayed match to sample in autistic children.' *Developmental Neuropsychology*, **11**, 53–69.

Bartolucci, G., Pierce, S.J., Streiner, D., Eppel, P.T. (1976) 'Phonological investigation of verbal autistic and mentally retarded subjects.' *Journal of Autism and Childhood Schizophrenia*, **6**, 303–316.

Bates, E. (1979) *The Emergence of Symbols: Cognition and Communication in Infancy*. New York: Academic Press.

—— Marchman, V.A. (1988) 'What is and is not universal in language acquisition.' *In:* Plum, F. (Ed.) *Language, Communication, and the Brain*. New York: Raven Press, pp. 19–38.

—— Thal, D., Janowsky, J.S. (1992) 'Early language development and its neural correlates.' *In:* Segalowitz, S.J., Rapin, I. (Eds.) *Handbook of Neuropsychology, Section 10, Vol. 7. Child Neuropsychology (Part 2)*. Amsterdam: Elsevier Science, pp. 69–110.

Bateson, G. (1955) 'A theory of play and fantasy.' *Psychiatric Research Reports*, **2**, 39–51.

Bauman, M.L. (1991) 'Microscopic neuroanatomic abnormalities in autism.' *Pediatrics*, **87**, 791–796.

—— (1992a) 'Motor dysfunction in autism.' *In:* Joseph, A.B., Young, R.R. (Eds.) *Movement Disorders in Neurology and Neuropsychiatry*. Boston, MA: Blackwell, pp. 658–661.

—— (1992b) 'Neuropathology of autism.' *In:* Joseph, A.B., Young, R.R. (Eds.) *Movement Disorders in Neurology and Neuropsychiatry*. Boston, MA: Blackwell, pp. 662–666.

—— Kemper, T.L. (1994) *The Neurobiology of Autism*. Baltimore, MD: Johns Hopkins University Press, pp. 119–145.

Bayley, N. (1969) *Bayley Scales of Infant Development*. Berkeley, CA: Psychological Corporation.

Beitchman, J.H., Nair, R., Clegg, M., Ferguson, B., Patel, P.G. (1986a) 'Prevalence of psychiatric disorders in children with speech and language disorders.' *Journal of the American Academy of Child Psychiatry*, **25**, 528–535.

—— —— —— Patel, P.G. (1986b) 'Prevalence of speech and language disorders in 5-year-old kindergarten children in the Ottawa–Carleton region.' *Journal of Speech and Hearing Disorders*, **51**, 98–110.

—— Tuckett, M., Batth, S. (1987) 'Language delay and hyperactivity in preschoolers: evidence for a distinct subgroup of hyperactives.' *Canadian Journal of Psychiatry*, **32**, 683–687.

—— Peterson, M., Clegg, M. (1988) 'Speech and language impairment and psychiatric disorder: the relevance of family demographic variables.' *Child Psychiatry and Human Development*, **18**, 191–207.

Belsky, J., Most, R.K. (1981) 'From exploration to play: a cross-sectional study of infant free play behavior.' *Developmental Psychology*, **17**, 630–639.

Bender, L. (1947) 'Childhood schizophrenia. Clinical study of one hundred schizophrenic children.' *American Journal of Orthopsychiatry*, **17**, 40–56.

Benton, A.L. (1959) 'Aphasia in children.' *Education*, **79**, 408–412.

—— (1964) 'Developmental aphasia and brain damage.' *Cortex*, **1**, 40–52.

Berk, R.A. (1984) *Screening and Diagnosis of Children with Learning Disabilities.* Springfield, IL: Charles C. Thomas.

Biederman, J., Munir, K., Knee, D., Habelow, W., Armentano, M., Autor, S., Hodge, S.K., Waternaux, C. (1986) 'A family study of patients with attention deficit disorder and normal controls.' *Journal of Psychiatric Research*, **4**, 263–274.

Biklen, D. (1990) 'Communication unbound: autism and praxis.' *Harvard Educational Review*, **60**, 291–314.

Bishop, D.V.M., Adams, C. (1989) 'Conversational characteristics of children with semantic–pragmatic disorder: II. What features lead to a judgement of inappropriacy?' *British Journal of Disorders of Communication*, **24**, 241–263.

—— —— (1990) 'A prospective study of the relationship between specific language impairment, phonological disorders and reading retardation.' *Journal of Child Psychology and Psychiatry*, **31**, 1027–1050.

—— Edmundson, A. (1987) 'Language-impaired 4-year-olds: distinguishing transient from persistent impairment.' *Journal of Speech and Hearing Research*, **52**, 156–173.

—— Rosenbloom, L. (1987) 'Childhood language disorders: classification and overview.' *In:* Yule, W., Rutter, M. (Eds.) *Language Development and Disorders. Clinics in Developmental Medicine No. 101/102.* London: Mac Keith Press, pp. 16–41.

Bloom, L. (1970) *Language Development: Form and Function in Emerging Grammars.* Cambridge, MA: MIT Press.

—— Lahey, M. (1978) *Language Development and Language Disorders.* New York: Wiley.

Boel, M., Casaer, P. (1989) 'Continuous spikes and waves during slow sleep: a 30 months follow-up study of neuropsychological recovery and EEG findings.' *Neuropediatrics*, **20**, 176–180.

Braverman, M., Fein, D., Lucci, D., Waterhouse, L. (1989) 'Affect comprehension in children with pervasive developmental disorders.' *Journal of Autism and Developmental Disorders*, **19**, 301–316.

Broman, S.H., Nichols, P.L., Kennedy, W.A. (1975) *Preschool IQ: Prenatal and Early Developmental Correlates.* New York: John Wiley.

—— —— Shaughnessy, P., Kennedy, W. (1987) *Retardation in Young Children: a Developmental Study of Cognitive Deficit.* Hillsdale, NJ: Lawrence Erlbaum.

Brookhouser, P.E., Goldgar, D.E. (1987) 'Medical profile of the language-delayed child: otitis-prone versus otitis-free.' *International Journal of Pediatric Otorhinolaryngology*, **12**, 237–271.

Brown, R. (1973) *A First Language: the Early Stages.* Cambridge, MA: Harvard University Press.

Brunquell, P.J., Russman, B.S., Lerer, T.J. (1991) 'Sources of information used in diagnosing childhood learning disabilities.' *Pediatric Neurology*, **7**, 342–346.

Bryson, S.E., Clark, B.S., Smith, I.M. (1988) 'First report of a Canadian epidemiological study of autistic syndromes.' *Journal of Child Psychology and Psychiatry*, **29**, 433–445.

Burd, L., Fisher, W., Kerbeshian, J., Arnold, M.E. (1987*a*) 'Is development of Tourette disorder a marker for improvement in patients with autism and other pervasive development disorders?' *Journal of the American Academy of Child and Adolescent Psychiatry*, **26**, 162–165.

—— —— Knowlton, D., Kerbeshian, J. (1987*b*) 'Hyperlexia: a marker for improvement in children with pervasive developmental disorder?' *Journal of the American Academy of Child Psychiatry*, **26**, 407–412.

—— —— Kerbeshian, J. (1989) 'Pervasive disintegrative disorder: are Rett syndrome and Heller dementia infantilis subtypes?' *Developmental Medicine and Child Neurology*, **31**, 609–616.

Cantwell, D.P., Baker, L., Rutter, M. (1978) 'A comparative study of infantile autism and specific developmental receptive language disorder—IV. Analysis of syntax and language function.' *Journal of Child Psychology and Psychiatry*, **19**, 351–362.

—— —— Mawhood, L. (1989) 'Infantile autism and developmental receptive dysphasia: a comparative follow-up into middle childhood.' *Journal of Autism and Developmental Disorders*, **19**, 19–31.

Cardon, L.R., Smith, S.D., Fulker, D.W., Kimberling, W.J., Pennington, B.F., DeFries, J.C. (1994) 'Quantitative trait locus for reading disability on chromosome 6.' *Science*, **266**, 276–279.

Casby, M.W. (1992) 'The cognitive hypothesis and its influence on speech–language services.' *Language, Speech, and Hearing Services in Schools*, **23**, 198–202.

Castelloe, P., Dawson, G. (1993) 'Subclassification of children with autism and pervasive developmental disorder: a questionnaire based on Wing's subgrouping scheme.' *Journal of Autism and Developmental Disorders*, **23**, 229–241.

231

Chess, S. (1944) 'Developmental language disability as a factor in personality distortion in childhood.' *American Journal of Orthopsychiatry*, **14**, 483–490.

Clinical Forum (1991) 'Specific language impairment as a clinical category.' *Language, Speech, and Hearing Services in Schools*, **22**, 65–88.

Cohen, D.J., Caparulo, B.K., Shaywitz, B.A. (1976) 'Primary childhood aphasia and childhood autism: clinical, biological, and conceptual observations.' *Journal of the American Academy of Child and Adolescent Psychiatry*, **15**, 604–645.

—— Paul, R., Volkmar, F.R. (1986) 'Issues in the classification of pervasive and other developmental disorders: toward DSM-IV.' *Journal of the American Academy of Child Psychiatry*, **25**, 213–220.

—— —— —— (1987) 'Issues in the classification of PDD and associated conditions.' *In:* Cohen, D.J., Donnellan, A.M., Paul, R. (Eds.) *Handbook of Autism and Pervasive Developmental Disorders.* New York: Wiley, pp. 20–40.

Cohen, M., Campbell, R., Yaghmai, F. (1989) 'Neuropathological abnormalities in developmental dysphasia.' *Annals of Neurology*, **25**, 567–570.

Cole, K., Dale, P., Mills, P. (1990) 'Defining language delay in young children by cognitive referencing: are we saying more than we know?' *Applied Psycholinguistics*, **11**, 291–302.

—— Mills, P., Kelley, D. (1994) 'Agreement of assessment profiles used in cognitive referencing.' *Language, Speech, and Hearing Services in Schools*, **25**, 25–31.

Coleman, M. (1990) 'Delineation of the subgroups of the autisic syndrome.' *Brain Dysfunction*, **3**, 208–217.

—— Gillberg, C. (1985) *The Biology of the Autistic Syndromes.* New York: Praeger.

Comings, D.E., Comings, B.G. (1991) 'Clinical and genetic relationships between autism–pervasive developmental disorder and Tourette syndrome: a study of 19 cases.' *American Journal of Medical Genetics*, **39**, 180–191.

Coplan, J. (1989) *ELM Scale: the Early Language Milestone Scale (Revised).* Austin, TX: Pro-Ed.

—— Gleason, J.R. (1990) 'Quantifying language development from birth to 3 years using the Early Language Milestone Scale.' *Pediatrics*, **86**, 963–971.

Courchesne, E. (1991) 'Neuroanatomic imaging in autism.' *Pediatrics*, **87**, 781–790.

—— Yeung-Courchesne, R., Press, G.A., Hesselink, J.R., Jernigan, T.L. (1988) 'Hypoplasia of cerebellar vermal lobules VI and VII in autism.' *New England Journal of Medicine*, **318**, 1349–1354.

—— Townsend, J., Saitoh, O. (1994) 'The brain in infantile autism: posterior fossa structures are abnormal.' *Neurology*, **44**, 214–223.

Creak, E.M. (1963) 'Childhood psychosis. A review of 100 cases.' *British Journal of Psychiatry*, **109**, 84–89.

—— *et al.* (1961) 'Schizophrenic syndrome in childhood. Progress report of a working party (April, 1961).' *Cerebral Palsy Bulletin*, **3**, 501–504.

Cromer, R. (1981) 'Developmental language disorders: cognitive processes, semantics, pragmatics, phonology, and syntax.' *Journal of Autism and Developmental Disorders*, **11**, 57–74.

—— (1983) 'Hierarchical planning disability in the drawings and constructions of a special group of severely aphasic children.' *Brain and Cognition*, **2**, 144–164.

Cummins, R.A., Prior, M.P. (1992) 'Autism and assisted communication: a response to Biklen.' *Harvard Educational Review*, **62**, 228–241.

Cunningham, C.C., Glenn, S.M., Wilkinson, P., Sloper, P. (1985) 'Mental ability, symbolic play and receptive and expressive language of young children with Down's syndrome.' *Journal of Child Psychology and Psychiatry*, **26**, 255–265.

Curtiss, S., Katz, W., Tallal, P. (1992) 'Delayed versus deviance in the language acquisition of language-impaired children.' *ASHA*, **35**, 373–383.

Dahl, E.K., Cohen, D.J., Provence, S. (1986) 'Clinical and multivariate approaches to the nosology of pervasive developmental disorders.' *Journal of the American Academy of Child Psychiatry*, **25**, 170–180.

Dalrymple, N.J., Ruble, L.A. (1992) 'Toilet training and behaviors of people with autism: parent views.' *Journal of Autism and Developmental Disorders*, **22**, 265–275.

Dawson, G., Lewy, A. (1989) 'Arousal, attention, and socioemotional impairments of individuals with autism.' *In:* Dawson, G. (Ed.) *Autism: Nature, Diagnosis, and Treatment.* New York: Guilford Press, pp. 49–74.

—— Klinger, L., Panatiotides, H., Lewy, A., Castelloe, P. (1996) 'Subgroups of autistic children based on social behavior display distinct patterns of brain activity.' *Journal of Abnormal Child Psychology. (In press.)*

de Ajuriaguerra, J., Jaeggi, A., Guignard, F., Kocher, F., Maquard, M., Roth, S., Schmid, E. (1976) 'The development and prognosis of dysphasia in children.' *In:* Morehead, D.M., Morehead, A.E. (Eds.) *Normal and Deficient Child Language.* Baltimore: University Park Press, pp. 345–385.

DeLong, G.R., Dwyer, J.T. (1988) 'Correlation of family history with specific autistic subgroups: Asperger's syndrome and bipolar affective disease.' *Journal of Autism and Developmental Disorders,* **18,** 593–600.

—— Bean, S.C., Brown, F.R. (1981) 'Acquired reversible autistic syndrome in acute encephalopathic illness in children.' *Archives of Neurology,* **38,** 191–194.

DeLong, R. (1994) 'Children with autistic spectrum disorder and a family history of affective disorder.' *Developmental Medicine and Child Neurology,* **36,** 674–688.

—— Nohria, C. (1994) 'Psychiatric family history and neurological disease in autistic spectrum disorders.' *Developmental Medicine and Child Neurology,* **36,** 441–448.

DeMyer, M.K., Alpern, G.D., Barton, S., DeMyer, W.E., Churchill, D.W., Hingtgen, J.N., Bryson, C.Q., Pontius, W., Kimberlin, C. (1972) 'Imitation in autistic, early schizophrenic, and non-psychotic sub-normal children.' *Journal of Autism and Childhood Schizophrenia,* **2,** 264–287.

Denckla, M.B. (1985) 'Revised neurological examination for subtle signs.' *Psychopharmacology Bulletin,* **21,** 773–789.

Deonna, T.W. (1991) 'Acquired epileptiform aphasia in children (Landau–Kleffner syndrome).' *Journal of Clinical Neurophsyiology,* **8,** 288–298.

—— Ziegler, A-L., Moura-Serra, J., Innocenti, G. (1993) 'Autistic regression in relation to limbic pathology and epilepsy: report of two cases.' *Developmental Medicine and Child Neurology,* **35,** 166–176.

Deuel, R.K. (1992) 'The neurologic examination of the school-age and adolescent child.' *In:* David, R.B. (Ed.) *Pediatric Neurology for the Clinician. 4th Edn.* Norwalk, CT: Appleton & Lange, pp. 81–95.

Deutsch, S.I., Campbell, M., Perry, R., Green, W.H., Poland, R.E., Rubin, R.T. (1986) 'Plasma growth hormone response to insulin-induced hypoglycemia in infantile autism: a pilot study.' *Journal of Autism and Developmental Disorders,* **16,** 59–68.

Deykin, E.Y., MacMahon, B. (1980) 'Pregnancy, delivery, and neonatal complications among autistic children.' *American Journal of Diseases of Children,* **134,** 860–864.

Dihoff, R.E., Hetznecher, W., Brosovic, G.M. (1993) 'Ordinal measurements of autistic behavior: a pre-liminary report.' *Bulletin of the Psychonomic Society,* **31,** 287–290.

DiLalla, D.L., Rogers, S.J. (1994) 'Domains of the Childhood Autism Rating Scale: relevance for diagnosis and treatment.' *Journal of Autism and Developmental Disorders,* **24,** 115–128.

Doll, E.A. (1965) *The Vineland Social Maturity Scale.* Circle Pines, MN: American Guidance Service.

Dunn, L.M., Dunn, L. (1981) *Peabody Picture Vocabulary Test—Revised.* Circle Pines, MN: American Guidance Service.

Dunn, M. (1994) 'Neurophysiologic observations in autism and implications for neurologic dysfunction.' *In:* Bauman, M.L., Kemper, T.L. (Eds.) *The Neurobiology of Autism.* Baltimore, MD: Johns Hopkins University Press, pp. 45–65.

—— Flax, J., Sliwinski, M., Aram, D. (1996) 'The use of spontaneous language measures as criteria in identifying children with specific language impairment: an attempt to reconcile clinical and research incongruence.' *Journal of Speech and Hearing Research. (In press.)*

du Verglas, G., Banks, S.R., Guyer, K.E. (1988) 'Clinical effects of fenfluramine on children with autism: a review of the research.' *Journal of Autism and Developmental Disorders,* **18,** 297–308.

Eberlin, M., McConnachie, G., Ibel, S., Volpe, L. (1993) 'Facilitated communication: a failure to replicate the phenomenon.' *Journal of Autism and Developmental Disorders,* **23,** 507–530.

Echenne, B., Cheminal, R., Rivier, F., Negre, C., Touchon, J., Billiard, M. (1992) 'Epileptic electroenceph-alographic abnormalities and developmental dysphasias: a study of 32 patients.' *Brain and Development,* **14,** 216–225.

Eisenson, J. (1968) 'Developmental aphasia (dyslogia): a postulation of a unitary concept of the disorder.' *Cortex,* **4,** 184–200.

Engel, J.J. (1989) *Seizures and Epilepsy.* Philadelphia: F.A. Davis.

Ewing, A. (1930) *Aphasia in Children.* London: Oxford University Press.

Fama, R., Fein, D., Waterhouse, L. (1992) 'Verbal and nonverbal short-term memory in autistic children.' *Journal of Clinical and Experimental Neuropsychology,* **14,** 114. *(Abstract.)*

Fay, W., Schuler, A.L. (1989) *Emerging Language in Autistic Children.* Baltimore, MD: University Park Press.

Fein, D., Waterhouse, L., Lucci, D., Pennington, B.F., Humes, M. (1985a) 'Handedness and cognitive functions in pervasive developmental disorders.' *Journal of Autism and Developmental Disorders*, **15**, 323–333.

—— —— —— Snyder, D. (1985b) 'Cognitive subtypes in developmentally disabled children: a pilot study.' *Journal of Autism and Developmental Disorders*, **15**, 77–95.

—— Pennington, B., Markowitz, P., Braverman, M., Waterhouse, L. (1986) 'Toward a neuropsychological model of infantile autism: are the social deficits primary?' *Journal of the American Academy of Child Psychiatry*, **25**, 198–212.

—— —— Waterhouse, L. (1987) 'The neurobiology of social deficits.' *In:* Schopler, E., Mesibov, G.B. (Eds.) *Neurobiology Issues in Autism.* New York: Plenum Press, pp. 127–144.

Fenson, L., Kagan, J., Kearsley, R.B., Zelazo, P.R. (1976) 'The developmental progression of manipulative play in the first two years.' *Child Development*, **47**, 232–236.

—— Dale, P.S., Reznick, S., Thal, D., Bates, E., Hartung, J.P., Pethick, S., Reilly, J.S. (1991) *Technical Manual for the MacArthur Communicative Development Inventories.* San Diego, CA: San Diego State University.

Filipek, P.A., Kennedy, D.N., Caviness, V.S.J. (1992a) 'Neuroimaging in child neuropsychology.' *In:* Rapin, I., Segalowitz, S.J. (Eds.) *Handbook of Neuropsychology. Volume 6: Child Neuropsychology. 11th Edn.* Amsterdam: Elsevier Science, pp. 301–329.

—— Rachelme, C., Kennedy, D.N., Rademacher, J., Pitcher, D.A., Zidel, S., Caviness, V.S. (1992b) 'Morphometric analysis of the brain in developmental language disorders and autism.' *Annals of Neurology*, **32**, 475. *(Abstract.)*

Finegan, J.A., Quarrington, B. (1979) 'Pre-, peri-, and neonatal factors and infantile autism.' *Journal of Child Psychology and Psychiatry*, **2**, 119–128.

Finucci, J.M., Guthrie, J.T., Childs, A.L., Abbey, H., Childs, B. (1976) 'The genetics of specific reading disability.' *Annals of Human Genetics*, **40**, 1–23.

Fish, B. (1977) 'Neurobiologic antecedents of schizophrenia in children. Evidence for an inherited, congenital neurointegrative defect.' *Archives of General Psychiatry*, **34**, 1297–1313.

Fletcher, J.M., Taylor, H.G. (1984) 'Neuropsychological approaches to children: towards a developmental neuropsychology.' *Journal of Clinical Neuropsychology*, **6**, 39–56.

—— Francis, D.J., Morris, R. (1988) 'Methodological issues in neuropsychology: classification, measurement, and the comparison of non-equivalent groups.' *In:* Boller, F., Grafman, J. (Eds.) *Handbook of Neuropsychology. Vol. 1.* Amsterdam: Elsevier, pp. 83–110.

Folstein, S.E., Piven, J. (1991) 'Etiology of autism: genetic influences.' *Pediatrics*, **87**, 767–775.

—— Rutter, M. (1977) 'Infantile autism: a genetic study of 21 twin pairs.' *Journal of Child Psychology and Psychiatry*, **18**, 297–321.

Frantzen, E., Lennox-Buchthal, M., Nygaard, A., Stene, J. (1970) 'A genetic study of febrile convulsions.' *Neurology*, **20**, 909–917.

Freeman, B.J., Ritvo, E.R., Schroth, P.C., Tonick, I., Guthrie, D., Wake, L. (1981) 'Behavioral characteristics of high- and low-IQ autistic children.' *American Journal of Psychiatry*, **138**, 25–29.

—— —— (1984) 'Behavior assessment of the syndrome of autism: behavior observation system.' *Journal of the American Academy of Child Psychiatry*, **23**, 588–594.

Frith, U. (Ed.) (1991) *Autism and Asperger Syndrome.* Cambridge: Cambridge University Press.

—— (1993) 'Autism: autistic individuals suffer from a biological defect. Although they cannot be cured, much can be done to make life more hospitable for them.' *Scientific American*, (June), 78–84.

Fyffe, C., Prior, M. (1978) 'Evidence for language recoding in autistic, retarded and normal children: a reexamination.' *British Journal of Psychology*, **69**, 393–402.

Galaburda, A.M. (1993) 'Neuroanatomic basis of developmental dyslexia.' *Neurologic Clinics*, **11**, 161–173.

—— Sherman, G.F., Rosen, G.D., Aboitiz, F., Geschwind, N. (1985) 'Developmental dyslexia: four consecutive patients with cortical anomalies.' *Annals of Neurology*, **18**, 222–233.

Gardner, M.F. (1979) *Expressive One-Word Picture Vocabulary Test.* Novato, CA: Academic Therapy Publications.

Geschwind, N., Galaburda, A.M. (1984) *Cerebral Dominance: the Biological Foundations.* Cambridge, MA: Harvard University Press.

Gillberg, C. (1984) 'Infantile autism and other childhood psychoses in a Swedish urban region. Epidemiological aspects.' *Journal of Child Psychology and Psychiatry*, **25**, 35–43.

—— (1989) 'Asperger syndrome in 23 Swedish children.' *Developmental Medicine and Child Neurology*, **31**, 520–531.

—— (1990) 'Autism and pervasive developmental disorders.' *Journal of Child Psychology and Psychiatry*, **31**, 99–119.

—— (1991) 'Clinical and neurobiological aspects of Asperger syndrome in six family studies.' *In:* Frith, U. (Ed.) *Autism and Asperger Syndrome.* Cambridge: Cambridge University Press, pp. 122–146.

—— (1992) 'Subgroups of autism: are there behavioural phenotypes typical of underlying medical conditions?' *Journal of Intellectual Disabilities Research*, **36**, 201–214.

—— Coleman, M. (1992) *The Biology of the Autistic Syndromes. 2nd Edn. Clinics in Developmental Medicine No. 126.* London: Mac Keith Press.

—— Gillberg, I.C. (1983) 'Infantile autism: a total population study of reduced optimality in the pre-, peri-, and neonatal periods.' *Journal of Autism and Developmental Disorders*, **13**, 153–166.

—— Schaumann, H. (1981) 'Infantile autism and puberty.' *Journal of Autism and Developmental Disorders*, **11**, 365–371.

—— Gillberg, I.C., Steffenburg, S. (1990) 'Reduced optimality in the pre-, peri-, and neonatal periods is not equivalent to severe peri- or neonatal risk: a rejoinder to Goodman's technical note.' *Journal of Child Psychology and Psychiatry*, **31**, 813–815.

—— Steffenburg, S., Schaumann, H. (1991) 'Autism: is autism more common now than ten years ago?' *British Journal of Psychiatry*, **158**, 403–409.

Golden, R.R., Mayer, M.M. (1995) 'Peaked indicators: a source of pseudo-taxonicity of a latent trait.' *In:* Lubinski, D., Dawis, R. (Eds.) *Assessing Individual Differences in Human Behavior: New Concepts, Methods, and Findings.* Palo Alto, CA: Davies-Black, pp. 93–115.

Goldfarb, W. (1964) 'An investigation of childhood schizophrenia. A retrospective view.' *Archives of General Psychiatry*, **11**, 620–634.

Goodall, D.W. (1966) 'Hypothesis-testing in classification.' *Nature*, **211**, 329–330.

Goodman, R., Stevenson, J. (1989) 'A twin study of hyperactivity—II. The aetiological role of genes, family relationships and perinatal adversity.' *Journal of Child Psychology and Psychiatry*, **30**, 691–709.

Gopnik, M., Crago, M.B. (1991) 'Familial aggregation of a developmental language disorder.' *Cognition*, **39**, 1–50.

Gould, S.J. (1994) 'Pride of place: science without taxonomy is blind.' *The Sciences*, **34**, 38–39.

Goulden, K.S., Shinnar, S., Koller, H., Katz, M., Richardson, S.A. (1991) 'Epilepsy in children with mental retardation: a cohort study.' *Epilepsia*, **32**, 690–697.

Graham, N.C. (1980) *Memory Constraints in Language Deficiency.* Baltimore, MD: University Park Press.

Green, W.H., Campbell, M., Hardesty, A.S., Grega, D.M., Padron-Gayol, M., Shell, J., Erlenmeyer-Kimling, L. (1984) 'A comparison of schizophrenic and autistic children.' *Journal of the American Academy of Child Psychiatry*, **23**, 399–409.

Group for the Advancement of Psychiatry (1966) *Psychopathological Disorders in Childhood: Theoretical Considerations and a Proposed Classification.* New York: GAP.

Hallgren, B. (1950) 'Specific dyslexia ("congenital word blindness"): a clinical and genetic study.' *Acta Psychiatrica Neurologica*, **65** (Suppl.), 1–287.

Happé, F.G.E. (1991) 'The autobiographical writings of three Asperger syndrome adults: problems of interpretation and implications for theory.' *In:* Frith, U. (Ed.) *Autism and Asperger Syndrome.* Cambridge: Cambridge University Press, pp. 207–242.

Hardy, W.G. (1965) 'On language disorders in young children: a reorganization of thinking.' *Journal of Speech and Hearing Disorders*, **30**, 3–16.

Haynes, C., Naidoo, S. (1991) *Children with Specific Speech and Language Impairment. Clinics in Developmental Medicine No. 119.* London: Mac Keith Press.

Hedrick, D.L., Prather, E.M., Tobin, A.R. (1984) *Sequenced Inventory of Communication Development (Revised Edition).* Seattle: University of Washington Press.

Hefner, L.T., Mednick, S.A. (1969) 'Reliability of developmental histories.' *Pediatrics Digest*, **8** (Aug.), 28–39.

Hermelin, B., O'Connor, N. (1970) *Psychological Experiments with Autistic Children.* Oxford: Pergamon Press.

—— —— (1975) 'The recall of digits by normal, deaf and autistic children.' *British Journal of Psychology*, **66**, 203–209.

235

Hiskey, M.S. (1966) *Hiskey–Nebraska Test of Learning Aptitude*. Lincoln, NE: University of Nebraska Press.

Ho, H-Z., Glahn, T.J., Ho, J-C. (1988) 'The fragile-X syndrome.' *Developmental Medicine and Child Neurology*, **30**, 257–261.

Hollingshead, A.B. (1975) *Four Factor Index of Social Status*. New Haven, CT: Yale University Press.

Howlin, P., Rutter, M. (1987) 'The consequences of language delay for other aspects of development.' *In:* Yule, W., Rutter, M. (Eds.) *Language Development and Disorders. Clinics in Developmental Medicine No. 101/102*. London: Mac Keith Press, pp. 271–294.

Hresko, W.P., Reid, D.K., Hammill, D.D. (1981) *The Test of Early Language Development*. Austin, TX: PRO-ED.

Huebner, R.A. (1992) 'Autistic disorder: a neuropsychological enigma.' *American Journal of Occupational Therapy*, **46**, 487–501.

Hurst, J.A., Baraitser, M., Auger, E., Graham, F., Norell, S. (1990) 'An extended family with a dominantly inherited speech disorder.' *Developmental Medicine and Child Neurology*, **32**, 352–355.

Hurtig, R., Ensrud, S., Tomblin, J.B. (1982) 'The communicative function of question production in autistic children.' *Journal of Autism and Developmental Disorders*, **12**, 57–69.

Hynd, G.W., Semrud-Clikeman, M., Lorys, A.R., Novey, E.S., Eliopulos, D. (1990) 'Brain morphology in developmental dyslexia and attention deficit disorder/hyperactivity.' *Archives of Neurology*, **47**, 919–926.

Ingram, T.T.S. (1959) 'Specific developmental disorders of speech in childhood.' *Brain*, **82**, 450–467.

—— Reid, J.F. (1956) 'Developmental aphasia observed in a department of child psychiatry.' *Archives of Disease in Childhood*, **31**, 161–172.

Inhelder, B. (1966) 'Cognitive development and its contribution to the diagnosis of some phenomena of mental deficiency.' *Merrill–Palmer Quarterly*, **12**, 299–319.

—— (1976) 'Observations on the operational and figurative aspects of thought in dysphasic children.' *In:* Morehead, D.M., Morehead, A.E. (Eds.) *Normal and Deficient Child Language*. Baltimore: University Park Press, pp. 335–343.

Jacobson, J.W., Ackerman, L.J. (1990) 'Differences in adaptive functioning among people with autism or mental retardation.' *Journal of Autism and Developmental Disorders*, **20**, 205–219.

Jayakar, P.B., Seshia, S.S. (1991) 'Electrical status epilepticus during slow-wave sleep: a review.' *Journal of Clinical Neurophysiology*, **7**, 299–311.

Johnson, W.G. (1982) 'Genetic heterogeneity of the hexosaminidase deficiency diseases.' *In:* Kety, S.S., Rowland, L.P., Sidman, R.L., Matthysse, S.W. (Eds.) *Genetics of Neurological and Psychiatric Disorders*. New York: Raven Press, pp. 215–237.

Johnston, J.R. (1982) 'Interpreting the Leiter IQ: performance profiles of young normal and language-disordered children.' *Journal of Speech and Hearing Research*, **25**, 291–296.

—— (1988) 'Specific language disorders in the child.' *In:* Lass, N.J., McReynolds, L.V., Northern, J.L., Yoder, D.E. (Eds.) *Handbook of Speech–Language Pathology and Audiology*. Philadelphia: B.C. Decker, pp. 685–715.

—— Ellis Weisman, S. (1983) 'Mental rotation abilities in language-disordered children.' *Journal of Speech and Hearing Research*, **26**, 340–397.

—— Kamhi, A. (1984) 'The same can be less: syntactic and semantic aspects of the utterances of language impaired children.' *Merrill–Palmer Quarterly*, **30**, 65–86.

—— Ramstad, V. (1983) 'Cognitive development in preadolescent language impaired children.' *British Journal of Disordered Communication*, **18**, 49–55.

—— Schery, T.K. (1976) 'The use of grammatical morphemes by children with communication disorders.' *In:* Morehead, D., Morehead, A. (Eds.) *Normal and Deficient Child Language*. Baltimore: University Park Press, pp. 239–258.

—— Kamhi, A., McDonald, J. (1981) 'Patterns of predicate use in language impaired children.' *Proceedings of the Symposium on Research in Child Language Disorders*, **2**, 17–28.

—— Blatchley, M., Streit, G. (1985) 'Miniature language system learning by normal and language disorded children.' *Proceedings of the Symposium on Research in Child Language Disorders*, **6**, 1–10.

Jones, K.L. (1988) *Smith's Recognizable Patterns of Human Malformation. 4th Edn.* Philadelphia: W.B. Saunders.

Jones, M.B., Szatmari, P. (1988) 'Stoppage rules and genetic studies of autism.' *Journal of Autism and Developmental Disorders*, **18**, 31–40.

Kamhi, A.G. (1981) 'Nonlinguistic symbolic and conceptual abilities of language-impaired and normally

developing children.' *Journal of Speech and Hearing Disorders*, **24**, 446–453.
—— Catts, H.W. (1986) 'Towards an understanding of developmental language and reading disorders.' *Journal of Speech and Hearing Disorders*, **51**, 337–347.
—— Johnston, J.R. (1982) 'Towards an understanding of retarded children's linguistic deficiencies.' *Journal of Speech and Hearing Research*, **25**, 435–445.
Kaminer, R.K., Jedrysek, E., Soles, B. (1984) 'Behavior problems of young retarded children.' *In:* Berg, J.M. (Ed.) *Perspectives and Progress in Mental Retardation. Vol. II —Biomedical Aspects.* Baltimore: University Park Press, pp. 289–298.
Kanner, L. (1943) 'Autistic disturbances of affective contact.' *Nervous Child*, **2**, 217–250.
—— (1973) 'The birth of infantile autism.' *Journal of Autism and Childhood Schizophrenia*, **2**, 93–95.
Karlin, I.W. (1951) 'Congenital verbal–auditory agnosia (word deafness).' *Pediatrics*, **7**, 60–68.
Kavanaugh, J.F. (1986) *Otitis Media and Child Development.* Parkton, MD: York Press.
Kemper, T.L., Bauman, M. (1992) 'Neuropathology of infantile autism.' *In:* Naruse, H., Ornitz, E.M. (Eds.) *Neurobiology of Infantile Autism. Excerpta Medica International Congress Series No. 965.* Amsterdam: Elsevier Science, pp. 43–57.
Kendell, R. (1982) 'The choice of diagnostic criteria for biological research.' *Archives of General Psychiatry*, **39**, 1334–1339.
Kilshaw, D., Annett, M. (1983) 'Right- and left-hand skill. I: Effects of age, sex and hand preference showing superior skill in left-handers.' *British Journal of Psychology*, **74**, 253–268.
Kirchner, D.M., Klatzky, R.L. (1985) 'Verbal rehearsal and memory in language-disordered children.' *Journal of Speech and Hearing Research*, **28**, 556–565.
Kirk, S.A., McCarthy, J.J., Kirk, W.D. (1968) *Examiner's Manual: Illinois Test of Psycholinguistic Abilities.* Urbana, IL: University of Illinois Press.
Klein, S.K., Rapin, I. (1988) 'Intermittent conductive hearing loss and language development.' *In:* Bishop, D., Mogford, K. (Eds.) *Language Development in Exceptional Circumstances. 6th Edn.* New York: Churchill Livingstone, pp. 96–109.
Knobloch, H., Pasamanick, B. (1959) 'Syndrome of minimal cerebral damage in infancy.' *Journal of the American Medical Association*, **170**, 1384–1387.
—— Stevens, F., Malone, A., Ellison, P., Risemberg, H. (1979) 'The validity of parental reporting of infant development.' *Pediatrics*, **63**, 872–878.
Kolvin, I. (1971) 'Studies in the childhood psychoses. I. Diagnostic criteria and classification.' *British Journal of Psychiatry*, **118**, 381–384.
Konstantareas, M.M., Hauser, P., Lennox, C., Homatidis, S. (1988) 'Season of birth in infantile autism.' *Journal of Child Psychiatry and Human Development*, **42**, 785–793.
Kotsopoulos, A., Boodoosingh, L. (1987) 'Language and speech disorders in children attending a day psychiatric programme.' *British Journal of Disorders of Communication*, **22**, 227–236.
Kurita, H. (1985) 'Infantile autism with speech loss before the age of thirty months.' *Journal of the American Academy of Child Psychiatry*, **24**, 191–196.
—— (1988) 'The concept and nosology of Heller's syndrome: review of articles and report of two cases.' *Japanese Journal of Psychiatry and Neurology*, **42**, 785–793.
—— Kita, M., Miyake, Y. (1992) 'A comparative study of development and symptoms among disintegrative psychosis and infantile autism with and without speech loss.' *Journal of Autism and Developmental Disorders*, **22**, 175–188.
Lahey, M. (1990) 'Who shall be called language disordered? Some reflections and one perspective.' *Journal of Speech and Hearing Disorders*, **55**, 612–620.
Landau, W.M., Kleffner, F.R. (1957) 'Syndrome of acquired aphasia with convulsive disorder in children.' *Neurology*, **7**, 523–530.
Leonard, L.B. (1979) 'Language impairment in children.' *Merrill–Palmer Quarterly*, **25**, 205–232.
—— (1982) 'The nature of specific language impairment in children.' *In:* Rosenberg, S. (Ed.) *Handbook of Applied Psycholinguistics: Major Thrusts of Research and Theory.* Hillsdale, NJ: Lawrence Erlbaum, pp. 295–327.
—— (1983) 'Discussion. Part II: Defining the boundaries of language disorders in children.' *In:* Miller, J., Yoder, D.E., Schiefelbusch, R. (Eds.) *Comtemporary Issues in Language Intervention.* Washington, DC: ASHA, pp. 107–114.
—— (1986) 'Conversational replies of children with specific language impairment.' *Journal of Speech and Hearing Research*, **29**, 114–119.

—— (1987) 'Is specific language impairment a useful construct?' *In:* Rosenberg, S. (Ed.) *Advances in Applied Psycholinguistics. Vol. I: Disorders of First Language Development.* New York: Cambridge University Press, pp. 1–39.

—— (1991) 'Specific language impairment as a clinical category.' *Language, Speech, and Hearing Services in Schools*, **22**, 66–88.

—— Camarata, S., Rowan, L., Chapman, K.L. (1982) 'The communicative functions of lexical usage by language impaired children.' *Applied Psycholinguistics*, **3**, 109–125.

Lerman, P., Lerman-Sagie, T., Kivity, S. (1991) 'Effect of early corticosteroid therapy for Landau–Kleffner syndrome.' *Developmental Medicine and Child Neurology*, **33**, 257–260.

Levine, M.D. (1980) 'The child with learning disabilities.' *In:* Scheiner, A.P., Abroms, I.F. (Eds.) *The Practical Management of the Developmentally Disabled Child.* St Louis, MO: C.V. Mosby, pp. 312–339.

Lewis, B.A. (1992) 'Pedigree analysis of children with phonology disorders.' *Journal of Learning Disabilities*, **25**, 586–597.

—— Thompson, L.A. (1992) 'A study of developmental speech and language disorders in twins.' *Journal of Speech and Hearing Research*, **35**, 1086–1094.

—— Ekelman, B.L., Aram, D.M. (1989) 'A familial study of severe phonological disorders.' *Journal of Speech and Hearing Research*, **32**, 713–724.

Lewis, V., Boucher, J. (1988) 'Spontaneous, instructed and elicited play in relatively able autistic children.' *British Journal of Developmental Psychology*, **6**, 325–339.

Lieberman, R.J., Michael, A. (1986) 'Content relevance and content coverage in tests of grammatical ability.' *Journal of Speech and Hearing Disorders*, **51**, 71–81.

Lincoln, A.J., Courchesne, E., Kilman, B.A., Elmasian, R., Allen, M.A. (1988) 'A study of intellectual abilities in high-functioning people with autism.' *Journal of Autism and Developmental Disorders*, **18**, 505–524.

Links, P. (1980) 'Minor physical anomalies in infantile autism. II: Their relationship to maternal age.' *Journal of Autism and Developmental Disorders*, **10**, 287–292.

Locke, J.L. (1994) 'Gradual emergence of developmental language disorders.' *Journal of Speech and Hearing Research*, **37**, 608–616.

Lombardino, L.J., Stein, J.E., Kricos, P.B., Wolf, M.A. (1986) 'Play diversity and structural relationships in the play and language of language-impaired and language-normal preschoolers: preliminary data.' *Journal of Communication Disorders*, **19**, 475–489.

Lord, C. (1985) 'Autism and the comprehension of language.' *In:* Schopler, E., Mesibov, G. (Eds.) *Communication Problems in Autism.* New York: Plenum Press, pp. 257–281.

—— Venter, A. (1992) 'Outcome and follow-up studies of high-functioning autistic individuals.' *In:* Schopler, E., Mesibov, G.B. (Eds.) *High-Functioning Individuals with Autism.* New York: Plenum Press, pp. 187–199.

—— Mulloy, C., Wendelboe, M., Schopler, E. (1991) 'Pre- and perinatal factors in high-functioning females and males with autism.' *Journal of Autism and Developmental Disorders*, **21**, 197–209.

—— Rutter, M., Le Couteur, A. (1994) 'Autism Diagnostic Interview—Revised: a revised version of a diagnostic interview for caregivers of individuals with possible pervasive developmental disorders.' *Journal of Autism and Developmental Disorders*, **24**, 659–685.

Lowe, M., Costello, A.J. (1976) *Manual of the Symbolic Play Test.* Windsor: NFER.

Ludlow, C.L., Cooper, J.A. (1983) 'Genetic aspects of speech and language disorders: current status and future directions.' *In:* Ludlow, C.L., Cooper, J.A. (Eds.) *Genetic Aspects of Speech and Language Disorders.* New York: Academic Press, pp. 1–18.

Majnemer, A., Rosenblatt, B. (1994) 'Reliability of parental recall of developmental milestones.' *Pediatric Neurology*, **10**, 304–308.

Marescaux, C., Hirsch, E., Finck, S., Maquet, P., Schlumberger, E., Sellal, F., Metz-Lutz, M.N., Alembik, Y., Salmon, E., *et al.* (1990) 'Landau–Kleffner syndrome: a pharmacologic study of five cases.' *Epilepsia*, **31**, 768–777.

Martineau, J., Roux, S., Adrien, J.L., Garreau, B., Barthélémy, C., Lelord, G. (1992) 'Electrophysiological evidence of different abilities to form cross-modal associations in children with autistic behavior.' *Electroencephalography and Clinical Neurophysiology*, **82**, 60–66.

Mason-Brothers, A., Ritvo, E.R., Pingree, C., Petersen, P.B., Jenson, W.R., McMahon, W.M., Freeman, B.J., Jorde, L.B., Spencer, M.J., *et al.* (1990) 'The UCLA–University of Utah epidemiologic survey of autism: prenatal, perinatal, and postnatal factors.' *Pediatrics*, **4**, 514–519.

Masterson, J.J. (1993) 'The performance of children with language–learning disabilities on two types of cognitive tasks.' *Journal of Psycholinguistic Research*, **36**, 1026–1036.

Maurer, R.G., DeMasio, A.R. (1982) 'Childhood autism from the point of view of behavioral neurology.' *Journal of Autism and Developmental Disorders*, **12**, 195–205.

Mayes, L., Volkmar, F., Hooks, M., Cicchetti, D. (1993) 'Differentiating Pervasive Developmental Disorder Not Otherwise Specified from autism and language disorders.' *Journal of Autism and Developmental Disorders*, **23**, 79–90.

Maytal, J., Shinnar, S., Moshé, S.L., Alvarez, L.A. (1989) 'Low morbidity and mortality of status epilepticus in children.' *Pediatrics*, **83**, 323–331.

McCall, R.B. (1974) *Exploratory Manipulation and Play in the Human Infant. Monographs of the Society for Research in Child Development, Vol. 39, No. 2.*

McCarthy, D. (1972) *McCarthy Scales of Children's Abilities.* Cleveland, OH: Psychological Corp.

McCauley, R.J., Swisher, L. (1984) 'Use and misuse of norm-referenced tests in clinical assessment: a hypothetical case.' *Journal of Speech and Hearing Disorders*, **49**, 338–348.

McCune-Nicolich, L. (1981) 'Toward symbolic functioning: structure of early pretend games and potential parallels with language.' *Child Development*, **52**, 785–797.

—— Bruskin, C. (1982) *Combinatorial Competency in Symbolic Play and Language.* Basel: Karger.

McGinnis, M.A. (1963) *Aphasic Children: Identification and Education by the Association Method.* Washington, DC: Alexander Graham Bell Association for the Deaf.

—— Kleffner, F.R., Goldstein, R. (1956) 'Teaching aphasic children.' *Volta Review*, **58**, 239–244.

McNemar, Q. (1969) *Psychological Statistics. 4th Edn.* New York: Wiley.

Meehl, P.E. (1986) 'Diagnostic taxa as open concepts: metatheoretical and statistical questions about reliability and construct validity in the grand strategy of nosological revision.' *In:* Millon, T., Klerman, G.L. (Eds.) *Contemporary Directions in Psychopathology: Toward the DSM-IV.* New York: Guilford Press, pp. 215–231.

Meiselas, K.D., Spencer, E.K., Oberfield, R., Peselow, E.D., Angrist, B., Campbell, M. (1989) 'Differentiation of stereotypies from neuroleptic-related dyskinesias in autistic children.' *Journal of Clinical Psychopharmacology*, **9**, 207–209.

Menyuk, P. (1978) 'Language: what's wrong and why.' *In:* Rutter, M., Schopler, E. (Eds.) *Autism: a Reappraisal of Concepts and Treatment.* New York: Plenum, pp. 105–116.

Miller, J.F. (1981) *Assessing Language Production in Children.* Austin, TX: Pro-Ed.

—— Chapman, R.S., MacKenzie, H. (1981) 'Individual differences in the language acquisition patterns of mentally retarded children.' *Proceedings of the Symposium on Research in Child Language Disorders*, **2**, 130–146.

Minshew, N.J. (1991) 'Indices of neural function in autism: clinical and biologic implications.' *Pediatrics*, **87**, 774–780.

—— Goldstein, G., Muenz, L.R., Payton, J.B. (1992) 'Neuropsychological functioning in nonmentally retarded autistic individuals.' *Journal of Clinical and Experimental Neuropsychology*, **14**, 749–761.

Mordecai, D.R., Palin, M.W., Palmer, C.B. (1985) *Lingquest I: Language Sample Analysis.* Columbus, OH: Charles E. Merrill.

Morehead, D.M., Ingram, D. (1973) 'The development of base syntax in normal and linguistically deviant children.' *Journal of Speech and Hearing Research*, **16**, 330–352.

Morley, M.E. (1957) *The Development and Disorders of Speech in Childhood.* Edinburgh: E & S Livingstone.

—— (1965) *The Development and Disorders of Speech in Childhood. 2nd Edn.* Edinburgh: E & S Livingstone.

—— (1972) *The Development and Disorders of Speech in Childhood. 3rd Edn.* Edinburgh: Churchill Livingstone.

Morris, R.D., Fletcher, J.M. (1988) 'Classification in neuropsychology: a theoretical framework and research paradigm.' *Journal of Clinical and Experimental Neuropsychology*, **10**, 640–658.

Mundy, P., Sigman, M.D., Ungerer, J.A., Sherman, T. (1987) 'Nonverbal communication and play correlates of language development in autistic children.' *Journal of Autism and Developmental Disorders*, **17**, 349–364.

—— —— Kasari, C. (1990) 'A longitudinal study of joint attention and language development in autistic children.' *Journal of Autism and Developmental Disorders*, **20**, 115–128.

239

Myklebust, H.R. (1954) *Auditory Disorders in Children: a Manual for Differential Diagnosis.* New York: Grune & Stratton.

Nation, J.E., Aram, D.M. (1990) *Diagnosis of Speech and Language Disorders. 3rd Edn.* San Diego, CA: Singular Press.

Nellhaus, G. (1968) 'Head circumference from birth to eighteen years. Practical composite international and interracial graphs.' *Pediatrics*, **41**, 106–114.

Nelson, K.B. (1991) 'Prenatal and perinatal factors in the etiology of autism.' *Pediatrics*, **87**, 761–766.

Nelson, L.K., Kamhi, A.G., Apel, K. (1987) 'Cognitive strengths and weaknesses in language-impaired children: one more look.' *Journal of Speech and Hearing Disorders*, **52**, 36–43.

Nye, C., Montgomery, J.K. (1989) 'Identification criteria for language disordered children: a national survey.' *Hearsay*, **1**, 26–33.

—— Weems, L. (1991) 'Identification criteria for children with language disorders.' *Hearsay*, **6**, 34–38.

Obler, L.K., Fein, D. (Eds.) (1988) *The Exceptional Brain: Neuropsychology of Talent and Special Abilities.* New York: Guilford Press.

Ornitz, E.M. (1994) 'A behavioral-based neurophysiological model for dysfunction of directed attention in infantile autism.' *In:* Naruse, H., Ornitz, E.M. (Eds.) *Neurobiology of Infantile Autism.* Amsterdam: Excerpta Medica, pp. 89–109.

Orton, S.T. (1937) *Reading, Writing and Speech Problems in Children: a Presentation of Certain Types of Disorders in the Development of the Language Faculty.* New York: W.W. Norton.

Overall, J.E., Campbell, M. (1988) 'Behavioral assessment of psychopathology in children: infantile autism.' *Journal of Clinical Psychology*, **44**, 708–716.

Ozonoff, S., Rogers, S.J., Pennington, B.F. (1991) 'Asperger's syndrome: evidence of an empirical distinction from high-functioning autism.' *Journal of Child Psychology and Psychiatry*, **32**, 1107–1122.

Parks, S.L. (1983) 'The assessment of autistic children: a selective review of available instruments.' *Journal of Autism and Developmental Disorders*, **13**, 255–267.

Paul, R. (1992) 'Communication.' *In:* Cohen, D.J., Donnellan, A.M., Paul, R. (Eds.) *Handbook of Autism and Pervasive Developmental Disorders.* New York: John Wiley, pp. 61–84.

—— Cohen, D.J. (1984*a*) 'Responses to contingent queries in adults with mental retardation and pervasive developmental disorders.' *Applied Psycholinguistics*, **5**, 349–357.

—— —— (1984*b*) 'Outcomes of severe disorders of language acquisition.' *Journal of Autism and Developmental Disorders*, **14**, 405–421.

—— Fischer, M.L., Cohen, D.J. (1988) 'Sentence comprehension strategies in children with autism and specific language disorders.' *Journal of Autism and Developmental Disorders*, **18**, 669–679.

Pearson, D.A., Aman, M.G. (1994) 'Ratings of hyperactivity and developmental indices: should clinicians correct for developmental level?' *Journal of Autism and Developmental Disorders*, **24**, 395–411.

Pehrsson, R.S., Robinson, H.A. (1985) *The Semantic Organizer Approach to Reading and Writing Instruction.* Rockville, MD: Aspen.

Pendergast, K., Dickey, S.E., Selmar, J.W., Soder, A.L. (1984) *Photo Articulation Test.* Chicago: Stoelting.

Pennington, B.F. (1991) 'Genetics of learning disabilities.' *Seminars in Neurology*, **11**, 28–34.

—— Smith, S.D. (1983) 'Genetic influences on learning disabilities and speech and language disorders.' *Child Development*, **54**, 369–387.

—— Gilger, J.W., Pauls, D., Smith, S.A., Smith, S.D., DeFries, J.C. (1991) 'Evidence for major gene transmission of developmental dyslexia.' *Journal of the American Medical Association*, **266**, 1527–1534.

Percy, A., Gillberg, C., Hagberg, B., Witt-Engerström, I. (1990) 'Rett syndrome and the autistic disorders.' *Neurologic Clinics*, **8**, 659–676.

Petty, L., Ornitz, E.M., Michelman, J., Zimmerman, E. (1985) 'Autistic children who become schizophrenic.' *In:* Chess, S., Thomas, A. (Eds.) *Annual Progress in Child Psychiatry and Child Development.* New York: Bruner/Mazel, pp. 452–469.

Piaget, J. (1962) *Play, Dreams and Imitation in Childhood.* New York: Norton.

Piven, J., Folstein, S. (1994) 'The genetics of autism.' *In:* Bauman, M.L., Kemper, T.L. (Eds.) *The Neurobiology of Autism.* Baltimore, MD: Johns Hopkins University Press, pp. 18–44.

—— Gayle, J., Chase, G.A., Fink, B., Landa, R., Wzorek, M.M., Folstein, S.E. (1990) 'A family history study of neuropsychiatric disorders in the adult siblings of autistic individuals.' *Journal of the American Academy of Child and Adolescent Psychiatry*, **29**, 177–183.

Potvin, A.R., Tourtellotte, W.W. (1985) *Quantitative Examination of Neurologic Functions. Vol. I:*

*Scientific Basis and Design of Instrumented Tests. Vol. II: Methodology for Test and Patient Assessments and Design of a Computer-Automated System.* Boca Raton, FL: CRC Press.

Power, T.J., Radcliffe, J. (1989) 'The relationship of play behavior to cognitive ability in developmentally disabled preschoolers.' *Journal of Autism and Developmental Disorders,* **19**, 97–107.

Pring, L., Hermelin, B. (1993) 'Bottle, tulip and wineglass: semantic and structural picture processing by savant artists.' *Journal of Child Psychology and Psychiatry,* **34**, 1365–1385.

Prior, M.R. (1979) 'Cognitive abilities and disabilities in infantile autism.' *Journal of Abnormal Child Psychology,* **7**, 357–380.

—— Hall, L.C. (1979) 'Comprehension of transitive and intransitive phrases by autistic, retarded, and normal children.' *Journal of Communication Disorders,* **12**, 103–111.

—— Perry, D., Gajzago, C. (1975) 'Kanner's syndrome and early-onset psychosis: a taxonomic analysis of 142 cases.' *Journal of Autism and Developmental Disorders,* **5**, 71–80.

Prizant, B.M., Rydell, P.J. (1984) 'Analysis of functions of delayed echolalia in autistic children.' *Journal of Speech and Hearing Research,* **27**, 183–192.

Pyles, M.K., Stolz, H.R., Macfarlane, J.W. (1935) 'The accuracy of mothers' reports on birth and developmental data.' *Child Development,* **6**, 165–176.

Quay, H.C. (1985) 'A critical analysis of DSM-III as a taxonomy of psychopathology in childhood and adolescence.' *In:* Miller, T., Klerman, G. (Eds.) *Contemporary Issues in Psychopathology.* New York: Guilford Press, pp. 151–165.

Rapin, I. (1985) 'Cortical deafness, auditory agnosia, and word-deafness: how distinct are they?' *Human Communication Canada,* **9**, 29–37.

—— (1987) 'Searching for the cause of autism: a neurologic perspective.' *In:* Cohen, D.J., Donnellan, A.M., Paul, R. (Eds.) *Autism and Pervasive Developmental Disorders.* Silver Spring, MD: V.H. Winston, pp. 710–717.

—— (1991) 'Autistic children: diagnosis and clinical features.' *Pediatrics,* **87**, 751–760.

—— (1992) 'On the classification of the developmental disorders of brain function.' *In:* Benton, A., Levin, H., Moretti, G., Riva, D. (Eds.) *Developmental Neuropsychology.* Milan: Franco Angeli, pp. 26–39.

—— (1994) 'Update on the genetics of the developmental disorders of verbal, non-verbal, and written communication.' *In:* Gajdusek, D.C., McKhann, G.M., Bolis, L.C. (Eds.) *Evolution and Neurology of Language.* Amsterdam: Elsevier Science, pp. 57–67.

—— (1995) 'Autistic regression and disintegrative disorder: how important the role of epilepsy?' *Seminars in Pediatric Neurology,* **2**, 150–162.

—— Allen, D.A. (1983) 'Developmental language disorders: nosologic considerations.' *In:* Kirk, U. (Ed.) *Neuropsychology of Language, Reading, and Spelling.* New York: Academic Press, pp. 155–184.

—— —— (1988) 'Syndromes in developmental dysphasia and adult aphasia.' *In:* Plum, F. (Ed.) *Language, Communication, and the Brain.* New York: Raven Press, pp. 57–75.

—— Tourk, L.M., Costa, L.D. (1966) 'Evaluation of the Purdue Pegboard as a screening test for brain damage.' *Developmental Medicine and Child Neurology,* **8**, 45–54.

—— Mattis, S., Rowan, A.J., Golden, G.G. (1977) 'Verbal auditory agnosia in children.' *Developmental Medicine and Child Neurology,* **19**, 192–207.

Records, N.L., Tomblin, J.B. (1994) 'Clinical decision making: describing the decision rules of practicing speech–language pathologists.' *Journal of Speech and Hearing Research,* **37**, 144–156.

Reichelt, K.L., Saelid, G., Lindback, T., Bøler, J.B. (1986) 'Childhood autism: a complex disorder.' *Biological Psychiatry,* **21**, 1279–1290.

Reichler, R.J., Lee, E.M.C. (1987) 'Overview of biomedical issues in autism.' *In:* Schopler, E., Mesibov, G.B. (Eds.) *Neurobiological Issues in Autism.* New York: Plenum Press, pp. 13–41.

Reiss, S. (1994) 'Issues in defining mental retardation.' *American Journal on Mental Retardation,* **99**, 1–7.

Reuter, J., Stancin, T., Craig, P. (1981) *Kent Scoring Adaptation of the Bayley Scales of Infant Development.* Kent, OH: Kent Developmental Metrics.

Richardson, S.A. (1981) 'Family characteristics associated with mild mental retardation.' *In:* Begab, M., Garber, H. (Eds.) *Psychosocial Influences in Retarded Performance. Vol. II.* Baltimore, MD: University Park Press, pp. 29–43.

Riquet, C.B., Taylor, N.D., Benroya, S., Klein, L.S. (1981) 'Symbolic play in autistic, Down's and normal children of equivalent mental age.' *Journal of Autism and Developmental Disorders,* **11**, 439–448.

Rissman, M., Curtis, S., Tallal, P. (1990) 'School placement outcomes of young language impaired children.' *Journal of Speech and Hearing Pathology and Audiology,* **14**, 49–58.

241

Ritvo, E.R., Spence, M.A., Freeman, B.J., Mason-Brothers, A., Mo, A., Marazita, M.L. (1985) 'Evidence for autosomal recessive inheritance in 46 families with multiple incidences of autism.' *American Journal of Psychiatry*, **142**, 187–192.

—— Creel, D., Crandall, A.S., Freeman, B.J., Pingree, C., Barr, R., Realmuto, G. (1986) 'Retinal pathology in autistic children—a possible biological marker for a subtype?' *Journal of the American Academy of Child Psychiatry*, **25**, 137.

—— Brothers, A.M., Freeman, B.J., Pingree, C. (1988) 'Eleven possibly autistic parents.' *Journal of Autism and Developmental Disorders*, **18**, 139–143.

—— Freeman, B.J., Pingree, C., Mason-Brothers, A., Jorde, L., Jenson, W.R., McMahon, W.M., Petersen, P.B., Mo, A., Ritvo, A. (1989a) 'The UCLA–University of Utah epidemiologic survey of autism: prevalence.' *American Journal of Psychiatry*, **146**, 194–199.

—— Jorde, L.B., Mason-Brothers, A., Freeman, B.J., Pingree, C., Jones, M.B., McMahon, W.M., Petersen, P.B., Jenson, W.R., Mo, A. (1989b) 'The UCLA–University of Utah epidemiologic survey of autism: recurrence risk estimates and genetic counseling.' *American Journal of Psychiatry*, **146**, 1032–1036.

Robinson, R.J. (1987) 'The causes of language disorder: introduction and overview.' *In: Proceedings of the First International Symposium on Specific Speech and Language Disorders in Children.* London: AFASIC, pp. 1–19.

Rogers, S.J., DiLalla, D.L. (1990) 'Age of symptom onset in young children with pervasive developmental disorders.' *Journal of the American Academy of Child and Adolescent Psychiatry*, **29**, 863–872.

—— Pennington, B. (1991) 'A theoretical approach to the deficits in infantile autism.' *Development and Psychopathology*, **3**, 137–162.

Rosen, G.D., Galaburda, A.M., Sherman, G.F. (1990) 'The ontogeny of anatomic asymmetry: constraints derived from basic mechanisms.' *In:* Scheibel, A.B., Wechsler, A.F. (Eds.) *Neurobiology of Higher Cognitive Functions.* New York: Guilford Press, pp. 215–238.

Roth, F.P., Clark, D.M. (1987) 'Symbolic play and social participation abilities of language-impaired and normally developing children.' *Journal of Speech and Hearing Disorders*, **52**, 17–29.

Roulet Perez, E., Davidoff, V., Despland, P-A., Deonna, T. (1993) 'Mental and behavioural deterioration of children with epilepsy and CSWS: acquired epileptic frontal syndrome.' *Developmental Medicine and Child Neurology*, **35**, 661–674.

Routh, D.K., Walton, M.D., Padan-Belkin, E. (1978) 'Development of activity level in children revisited: effects of mother presence.' *Developmental Psychology*, **14**, 571–581.

Rowan, L.E., Leonard, L.B., Chapman, K., Weiss, A.L. (1983) 'Performative and presuppositional skills in language-disordered and normal children.' *Journal of Speech and Hearing Research*, **26**, 97–106.

Rubin, K.H., Fein, G.G., Vandenberg, B. (1983) 'Play.' *In:* Mussin, P. (Ed.) *Handbook of Child Psychology. Vol 4: Socialization, Personality and Social Behavior.* New York: Wiley, pp. 693–774.

Rutter, M. (1974) 'The development of infantile autism.' *Psychological Medicine*, **4**, 147–163.

—— (1979) 'Language, cognition, and autism.' *In:* Katzman, R. (Ed.) *Congenital and Acquired Cognitive Disorders.* New York: Raven Press, pp. 247–264.

—— (1983) 'Developmental psychopathology.' *In:* Hetherington, E.M. (Ed.) *Mussen's Handbook of Child Psychology. 4th Edn.* New York: Wiley, pp. 775–911.

—— Schopler, E. (1988) 'Autism and pervasive developmental disorders.' *In:* Rutter, M., Tuma, A.H., Lann, I.S. (Eds.) *Assessment and Diagnosis in Child Psychopathology.* London: David Fulton, pp. 408–434.

Sarimski, K., Hoffmann, W., Süss, H. (1985) 'Entwicklungsdysphasie und Symbolgebrauch im Spiel.' *Zeitschrift für Kinder- und Jugendpsychiatrie*, **13**, 354–361.

Schopler, E., Reichler, R.J., Renner, B.R. (1986) *The Childhood Autism Rating Scale (CARS) for Diagnostic Screening and Classification in Autism.* New York: Irvington.

Segalowitz, S.J., Hiscock, M. (1992) 'The emergence of a neuropsychology of normal development: rapprochement between neuroscience and developmental psychology.' *In:* Rapin, I., Segalowitz, S.J. (Eds.) *Handbook of Neuropsychology. Vol. 6: Child Neuropsychology.* Amsterdam: Elsevier, pp. 45–71.

Segawa, M., Katoh, J., Nomura, Y. (1992a) 'Neurology: as a window to brainstem dysfunction.' *In:* Naruse, H., Ornitz, E.M. (Eds.) *Neurobiology of Infantile Autism.* Amsterdam: Excerpta Medica, pp. 187–200.

—— Katoh, M., Katoh, J., Nomura, Y. (1992b) 'Early modulation of sleep parameters and its importance in later behavior.' *Brain Dysfunction*, **5**, 211–223.

Shapiro, T., Fish, B., Ginsberg, G.L. (1972) 'The speech of a schizophrenic child from two to six.'

*American Journal of Psychiatry,* **128**, 1408–1414.

Shatz, M., Bernstein, D., Shulman, M. (1980) 'The responses of language disordered children to indirect directives in varying contexts.' *Applied Psycholinguistics,* **1**, 295–306.

Shaywitz, S.E., Escobar, M.D., Shaywitz, B.A., Fletcher, J.M., Makuch, R. (1992) 'Evidence that dyslexia may represent the lower tail of a normal distribution of reading ability.' *New England Journal of Medicine,* **326**, 145–150.

Sheslow, D., Adams, W. (1990) *Wide Range Assessment of Memory and Learning.* New York: Psychological Corporation.

Siegel, B., Anders, T.F., Ciaranello, R.D., Bienenstock, B., Kraemer, H.C. (1986) 'Empirically derived subclassification of the autistic syndrome.' *Journal of Autism and Developmental Disorders,* **16**, 275–293.

Silva, P.A. (1980) 'The prevalence, stability and significance of developmental language delay in preschool children.' *Developmental Medicine and Child Neurology,* **22**, 768–777.

Simko, A., Hornstein, L., Soukup, S., Bagamery, N. (1989) 'Fragile X syndrome: recognition in young children.' *Pediatrics,* **83**, 547–552.

Simmons, J.Q., Baltaxe, C. (1975) 'Language patterns of adolescent autistics.' *Journal of Autism and Childhood Schizophrenia,* **5**, 333–351.

Skinner, H.A. (1981) 'Toward the integration of classification theory and methods.' *Journal of Abnormal Psychology,* **90**, 68–87.

Smalley, S.L. (1991) 'Genetic influences in autism.' *Psychiatric Clinics of North America,* **14**, 125–139.

—— Asarnow, R.F. (1990) 'Cognitive subclinical markers in autism.' *Journal of Autism and Developmental Disorders,* **20**, 271–278.

Smith, S.D., Kimberling, W.J., Pennington, B.F., Lubs, H.A. (1983) 'Specific reading disability: identification of an inherited form through linkage analysis.' *Science,* **219**, 1345–1347.

Snyder, L. (1978) 'Communicative and cognitive abilities and disabilities in the sensory-motor period.' *Merrill–Palmer Quarterly,* **24**, 161–180.

Soper, H.V., Satz, P., Orsini, D.L., Henry, R.R., Zvi, J.C., Schulman, M. (1986) 'Handedness patterns in autism suggest subtypes.' *Journal of Autism and Developmental Disorders,* **16**, 155–167.

Sparrow, S.S., Cicchetti, D.V. (1984) 'The Behavior Inventory for Rating Development (BIRD): assessments of reliability and factorial validity.' *Applied Research in Mental Retardation,* **5**, 219–231.

—— Balla, D.A., Cicchetti, D.V. (1984) *Vineland Adaptive Behavior Scales.* Circle Pines, MN: American Guidance Service.

Stanovich, K.E. (1991) 'Discrepancy definitions of reading disability: has intelligence led us astray?' *Reading Research Quarterly,* **26**, 7–29.

Stark, R.E., Tallal, P. (1981) 'Selection of children with specific language deficits.' *Journal of Speech and Hearing Disorders,* **46**, 114–122.

—— —— Kallman, C., Mellits, E.D. (1983) 'Cognitive abilities of language-delayed children.' *Journal of Psychology,* **114**, 9–19.

Steckol, K., Leonard, L.B. (1979) 'The use of grammatical morphemes by normal and language impaired children.' *Journal of Communication Disorders,* **12**, 291–301.

Steffenburg, S. (1991) 'Neuropsychiatric assessment of children with autism: a population-based study.' *Developmental Medicine and Child Neurology,* **33**, 495–511.

Stevenson, J., Richman, N. (1976) 'The prevalence of language delay in a population of three-year-old children and its association with general retardation.' *Developmental Medicine and Child Neurology,* **18**, 431–441.

Stone, W.L., Rosenbaum, J.L.A. (1988) 'A comparison of teacher and parent views of autism.' *Journal of Autism and Developmental Disorders,* **18**, 403–414.

—— Hoffman, E.L., Lewis, S.E., Ousley, O.Y. (1994) 'Early recognition of autism. Parental reports vs clinical observation.' *Archives of Pediatric and Adolescent Medicine,* **148**, 174–179.

Strauss, A.A. (1954) 'Aphasia in children.' *American Journal of Physical Medicine,* **33**, 93–99.

Sturmey, P. (1994) 'Assessing the functions of aberrant behaviors: a review of psychometric instruments.' *Journal of Autism and Developmental Disorders,* **24**, 293–304.

Stutsman, R. (1931) *Mental Measurement of Pre-school Children. With a Guide for the Administration of the Merrill–Palmer Scale of Mental Tests.* Yonkers, NY: World Book Co.

Sugiyama, T., Abe, A. (1989) 'The prevalence of autism in Nagoya, Japan: a total population study.' *Journal of Autism and Developmental Disorders,* **19**, 87–96.

243

—— Takei, Y., Abe, T. (1992) 'The prevalence of autism in Nagoya, Japan. II: A total population study for 10 years.' *In:* Naruse, H., Ornitz, E.M. (Eds.) *Neurobiology of Infantile Autism. Excerpta Medica International Congress Series No. 965.* Amsterdam: Excerpta Medica, pp. 181–184.

Sverd, J. (1991) 'Tourette syndrome and autistic disorder: a significant relationship.' *American Journal of Medical Genetics*, **39**, 173–179.

Swisher, L., Demetras, M.J. (1985) 'The expressive language characteristics of autistic children compared with mentally retarded or specific language-impaired children.' *In:* Schopler, E., Mesibov, G. (Eds.) *Communication Problems in Autism.* New York: Plenum Press, pp. 147–162.

Szatmari, P., Bartolucci, G., Bremner, R. (1989*a*) 'Asperger's syndrome and autism: comparison of early history and outcome.' *Developmental Medicine and Child Neurology*, **31**, 709–720.

—— Bremner, R., Nagy, J. (1989*b*) 'Asperger's syndrome: a review of clinical features.' *Canadian Journal of Psychiatry*, **34**, 554–560.

—— Archer, L., Fisman, S., Streiner, D.L. (1994) 'Parent and teacher agreement in the assessment of Pervasive Developmental Disorders.' *Journal of Autism and Developmental Disorders*, **6**, 703–717.

Taft, L.T., Cohen, H.J. (1971) 'Hypsarrhythmia and infantile autism: a clinical report.' *Journal of Autism and Childhood Schizophrenia*, **1**, 327–336.

Tager-Flusberg, H. (1981) 'On the nature of linguistic functioning in early infantile autism.' *Journal of Autism and Developmental Disorders*, **11**, 45–54.

—— (1985) 'Psycholinguistic approaches to language and communication in autism.' *In:* Schopler, E., Mesibov, G. (Eds.) *Communication Problems in Autism.* New York: Plenum Press, pp. 69–87.

—— (1989) 'A psycholinguistic perspective on language development in the autistic child.' *In:* Dawson, G. (Ed.) *Autism: Nature, Diagnosis, and Treatment.* New York: Guilford Press, pp. 92–109.

—— (1991) 'Semantic processing in the free recall of autistic children: further evidence for a cognitive deficit.' *British Journal of Developmental Psychology*, **9**, 417–430.

Tallal, P. (1988) 'Developmental language disorders.' *In:* Kavanagh, J.F., Truss, T.J. (Eds.) *Learning Disabilities: Proceedings of the National Conference.* Parkton, MD: York Press, pp. 181–272.

—— Miller, S., Fitch, R.H. (1993) 'Neurobiological basis of speech: a case for the preeminence of temporal processing.' *In:* Tallal, P., Galaburda, A.M., Llinás, R.R., von Euler, C. (Eds.) *Temporal Information Processing in the Nervous System. Special Reference to Dyslexia and Dysphasia.* New York: Academy of Sciences, pp. 27–49.

—— Stark, R. (1981) 'Speech acoustic cue discrimination abilities of normally developing and language impaired children.' *Journal of the Acoustical Society of America*, **69**, 568–574.

—— Townsend, J., Curtiss, S., Wulfeck, B. (1991) 'Phenotypic profiles of language-impaired children based on genetic/family history.' *Brain and Language*, **41**, 81–95.

Tanguay, P.E. (1984) 'Toward a new classification of serious psychopathology in children.' *Journal of the American Academy of Child Psychiatry*, **23**, 373–384.

Teal, M.B., Wiebe, M.J. (1986) 'A validity analysis of selected instruments used to assess autism.' *Journal of Autism and Developmental Disorders*, **16**, 485–494.

Terrell, B.Y., Schwartz, R.C., Prelock, P.A., Messick, C.K. (1984) 'Symbolic play in normal and language-impaired children.' *Journal of Speech and Hearing Research*, **27**, 424–429.

Thorndike, R.L., Hagen, E.P., Sattler, J.M. (1986) *Stanford–Binet Intelligence Scale, Revised.* Chicago: Riverside.

Tomblin, J.B. (1983) 'An examination of the concept of disorder in the study of language variation.' *Proceedings of the Symposium on Research in Child Language Disorders*, **4**, 81–109.

—— Buchwalter, P.R. (1994) 'Preliminary results of a twin study of SLI.' *Paper presented at the Symposium of Research in Child Language Disorders, Madison, WI, June 3, 1994.*

Tonge, B.J., Dissanayake, C., Brereton, A.V. (1994) 'Autism: fifty years on from Kanner.' *Journal of Paediatric and Child Health*, **30**, 102–107.

Touwen, B.C.L. (1979) *Examination of the Child with Minor Neurological Dysfunction. 2nd Edn. Clinics in Developmental Medicine No. 71.* London: Spastics International Medical Publications.

Town, C.H. (1911) 'Congenital aphasia.' *The Psychological Clinic*, **5**, 167–179.

Treffert, D.A. (1989) *Extraordinary People: Understanding "Idiot Savants".* New York: Harper & Row.

Tsai, L. (1992) 'Diagnostic issues in high functioning autism.' *In:* Schopler, E., Mesibov, G. (Eds.) *High Functioning Individuals with Autism.* New York: Plenum, pp. 11–40.

—— Stewart, M.A., August, G. (1981) 'Implications of sex differences in the familial transmission of infantile autism.' *Journal of Autism and Developmental Disorders*, **11**, 165–172.

—— Tsai, M.C., August, G.J. (1985) 'Brief report: implication of EEG diagnoses in the subclassification of infantile autism.' *Journal of Autism and Developmental Disorders*, **15**, 339–344.

Tuchman, R.F., Rapin, I., Shinnar, S. (1991*a*) 'Autistic and dysphasic children. I: Clinical characteristics.' *Pediatrics*, **88**, 1211–1218.

—— —— (1991*b*) 'Autistic and dysphasic children. II: Epilepsy.' *Pediatrics*, **88**, 1219–1225.

Udwin, O., Yule, W. (1983) 'Imaginative play in language disordered children.' *British Journal of Disorders of Communication*, **18**, 197–205.

Ungerer, J.A., Sigman, M. (1981) 'Symbolic play and language comprehension in autistic children.' *Journal of the American Academy of Child Psychiatry*, **20**, 318–337.

Urion, D.K. (1988) 'Nondextrality and autoimmune disorders among relatives of language-disabled boys.' *Annals of Neurology*, **24**, 267–269.

US Department of Health and Human Services, Agency for Health Care Policy and Research (1994) *Clinical Practice Guideline: Otitis Media with Effusion in Young Children.* Washington, DC: Government Printing Office.

Van Bourgondien, N.E., Mesibov, G.B., Dawson, G. (1987) 'Autism.' *In:* Wolraich, M.L. (Ed.) *The Practical Assessment and Management of Children with Disorders of Development and Learning.* Chicago: Year Book Medical Publishers, pp. 328–351.

Vargha-Khadem, F., Passingham, R.E. (1990) 'Speech and language defects.' *Nature*, **346**, 226. *(Letter.)*

Volkmar, F.R. (1992) 'Childhood disintegrative disorder: issues for DSM-IV.' *Journal of Autism and Developmental Disorders*, **22**, 625–642.

—— Cohen, D.J. (1989) 'Disintegrative disorder or "late onset" autism.' *Journal of Child Psychology and Psychiatry*, **30**, 717–724.

—— —— Bregman, J.D., Hooks, M.Y., Stevenson, J.M. (1989) 'An examination of social typologies in autism.' *Journal of the American Academy of Child and Adolescent Psychiatry*, **28**, 82–86.

—— Cicchetti, D.V., Cohen, D.J., Bregman, J. (1992) 'Developmental aspects of DSM-III-R criteria for autism.' *Journal of Autism and Developmental Disorders*, **22**, 657–662.

—— Carter, A., Sparrow, S.S., Cicchetti, D.V. (1993) 'Quantifying social development in autism.' *Journal of the American Academy of Child and Adolescent Psychiatry*, **32**, 627–632.

Volpe, J.J. (1995) *Neurology of the Newborn. 3rd Edn.* Philadelphia: W.B. Saunders.

Volpe, J.J. (1991) 'Cognitive deficits in premature infants.' *New England Journal of Medicine*, **325**, 276–278.

Vygotsky, L.S. (1978) *Mind in Society.* Cambridge MA: Harvard University Press.

Wallace, I.F., Gravel, J.S., McCarton, C.M., Ruben, R.J. (1988) 'Otitis media and language development at one year of age.' *Journal of Speech and Hearing Disorders*, **53**, 245–251.

Waterhouse, L. (1994) 'Severity of impairment in autistic spectrum disorders.' *In:* Broman, S.H., Grafman, J. (Eds.) *Atypical Cognitive Deficits in Developmental Disorders: Implications for Brain Function.* Hillsdale, NJ: Lawrence Erlbaum, pp. 159–182.

—— Fein, D. (1982) 'Language skills in developmentally disabled children.' *Brain and Language*, **15**, 307–333.

—— —— (1984) 'Developmental trends in cognitive skills for children diagnosed as autistic and schizophrenic.' *Child Development*, **55**, 236–248.

—— —— Nath, J., Snyder, D. (1987) 'Pervasive developmental disorders and schizophrenia occurring in childhood: a review of critical commentary.' *In:* Tischler, G.L. (Ed.) *Diagnosis and Classification in Psychiatry: a Critical Appraisal of DSM III.* New York: Cambridge University Press, pp. 335–368.

—— Wing, L., Fein, D. (1989) 'Reevaluating the syndrome of autism in the light of empirical research.' *In:* Dawson, G., Segalowitz, S. (Eds.) *Autism.* New York: Guilford Press, pp. 263–281.

—— —— Spitzer, R., Siegel, B. (1992) 'Pervasive Developmental Disorders: from DSM-III to DSM-III-R.' *Journal of Autism and Developmental Disorders*, **22**, 525–549.

—— Feinstein, C., Allen, D.A., Morris, R. (1993) 'Behavior in high and low functioning autistic spectrum preschool children.' Paper presented in the symposium: Autism and Language Disorder Collaborative Project: Preschool Study, International Neuropsychology Society, Galveston TX.

—— Fein, D., Modahl, C. (1996) 'Neurofunctional mechanisms for social interaction: model of impairment in autism.' *Psychological Review. (In press.)*

—— Morris, R., Allen, D.A., Dunn, M., Fein, D., Feinstein, C., Rapin, I., Wing, L. (1996) 'Diagnosis and classification of autism.' *Journal of Autism and Developmental Disorders*, **26**, 59–86.

Watson, R.T., Gonzales Rothi, L.J., Heilman, K.M. (1992) 'Apraxia: a disorder of motor programming.'

245

*In:* Joseph, A.B., Young, R.R. (Eds.) *Movement Disorders in Neurology and Neuropsychiatry.* Oxford: Blackwell Scientific, pp. 681–690.

Weiner, P.S. (1974) 'A language-delayed child at adolescence.' *Journal of Speech and Hearing Disorders,* **39**, 202–212.

—— (1985) 'The value of follow-up studies.' *Topics in Language Disorders,* **5**, 78–92.

Werner, H., Kaplan, B. (1962) *Symbol Formation.* New York: Wiley.

Wetherby, A.M., Prizant, B.M. (1985) 'Intentional communicative behavior of children with autism: theoretical and practical issues.' *Australian Journal of Human Communication Disorders,* **13**, 21–59.

Whitehurst, G.J., Fischel, J.E. (1994) 'Practitioner review: early developmental language delay: what, if anything, should the clinician do about it?' *Journal of Child Psychology and Psychiatry,* **35**, 613–648.

Wiig, E.H., Semel, E.M. (1980) *Language Assessment and Intervention for the Learning Disabled.* Columbus, OH: Charles E. Merrill.

—— —— Nystrom, L.A. (1982) 'Comparison of rapid naming abilities in language-learning-disabled and academically achieving 8 year olds.' *Language, Speech, and Hearing Services in Schools,* **1**, 11–23.

Wilson, B.C. (1986) 'An approach 'to the neuropsychological assessment of the preschool child with developmental deficits.' *In:* Filskov, S.B., Boll, T.J. (Eds.) *Handbook of Clinical Neuropsychology. Vol. 2.* New York: John Wiley, pp. 121–171.

—— Risucci, D.A. (1986) 'A model for clinical–quantitative classification. Generation I: Application to language-disordered preschool children.' *Brain and Language,* **27**, 281–309.

Wing, L. (1981) 'Language, social and cognitive impairments in autism and severe mental retardation.' *Journal of Autism and Developmental Disorders,* **11**, 31–44.

—— (1988) 'The continuum of autistic characteristics.' *In:* Schopler, E., Mesibov, G. (Eds.) *Diagnosis and Assessment in Autism.* New York: Plenum Press, pp. 91–110.

—— (1991) 'The relationship between Asperger's syndrome and Kanner's autism.' *In:* Frith, U. (Ed.) *Autism and Asperger Syndrome.* Cambridge: Cambridge University Press, pp. 93–121.

—— (1993) 'The definition and prevalence of autism: a review.' *European Journal of Child and Adolescent Psychiatry,* **2**, 61–74.

—— Atwood, A. (1987) 'Syndromes of autism and atypical development.' *In:* Cohen, D.J., Donnellan, A.M., Paul, R. (Eds.) *Handbook of Autism and Pervasive Developmental Disorders.* New York: John Wiley, pp. 3–19.

—— Gould, J. (1979) 'Severe impairments of social interaction and associated abnormalities in children: epidemiology and classification.' *Journal of Autism and Developmental Disorders,* **9**, 11–30.

Wood, L.C., Cooper, D.S. (1992) 'Autoimmune thyroid disease, left-handedness, and developmental dyslexia.' *Psychoneuroendocrinology,* **17**, 95–99.

Wood, N.E. (1964) *Delayed Speech and Language Development.* Englewood Cliffs, NJ: Prentice–Hall.

World Health Organization (1978) *Mental Disorders: Glossary and Guide to their Classification in Accordance with the Ninth Revision of the International Classification of Diseases.* Geneva: WHO.

—— (1993) *Mental Disorders: Glossary and Guide to their Classification in Accordance with the Tenth Revision of the International Classification of Diseases.* Geneva: WHO.

Worster-Drought, C., Allen, I.M. (1930) 'Congenital auditory imperception (congenital word-deafness): and its relation to idioglossia and other speech defects.' *Journal of Neurology and Psychopathology,* **10**, 193–236.

Wulff, S.B. (1985) 'The symbolic and object play of children with autism: a review.' *Journal of Autism and Developmental Disorders,* **15**, 139–148.

Wyke, M.A., Asso, D. (1979) 'Perception and memory for spatial relations in children with developmental dysphasia.' *Neuropsychologia,* **17**, 231–239.

Zinkus, P.W., Gottlieb, M.I. (1980) 'Patterns of perceptual and academic deficits related to early chronic otitis media.' *Pediatrics,* **66**, 246–253.

# APPENDIX 1

## WING AUTISTIC DISORDER INTERVIEW CHECKLIST (WADIC)

*Lorna Wing*

N.B. All features must be evaluated for their significance in the light of the subject's mental age.

### SECTION A
**Qualitative impairment in reciprocal social interaction**

**Item A1.** Absence or impairment of use of body language to initiate and modulate reciprocal social interaction

—a. Does not anticipate being held (*e.g.* by lifting arms, changing posture, showing eagerness in facial expression).

—b. Does not adapt posture, cuddle in when held. May stiffen and resist when held.

—c. Does not look or smile when making a social approach.

—d. Does not use eye contact to get someone's attention. May make eye contact in brief glances only, but not for the purpose of gaining another's attention.

—e. Does make eye contact, but does so inappropriately (*e.g.* stares too long and hard; holds someone's face and looks closely into their eyes when wanting their attention).

—f. Does make social approaches, but does not use variations in eye-to-eye gaze, etc., or vocalizations such as 'um' or 'ah' to punctuate conversations and to guide turn-taking.

**Item A2.** Absence or impairment of greeting behaviour

—a. Does not rush to greet parent after a period of separation.

—b. Does not spontaneously wave to greet or when saying goodbye.

—c. Ignores visitors to the house, classroom, etc. (not just because absorbed in some activity).

—d. Says 'hello' or some stereotyped phrase but only when prompted, or because of previous training.

—e. Makes approaches indiscriminately and inappropriately to familiar people and strangers alike.

**Item A3.** Impairment of seeking comfort

—a. Never seeks comfort. Appears to ignore pain, heat or cold.

—b. Seeks comfort, but only in a mechanical way (*e.g.* sits on human lap as if the person were a chair).

—c. Shows distress if hurt, but does not come for comfort.

—d. Approaches others if hurt, but in a stereotyped way, and does not seek or respond to comforting (*e.g.* always demands 'put plaster on it' regardless of cause of pain).

—e. Approaches others, intrudes upon them, may cling tightly to them regardless of the needs and feelings of the person approached. May superficially appear to be seeking comfort or affection, but behaviour has a bizarre, repetitive quality.

**Item A4.** Impairment in giving comfort to others

—a. Ignores existence of and walks through and over other people, regardless of their feelings. Is unaware of others' 'personal space'.

—b. Indifferent to others' pain or distress or may laugh at others' distress (*e.g.* if someone falls over or is scolded).

—c. Is distressed by injury or illness in another person, but only because of change of appearance or routine. Does not offer comfort or sympathy.

—d. No intuitive sympathy with others' pain or distress, but has some understanding on an intellectual level if problem is explained. May then try to offer comfort and sympathy, but may do this in a naive and inappropriate manner.

**Item A5.** Impairment of ability to make friendships and to share interests and emotions
—a. No peer friendships despite ample opportunities.
—b. Poor relationships with peers—other children tend to tease and bully.
—c. Wants friends but has poor grasp of the concept of friendship. May refer to all acquaintances, however slight, as 'friends'.
—d. Has one 'friend', but has a limited, passive role in the partnership.
—e. Has a friend with the same circumscribed interest; they talk 'at' each other mainly concerning this interest.

**Item A6.** Impairment of awareness of social rules
—a. Lack of awareness of need for personal modesty (*e.g.* will remove clothing or appear naked in any company, in complete innocence).
—b. Lack of awareness of psychological barriers (*e.g.* invades other people's 'personal space'; walks behind counters in shops; enters other people's houses to 'collect' a particular object).
—c. Lack of awareness of social taboos in conversation (*e.g.* makes naive, embarrassing personal remarks in public; talks about delicate subjects in a loud voice in company; asks strangers inappropriate, embarrassing questions).
—d. Lack of awareness of correct behaviour in public (*e.g.* screams in public; removes objects from shelves in shops; sits down in puddles in middle of road).

**Item A7.** Impairment of joint referencing and interactive play
—a. Does not reciprocate in lap play (*e.g.* if mother touches and names child's nose and mouth, the child ignores, or may show some signs of pleasure, but does not reciprocate by touching mother's nose and mouth in his turn).
—b. Does not point things out to others and use eye contact in order to share the pleasure of seeing something interesting (not to be confused with pointing to indicate the desire to obtain an object).
—c. Does not spontaneously bring toys or other possessions to show other people to share pleasure and interest. Does not spontaneously offer others pretend food or drink.
—d. Self-chosen play activities are solitary.
—e. Involves other children only as mechanical aids (*e.g.* to bring objects to add to a construction).
—f. Directs other children as 'puppets' in a repetitive game. No interest in other children's suggestions.
—g. Amiably accepts passive role in other children's play (*e.g.* as baby in a game of 'mothers and fathers'), but makes little or no contribution.
—h. Engages with one other specific person who has the same circumscribed interest (*e.g.* train or aeroplane spotting, playing chess). The social interaction is dominated by the one theme.

**Item A8.** Impairment of imitation
—a. No spontaneous imitation of others' actions (though may be taught by having limbs moved for him/her).
—b. Automatic, mechanical imitation of others' actions without real appreciation of the meaning, sometimes amounting to echopraxia equivalent to echolalia in speech.
—c. May imitate simple movements, but fails to engage in imitative make-believe play (*e.g.* does not pretend to be mother or father, teacher, doctor or nurse).
—d. Does imitate actions of one person, animal or object (*e.g.* a character seen on television, a horse, a train, a robot), but does this repetitively in a stereotyped fashion and is difficult to divert from this activity.

—e. Does try to imitate other people's actions, and is aware of necessity for correct social behaviour, but gets details wrong in a naive, even bizarre fashion. (May be able to learn a sequence of actions, *e.g.* for a stage performance, but only if taught each step in detail.)

**Item A9.** <u>Impairment of social aspects of pretend play</u>
—a. Fails to 'animate' toy animals and dolls or objects (*e.g.* does not show tender care of and feed toy animals or dolls, or walk them along, make noises or talk in the animal's or doll's voices).
—b. Does appear to 'animate' one or a few toys or other objects, but does so in a limited, repetitive way and continues with the same activity for long periods. 'Play' does not become more elaborate with time.
—c. Invents a fantasy person or people, even an entire imaginary world, but the fantasy activities are concentrated on one or a few limited themes and are repetitive in quality (*e.g.* invents a fantasy family of people, but is concerned solely with talking about the details of the family tree—who is related to whom, and how—all of which are remembered with complete precision).

## SECTION B
### Qualitative impairments in communication and imagination

**Item B1.** <u>Impairment of use of language for communication</u>
—a. In the preverbal stages of development, no meaningful intoned vocalizations, or communicative babbling, plus failure to compensate by alternative methods of communication such as facial expression and simple gestures.
—b. At stage when speech should be present, has no spoken language (often with a history as in *a* above), and fails to compensate with gesture and mime, apart from pulling others' hands or arms in a mechanical way.
—c. Has speech, but neither initiates nor sustains a conversation with others.
—d. Makes approaches to others, but content of speech is one-sided, repetitive, without appropriate conversational turn-taking.

**Item B2.** <u>Impairment of comprehension of language</u>
—a. No response to communication from others (*e.g.* does not respond to own name).
—b. Responds to communication of simple instructions, but only in a familiar context; actions due to learned habits rather than to understanding of words.
—c. Responds to single words or phrases out of context, rather than the meaning of a whole statement (*e.g.* mother, while doing dishes, says, 'I've torn my glove, would you get me another pair please.' Child goes out of kitchen and returns with a pair of woollen gloves).
—d. Understands a wide range of words and grammatical constructions, but has marked tendency to interpret information in a literal way, failing to take the context into account, leading to naive mistakes (*e.g.* mother, making a cake, says to her 15-year-old autistic son, 'I need some cloves. Take some money from my purse and buy me some.' Boy mishears, but asks no questions and returns some hours later with bag full of teen-age girl's clothes).

**Item B3.** <u>Impairment of use of speech (if present)</u>
—a. Stereotyped and repetitive use of speech; immediate echolalia and/or repetition of phrases in a mechanical way The latter can vary from a vocabulary of a few words only used repetitively without meaning, to television commercials or even whole conversations repeated in the tones and accents of the original speakers. Such stereotyped phrases may also be used to obtain simple needs.
—b. Problems with words that change in meaning with the context (pronouns, prepositions, words relating to time, etc.). Most obviously shown in reversal of pronouns (*e.g.* 'you want cookie').
—c. Idiosyncratic use of words or phrases; these may be incorrect, concrete, literal, inverted or neologisms (*e.g.* 'earring plugs' for 'earphones'; 'shake-milk' for 'milk-shake'; 'go on

green ridings' for 'go on the swing in the park'; 'cushin' for apple puree).

—d. Grammatical speech and large vocabulary, but use of speech long-winded, pedantic, lacking in colloquialisms, repetitive (*e.g.* 'I wish to thank you for the hospitality you have extended to me this afternoon' instead of 'thanks for the cup of tea').

**Item B4.** Impairment of prosody

—a. Abnormalities in pitch, stress, rate, rhythm, volume or intonation of speech (*e.g.* speech monotonous; voice inappropriately high- or low-pitched; statements always have a questioning melody regardless of content).

**Item B5.** Impairment of symbolic development as shown in imaginative activities
(N.B. Evaluate behaviour in light of language comprehension age.)

—a. No appropriate use of miniature objects, despite language comprehension age of 2 years or above (*e.g.* handles toys only to obtain simple sensory stimuli, does not lay toy tea table with toy crockery, does not imitate car noises and pretend to drive toy car).

—b. Shows appropriate use of miniature objects when presented in test situation, but does so in a limited mechanical fashion without elaboration of pretence and does not choose to play with toys spontaneously.

—c. Uses some toys spontaneously in an appropriate way, but play is repetitive and does not include the use of one object to represent another of a quite different kind (*e.g.* a banana to represent a telephone).

—d. Has representational play, which may be elaborate (*e.g.* using wooden blocks to build a complex network of roads and bridges), but this is limited to the one theme and is markedly repetitive.


## SECTION C
### Restricted, repetitive pattern of self-chosen behaviour

**Item C1.** Stereotypic, repetitive postures or bodily movements

—a. Tends to stay in one position with little or no spontaneous activity (*e.g.* sits with legs tucked up and head bowed).

—b. Moves around aimlessly (*e.g.* wanders, runs, makes rapid darting movements, paces to and fro).

—c. Simple repetitive bodily movements (*e.g.* rocking, teeth grinding, tapping parts of own body).

—d. More complex repetitive movements (*e.g.* hand and finger twisting or flicking; complex whole body movements).

**Item C2.** Stereotypic repetitive activities related to bodily functions or sensations

—a. Smearing or other manipulation of saliva or excreta.

—b. Searches for and swallows inedible objects (*e.g.* cigarette ends, small pieces of metal, paper).

—c. Repetitive self-injury (*e.g.* head banging, eye poking, hand biting, self-induced vomiting).

—d. Preoccupation with visual, auditory, olfactory or tactile sensations (*e.g.* looks through fingers at lights; fascinated by watching things spin; listens to sounds made by water in radiators; deliberately plays records at the wrong speed; smells objects and/or people; feels, or scratches, or taps on different surfaces).

**Item C3.** Preoccupation with objects, regardless of their function

—a. Unusual attachment to objects (*e.g.* insists on carrying round a particular object such as a belt, a toy car, a stone, an empty detergent packet). Tends to be angry or distressed if object is mislaid.

—b. 'Collects' certain kinds of objects for no apparent purpose (*e.g.* dead holly leaves; wrappers from one brand of chocolate; small tea pots; books on a specific subject which may remain unread; toy trains). Tends to notice and react if even one item is missing.

—c. Arranges objects in straight lines or patterns—upset if arrangements are disturbed.

—d. Preoccupation with parts of objects, animals or people (*e.g.* fascinated by animal's fur, people's teeth, church steeples, one or two bars of music out of a complete recording).

—e. Preoccupied with repetitive actions involving objects (*e.g.* flicks pieces of string or other materials; turns light switches on and off; spins the wheels of toy cars; pours water from one vessel to another).

—f. Preoccupation with specific abstract attributes of objects or people, such as colour, shape, sound, number (*e.g.* fascinated with anything that is yellow, or round in shape, regardless of its practical function; identifies people by their numerical attributes such as age, house number).

**Item C4.** Maintenance of sameness of environment

—a. Preoccupied with the maintenance of small details of the familiar environment (*e.g.* disproportionately upset if things are broken or blemished; resists changes in arrangements of ornaments; upset if given a different brand of a particular food or drink; refuses to wear new shoes or other new clothes).

**Item C5.** Maintenance of sameness of routines

—a. Preoccupied with the maintenance of certain familiar routines (*e.g.* upset if different route taken to a familiar place; insists on following a complicated bedtime ritual before going to sleep; insists that cutlery, crockery, etc., must be placed on the table in precisely the same order for each meal; eats only a few types of food; always stands up and turns round three times before starting next course at each meal).

**Item C6.** Restricted and repetitive patterns of interests of a verbal or intellectual kind

a. Asks the same questions or series of questions repeatedly, regardless of the replies received (*e.g.* 'How old are you?' 'What colour is your car?' 'Where do you live?'), or talks repetitively on one or two themes regardless of suggestions from others.

—b. Acts the role of an object, animal, fictional character or real person in a repetitive, stereotyped way regardless of suggestions from other children.

—c. Preoccupied with special interests dependent on good rote memory, ability to calculate, or musical ability (*e.g.* timetables; routes to places; calendars; arithmetical calculations; computers; games depending on numbers; the music of a specific composer).

—d. Preoccupied with particular subjects; tends to amass facts but usually lacks depth of understanding (*e.g.* methods of transport; meteorology; genealogy of royal families; the legends of King Arthur; military uniforms; specific imaginary or real people. The subjects may be lurid or frightening, such as details of murders or monsters from outer space).

**Item C7.** Impairment of spontaneous activities

—a. Lifestyle is restricted, empty, routine-bound. Has virtually no spontaneous activities apart from those related to the daily routine.

# APPENDIX 2

## SOCIAL ABNORMALITIES SCALES

These scales should be completed after direct observation of the child. If the behaviors are not observed, the examiner should attempt to discern through interview with a familiar adult whether these behaviors have been observed by others. Scoring is on a three-point scale as follows: 0 = No or very rarely; 1 = Yes, occasionally; 2 = Yes, often (the child's usual way of behaving).

**Social Abnormalities: Scale I**

Does the child:                                                                0  1  2

1. Seem very 'hard to reach' or to be 'in a shell'?
2. Walk through or over people as if they do not exist?
3. Respond to affection or touching by active withdrawal, or by becoming rigid or limp?
4. Show aversion to being with people, preferring to engage in solitary activity?
5. Have difficulty maintaining eye contact; avoid looking at people, or 'look through them'?
6. Lack empathy for other people's needs, interests, or ideas; continue to pursue his/her own favorite preoccupations despite all attempts to dissuade?
7. Fail to initiate interactions with adults solely for social purposes (aside from need fulfillment)?
8. React to strangers and familiar persons indiscriminately?
9. Show many attachment behaviors to mother (and possibly a few other familiar people), but no social behavior in relation to most adults and children?
10. Have intense, prolonged 'temper outbursts' or 'panic attacks' with little or no visible motivation and inability to be soothed or consoled by familiar persons?

**Social Abnormalities: Scale II**

Does the child:                                                                0  1  2

1. Exhibit excessive and/or unusual fears?
2. Seem unaware or 'social rules' of interpersonal physical contact?
3. Exhibit or repeatedly discuss unusual preoccupations?
4. Masturbate or undress in public with no apparent awareness of inappropriateness?
5. Tend to be excessively clingy and overdependent, unable to tend to his/her own basic needs, or to become socially engaged without constant support from a familiar adult?
6. Repeat words or phrases from the past which have no discernible connection with the present social context?
7. While 'interacting' have a 'not really there' quality?
8. Become excessively excited or overstimulated by social contact or interactive play?
9. Seem unable to become fully engaged in reciprocal dialogue initiated by a conversational partner?
10. Engage in obsessive rituals without apparent awareness of possible reactions of others?

# APPENDIX 3

## HISTORY QUESTIONNAIRE

**Critique**

This appendix reproduces the family questionnaire we used to collect demographic, birth, developmental, medical and family histories from the 556 children originally entered in the study\*. Besides desirable features, the form has flaws. We provide here some critical comments to enable anyone wanting to use the form or one like it to profit from our experience.

1. Ideally, design a form that can be read optically into a computer, to bypass the transcribing of scores onto a screen, which is time-consuming and adds another layer of potential errors.

2. Expand and make more specific the section on complications of pregnancy. Specify in which trimester of the pregnancy there was bleeding. Be more specific on the amount of alcohol used.

3. Be more specific about breech delivery and the child's stay in the neonatal intensive care unit.

4. Delete some of the developmental milestones that parents do not remember, *e.g.* age at sitting, crawling. Add items like pointing, shaking head to indicate 'no'. Asking routinely about regression of milestones is critical, as at least a third and possibly more of parents of autistic children report regression of language, sociability and play.

5. Section D, a series of questions about aberrant development, virtually dichotomizes the non-autistic from the autistic, regardless of intellectual level, and turned out to be more sensitive than the neurologists' observations, especially in high-functioning and mildly autistic children whose abnormal behaviors may not be apparent in a highly structured neurological examination.

6. Drawing a family tree takes time but is important if one is interested in the genetics of developmental disorders. The reporting form for family members can be simplified. In order to collect reliable prevalence data, it is necessary to have a denominator (*i.e.* number of persons at risk) if one wants to evaluate the genetic data more than anecdotally. A serious genetic study requires personal evaluation of all family members.

\*This form is not suitable for children with known or suspected progressive conditions, or focal or diffuse brain diseases, because such children were excluded from the study.

## HISTORY INTERVIEW

The following questionnaire is designed to provide us with some basic information about your child and family. Please fill it out as completely as possible. We will go over it with you in order to fill in portions which are more difficult (*i.e.* family history charts), and to allow you to clarify your responses. Because of revisions in this form, numbering may be inconsistent. Thank you.

|                        |                 |                  |
|------------------------|-----------------|------------------|
| To be completed        | Subject Number  | \|_\|_\|_\|       |
| by examiner            | Examiner Code   | \|_\|_\|          |
|                        | Date            | \|__/__/__\|     |
|                        | Respondent      | \|_\|            |

## I. BASIC INFORMATION

A. Information about Child

1  Child's Date of Birth  |_ _ / _ _ / _ _|

2. Child's Sex:  Male |_|  Female |_|

3. Child's Race (enter correct code)  |_|

       Caucasian —1
       Black     —2
       Hispanic —3
       Oriental —4
       Other     —5

4. Birthweight |_ _| pounds, |_ _| ounces

6. Is child adopted?  Yes |_|  No |_|

7. Date of Adoption  |_ _ / _ _ / _ _|

B. Information About Parents

1. Marital Status (enter correct code) |_|

       Married   —1
       Single    —2
       Separated —3
       Divorced —4

2. Date of Birth of Father  |_ _ / _ _ / _ _|

3. Date of Birth of Mother  |_ _ / _ _ / _ _|

4. Father's Education (enter correct code, as below)  |_|

| | |
|---|---|
| Less than seventh grade | —1 |
| Junior high school (9th grade) | —2 |
| Partial high school (10th or 11th grade) | —3 |
| High school graduate (whether private preparatory, parochial, trade or public school | —4 |
| Partial college (at least one year) or specialized training | —5 |
| Standard college or university graduate | —6 |
| Graduate professional training (graduate degree) | —7 |

5. Mother's Education (use codes from question 4) |_|

6. Father's Current Occupation _____
    Code to be filled in by examiner  |_|_|_|_|_|
    (use Hollingshead codes)

7. Mother's Current Occupation _____
    Code to be filled in by examiner  |_|_|_|_|_|
    (use Hollingshead codes)

8. Language(s) spoken at home (enter correct code):  1. |_|
                                       2. |_|

       English —1
       Spanish —2
       Other    —3, specify: _____

9. Child's Siblings—use the following chart to include information on the child's siblings. Begin with the oldest sibling.

(Use the following codes for 'Relation to this child')

Full sibling —1    Adopted sibling    —3
Half sibling —2    Step sibling —4

| Initials | Date of birth mo/yr | Sex M/F | Birth-weight lbs/oz. | Relation to this child | Age in months of first words | Age in months of first sentences | Handed-ness R/L |
|----------|------|-----|------|------|------|------|------|
| 1. | | | | | | | |
| 2. | | | | | | | |
| 3. | | | | | | | |
| 4. | | | | | | | |
| 5. | | | | | | | |
| 6. | | | | | | | |
| 7. | | | | | | | |
| 8. | | | | | | | |

(Note: More family information is obtained at the end of the questionnaire.)

## II. CHILD'S DEVELOPMENT

A. <u>Prenatal and Birth Information</u>

1. Number of the following you have had:    How many
   a. Pregnancies besides this one    |_ _|
   b. Miscarriages    |_ _|
   c. Abortions    |_ _|
   e. Premature births    |_ _|

2. During your pregnancy with this child, did you use any of the following drugs or medicines?
   Yes |_| No |_|

   (circle)    Alcohol    Tobacco    Marijuana    Cocaine    Heroin
   LSD    Amphetamines    Methadone    Other _____

3. Did you have any of the following during this child's pregnancy?

| | Yes | No | Don't know |
|---|---|---|---|
| a. Toxemia (high blood pressure, eclampsia, etc. | \|_\| | \|_\| | \|_\| |
| b. Significant bleeding from the vagina | \|_\| | \|_\| | \|_\| |
| d. Hospitalization (describe on back) | \|_\| | \|_\| | \|_\| |
| e. Any illness with fever and rash (German measles, etc.) | \|_\| | \|_\| | \|_\| |
| f. Diabetes | \|_\| | \|_\| | \|_\| |
| h. X-rays | \|_\| | \|_\| | \|_\| |
| i. Amniocentesis | \|_\| | \|_\| | \|_\| |
| j. Other serious complications (describe on back) | \|_\| | \|_\| | \|_\| |

4. Duration of this pregnancy: |_ _| weeks

5. Birth history and neonatal difficulties (for this child)

| | Yes | No | Don't know |
|---|---|---|---|
| a. Was a caesarean birth performed? | \|_\| | \|_\| | \|_\| |
| b. Were you under anesthesia? (Type: general \|_\| Spinal \|_\| Other \|_\| ) | | | |
| c. Was labor induced? | \|_\| | \|_\| | \|_\| |
| d. Was your baby considered premature? | \|_\| | \|_\| | \|_\| |

|  | Yes | No | Don't know |
|---|---|---|---|

e. Was your baby considered small for his/her gestational age (small for term birth)? |_| |_| |_|

f. Was labor longer than 24 hours? |_| |_| |_|

g. Was your baby born head first? |_| |_| |_|

h. Were forceps used? (high |_| low |_|) |_| |_| |_|

i. Was the cord wrapped around your baby's neck? |_| |_| |_|

j. Was your fluid stained with your baby's meconium (baby moved his/her bowels before birth)? |_| |_| |_|

k. Did your baby cry immediately? |_| |_| |_|

l. Was your baby blue? |_| |_| |_|

m. Did your baby require oxygen? |_| |_| |_|

n. 1) Do you remember your baby's Apgar score? |_| |_| |_|
   2) What was it?   1 min. |_|
                     5 min. |_|

o. Was your baby placed in a special intensive care unit? |_| |_| |_|

p. Did your baby require transfusions (exchange transfusions)? |_| |_| |_|

q. Did your baby require phototherapy (lights)? |_| |_| |_|

r. Was your baby placed in an isolette or incubator? |_| |_| |_|

s. Did your baby have unusual movements of the head, arms or limbs? |_| |_| |_|

t. Did your baby have seizures or convulsions? |_| |_| |_|

v. Did your baby have breathing problems? |_| |_| |_|

w. Was your baby placed on a ventilator? |_| |_| |_|

x. Were there concerns about your baby's heart rate? |_| |_| |_|

y. Did your baby have sucking problems? |_| |_| |_|

z. Did your baby have swallowing problems? |_| |_| |_|

aa. Did your baby have feeding difficulties? |_| |_| |_|

bb. Was your baby limp? |_| |_| |_|

cc. Was your baby stiff? |_| |_| |_|

dd. Did your baby stay in the hospital after you left to go home? |_| |_| |_|

B. Medical Treatment Information

|  | Yes | No | Don't know |
|---|---|---|---|

1. Has this child had any of the following

a. Otitis media (ear infections, fluid in the ears)? |_| |_| |_|
   If yes, number of times:  1–2 |_|  3–6 |_|  6 or more |_|

b. Encephalitis |_| |_| |_|

c. Meningitis |_| |_| |_|

d. Poisoning or drug intoxication |_| |_| |_|

e. Coma |_| |_| |_|

f. Febrile seizures (convulsions with fever) |_| |_| |_|

g. Generalized seizures (without fever) |_| |_| |_|

h. Staring spells |_| |_| |_|

i. Infantile spasms |_| |_| |_|

j. Status epilepticus (seizures lasting 1 hour or more) |_| |_| |_|

k. Difficulty falling asleep |_| |_| |_|

l. Waking in the middle of the night |_| |_| |_|

m. Getting up extra early in the morning |_| |_| |_|

n. Visual defects |_| |_| |_|

o. Significant head injury with altered consciousness |_| |_| |_|

p. Other significant illness |_| |_| |_|
   (describe) _____

256

2. Has your child received any of the following (list reasons on back if not previously described)

|  | Yes | Date mo/yr | Where? | Results |
|---|---|---|---|---|
| a. Myringotomy and tubes | \|_\| | __ / __ | | _____ |
| c. CT scan (or MRI/NMR) | \|_\| | __ / __ | | _____ |
| e. EEG (brain wave) | \|_\| | __ / __ | | _____ |
| f. Hearing test | \|_\| | __ / __ | | _____ |
| g. Vision testing | \|_\| | __ / __ | | _____ |
| h. Brainstem evoked potentials | \|_\| | __ / __ | | _____ |
| i. Language therapy | \|_\| | __ / __ | | _____ |

Briefly describe _____

j. Sign language or lip reading
   training   \|_\|   \|__/__\|   _____

Briefly describe _____

k. Training in special education
   class   \|_\|   \|__/__\|   _____

Duration of training _____

Briefly describe _____

| | Yes | No | Don't know |
|---|---|---|---|
| 3. Has your child received one or more of the following medications for hyperactivity or behavior problems? (Circle all applicable) | \|_\| | \|_\| | \|_\| |

Cylert    Ritalin    Dexedrine    Imipramine (Tofranil)
Thioridazine (Mellaril)    Haloperidol (Haldol)    Fenfluramine
Other (specify) _____

| | Yes | No | Don't know |
|---|---|---|---|
| 3b. Is your child on medication now? (Specify) _____ | \|_\| | \|_\| | \|_\| |
| 4. Has you child received one or more of the following medications for seizures? (Circle all applicable) | \|_\| | \|_\| | \|_\| |

Clonopin    Mebaral    Diazepam (Valium)
Ethosuximide (Zarontin)    Carbamazepine (Tegretol)
Valproate (Depakene)    Primidone (Mysoline)    Phenobarbital
Phenytoin (Dilantin)
Other (specify ) _____

| | Yes | No | Don't know |
|---|---|---|---|
| 4k. Is your child on anticonvulsants now? (Specify) _____ | \|_\| | \|_\| | \|_\| |
| 5. Has your child ever been hospitalized beyond his stay at birth? (Answer yes if s/he had a prolonged stay in the premature or special care nursery.) Provide details below: | \|_\| | \|_\| | \|_\| |

_____
_____
_____

## C. Young Child

| Has your child done the following: | Age at onset in months | Was the skill lost? Yes | No | Don't know | Doesn't have skill |
|---|---|---|---|---|---|
| 1. Smiled at you? | \|__\| | \|_\| | \|_\| | \|_\| | \|_\| |
| 2. Followed you with his/her eyes? | \|__\| | \|_\| | \|_\| | \|_\| | \|_\| |
| 3. Looked at you when you held him/her? | \|__\| | \|_\| | \|_\| | \|_\| | \|_\| |
| 4. Reached for objects? | \|__\| | \|_\| | \|_\| | \|_\| | \|_\| |
| 5. Rolled over? | \|__\| | \|_\| | \|_\| | \|_\| | \|_\| |
| 6. Sat without support? | \|__\| | \|_\| | \|_\| | \|_\| | \|_\| |
| 7. Crawled? | \|__\| | \|_\| | \|_\| | \|_\| | \|_\| |
| 8. Walked alone? | \|__\| | \|_\| | \|_\| | \|_\| | \|_\| |

257

| | Age at onset in months | Was the skill lost? Yes | No | Don't know | Doesn't have skill |
|---|---|---|---|---|---|
| 9. Responded consistently to sounds? | \|__\| | \|_\| | \|_\| | \|_\| | \|_\| |
| 10. Babbled? | \|__\| | \|_\| | \|_\| | \|_\| | \|_\| |
| 12. Used single words? | \|__\| | \|_\| | \|_\| | \|_\| | \|_\| |
| 13. Combined words or 2-word phrases? | \|__\| | \|_\| | \|_\| | \|_\| | \|_\| |
| 14. Spoke in sentences? | \|__\| | \|_\| | \|_\| | \|_\| | \|_\| |
| 15. Asked questions which began with who/what/where/when/why/how? | \|__\| | \|_\| | \|_\| | \|_\| | \|_\| |
| 16. Named familiar objects/people? | \|__\| | \|_\| | \|_\| | \|_\| | \|_\| |
| 17. Understood most of what you say to him/her? | \|__\| | \|_\| | \|_\| | \|_\| | \|_\| |
| 18. Used speech which you can understand? | \|__\| | \|_\| | \|_\| | \|_\| | \|_\| |
| 19. Followed simple directions (one step)? | \|__\| | \|_\| | \|_\| | \|_\| | \|_\| |
| 20. Followed series of directions (2 or more steps)? | \|__\| | \|_\| | \|_\| | \|_\| | \|_\| |
| 21. Had pretend play? | \|__\| | \|_\| | \|_\| | \|_\| | \|_\| |
| 22. Carried a security blanket, teddy or doll? | \|__\| | \|_\| | \|_\| | \|_\| | \|_\| |
| 23. Initiated play with another child? | \|__\| | \|_\| | \|_\| | \|_\| | \|_\| |
| 24. Understood rules of games? | \|__\| | \|_\| | \|_\| | \|_\| | \|_\| |
| 25. Bladder trained—day? | \|__\| | \|_\| | \|_\| | \|_\| | \|_\| |
| 26. Bladder trained—night? | \|__\| | \|_\| | \|_\| | \|_\| | \|_\| |
| 27. Bowel trained—day? | \|__\| | \|_\| | \|_\| | \|_\| | \|_\| |
| 28. Bowel trained—night? | \|__\| | \|_\| | \|_\| | \|_\| | \|_\| |

## D. Childhood Behaviors

Each of the items below describe behaviors which may be seen in young children. Please indicate which behaviors you have observed in your child, the age in months at which the behaviors occurred, and the frequency with which they occurred. Use the codes below for 'frequency'. If these behaviors have not occurred, please place a 0 in the age column.

Frequency (when behavior was at its peak):    No or very rarely    —0
Yes, occasionally    —1
Yes, often or usually —2

| Does/did your child: | Age initiated in months | Peak frequency | Has this behavior disappeared? Yes | No |
|---|---|---|---|---|
| 1. Child's voice sound differently from that of other children? (Circle as applicable) Very loud  Very soft  Hoarse  Nasal  High or low in pitch for age/sex  Congested | \|__\| | \|_\| | \|_\| | \|_\| |
| 2. Repeat TV commercials, songs, or pieces of conversation heard earlier, for no apparent reason? | \|__\| | \|_\| | \|_\| | \|_\| |
| 2a. Appear to be very quiet as a baby (did not babble and coo as much as most babies)? | \|__\| | \|_\| | \|_\| | \|_\| |
| 3. Respond to questions by repeating the question or fail to respond? | \|__\| | \|_\| | \|_\| | \|_\| |
| 4. Have play that is limited to mouthing, banging, throwing or visually inspecting toys? | \|__\| | \|_\| | \|_\| | \|_\| |
| 5. Lack interest in, or show active dislike of interactive games such as ball play or games requiring turn-taking? | \|__\| | \|_\| | \|_\| | \|_\| |
| 6. Use toys inappropriately or non-functionally, such as lining up, pulling back and forth, spinning wheels, or flipping through the pages of a book? | \|__\| | \|_\| | \|_\| | \|_\| |
| 7. Prefer activities such as jigsaw puzzles, or shape matching or blocks instead of more creative games? | \|__\| | \|_\| | \|_\| | \|_\| |

|                                                                                                                                                                                   | Age initiated in months | Peak frequency | Has this behavior disappeared? | |
|---|:---:|:---:|:---:|:---:|
|                                                                                                                                                                                   |                         |                | Yes | No |
| 8. Have one line of pretend play that s/he goes over and over with little or no variation unless assisted by adult direction?                                                      | \|_ _\|                 | \|_\|          | \|_\| | \|_\| |
| 9. Become very upset or excited by slight or sudden change in routine or location?                                                                                                 | \|_ _\|                 | \|_\|          | \|_\| | \|_\| |
| 10. Make the same gesture(s) frequently, as finger rubbing, hand flapping, repeated touching of one place on his/her own body?                                                     | \|_ _\|                 | \|_\|          | \|_\| | \|_\| |
| 11. Engage in repetitive activities such as opening and closing of doors, touching all doorknobs, running hands along walls or fences, imaginary writing in the air?               | \|_ _\|                 | \|_\|          | \|_\| | \|_\| |
| 12. Becomes very upset when interrupted at what s/he is doing?                                                                                                                     | \|_ _\|                 | \|_\|          | \|_\| | \|_\| |
| 13. Seem unable to stop repetitive activity?                                                                                                                                       | \|_ _\|                 | \|_\|          | \|_\| | \|_\| |
| 14. Have abnormally long attention span for a preferred activity?                                                                                                                  | \|_ _\|                 | \|_\|          | \|_\| | \|_\| |
| 15. Tend to be remote from familiar persons, including family members?                                                                                                             | \|_ _\|                 | \|_\|          | \|_\| | \|_\| |
| 16. Stare into space as if seeing something that is not there or tuning out the environment?                                                                                       | \|_ _\|                 | \|_\|          | \|_\| | \|_\| |
| 17. Seem unaware of painful falls and bumps?                                                                                                                                       | \|_ _\|                 | \|_\|          | \|_\| | \|_\| |
| 18. Respond to affection by ignoring it?                                                                                                                                           | \|_ _\|                 | \|_\|          | \|_\| | \|_\| |
| 19. Show tremendous interest in mechanical objects such as vacuum cleaners or record players?                                                                                      | \|_ _\|                 | \|_\|          | \|_\| | \|_\| |
| 20. Seem underactive?                                                                                                                                                              | \|_ _\|                 | \|_\|          | \|_\| | \|_\| |
| 21. Eat or mouth objects such as dirt, plastic, paint?                                                                                                                             | \|_ _\|                 | \|_\|          | \|_\| | \|_\| |
| 22. Have catastrophic reactions and/or unexplained panics?                                                                                                                         | \|_ _\|                 | \|_\|          | \|_\| | \|_\| |
| 23. Have inability to be consoled when upset?                                                                                                                                      | \|_ _\|                 | \|_\|          | \|_\| | \|_\| |
| 24. Have unprovoked rage and/or unexplained aggressive outbursts?                                                                                                                  | \|_ _\|                 | \|_\|          | \|_\| | \|_\| |
| 25. Laugh or cry unexpectedly (without apparent reason)?                                                                                                                           | \|_ _\|                 | \|_\|          | \|_\| | \|_\| |
| 26. Have quick and drastic mood changes?                                                                                                                                           | \|_ _\|                 | \|_\|          | \|_\| | \|_\| |
| 27. Have severe temper tantrums and/or many minor tantrums?                                                                                                                        | \|_ _\|                 | \|_\|          | \|_\| | \|_\| |
| 28. Seem unaware of his/her mother's absence or leaving?                                                                                                                           | \|_ _\|                 | \|_\|          | \|_\| | \|_\| |
| 29. Become attached to an inanimate object (not a toy)?                                                                                                                            | \|_ _\|                 | \|_\|          | \|_\| | \|_\| |
| 30. Often seem nervous, tense, frightened or anxious?                                                                                                                              | \|_ _\|                 | \|_\|          | \|_\| | \|_\| |
| 31. Have special fears?                                                                                                                                                            | \|_ _\|                 | \|_\|          | \|_\| | \|_\| |

(Specify) _____

_____

_____

32. Has your child demonstrated ability which is clearly beyond what s/he can do in most other areas? Please specify and describe on the back of this page.

|_|  a. Memory
|_|  b. Musical ability
|_|  c. Puzzles or other spatial activities
|_|  d. Numbers/calculations/dates
|_|  e. Fine motor skills
|_|  f. Writing letters or numbers
|_|  g. Other (describe) _____

_____

_____

33. Has your child's behavior ever improved with a fever?    Yes    No    Don't know

                                                                \|_\|    \|_\|    \|_\|

### III. FAMILY HISTORY

A. Immediate Family

On the chart below, please fill in the person's initials or first name and the requested information.

| | Initial/first name | Sex M/F | Handedness R/L/Both |
|---|---|---|---|
| 1. Child's father | | M | |
| 2. Child's mother | | F | |
| 3. Oldest sibling | | | |
| 4. Second sibling | | | |
| 5. Third sibling | | | |
| 6. Fourth sibling | | | |
| 7. Fifth sibling | | | |
| 8. Sixth sibling | | | |
| 9. Seventh sibling | | | |
| 10. Eighth sibling | | | |

Child's Family History

Please indicate the number of affected individuals in each box. Place a 0 in all boxes that contain no family members affected so that there are no empty boxes. Please use the first initials on the genogram to identify members and write details about them on the back of the page.

| | Child's Father | Child's Mother | Child's Sisters | Child's Brothers |
|---|---|---|---|---|
| A. Stuttering | | | | |
| B. Speech/language delay/disorder | | | | |
| C. Motor difficulties | | | | |
| D. Learning/behavioral/ developmental problems | | | | |
|     Reading | | | | |
|     Spelling | | | | |
|     Writing | | | | |
|     Mathematics | | | | |
|     Mental retardation | | | | |
|     Hyperactivity | | | | |
|     Attention deficit | | | | |
|     Conduct disorder | | | | |
|     Eating disorder | | | | |
|     Other (specify on back) | | | | |
| E. Psychiatric disorders | | | | |
|     Schizophrenia | | | | |
|     Major depression | | | | |
|     Manic depression | | | | |
|     Anxiety disorders | | | | |
|     Psychiatric hospitalization | | | | |
|     Other (specify on back) | | | | |
| F. Neurological disorders | | | | |
|     Tourette syndrome/tics | | | | |
|     Seizure disorders | | | | |
|     Brain damage/head injuries | | | | |
|     Other (specify on back) | | | | |
| G. Autoimmune and other diseases | | | | |
|     Cancer | | | | |
|     Asthma | | | | |
|     Crohn's disease—colitis | | | | |
|     Migraine headaches | | | | |
|     Thyroid disease | | | | |
|     Diabetes | | | | |
|     Other (specify on back) | | | | |
| H. Died | | | | |

PATERNAL GENOGRAM (to be completed with interviewer)

Please include only the child's paternal grandparents, father, paternal aunts and uncles (father's sisters and brothers), and their children—first cousins (*i.e.* children of aunts and uncles only). Please mark the first initial of each family member in the box representing him/her so that individuals with important abnormalities can be identified in later questions about the family. Do not forget to include deceased family members in the genogram and in all subsequent questions; mark them with an oblique line across the box. Do not forget to mark the child (propositus) with an arrow.

Paternal Family History

Please indicate the number of individuals having the characteristic in each box. Place a zero (0) in all boxes containing no family member so that there are no empty boxes. Please include deceased family members in the count.

|  | Handedness | | | |
|---|---|---|---|---|
| Child's: | Right | Left | Both | Don't know |
| Grandfather |  |  |  |  |
| Grandmother |  |  |  |  |
| Aunts |  |  |  |  |
| Uncles |  |  |  |  |
| Female first cousins |  |  |  |  |
| Male first cousins |  |  |  |  |

261

Paternal Family History

Please indicate the number of affected individuals in each box. Place a zero (0) in all boxes containing no family members with that condition so that there are no empty boxes. Please use the first initials on the genogram to identify members and write details about them on the back of the page.

| | Child's | | | | | |
| --- | --- | --- | --- | --- | --- | --- |
| | Grandpa | Grandma | Aunts | Uncles | First cousins | |
| | | | | | Male | Female |
| A. Stuttering | | | | | | |
| B. Speech/language delay/disorder | | | | | | |
| C. Motor difficulties | | | | | | |
| D. Learning/behavioral/developmental problems | | | | | | |
|    Reading | | | | | | |
|    Spelling | | | | | | |
|    Writing | | | | | | |
|    Mathematics | | | | | | |
|    Autism | | | | | | |
|    Mental retardation | | | | | | |
|    Hyperactivity | | | | | | |
|    Attention deficit | | | | | | |
|    Conduct disorder | | | | | | |
|    Eating disorder | | | | | | |
|    Other (specify on back) | | | | | | |
| E. Psychiatric disorders | | | | | | |
|    Schizophrenia | | | | | | |
|    Major depression | | | | | | |
|    Manic depression | | | | | | |
|    Anxiety disorders | | | | | | |
|    Psychiatric hospitalizations | | | | | | |
|    Other (specify on back) | | | | | | |
| F. Neurological disorders | | | | | | |
|    Tourette syndrome/tics | | | | | | |
|    Seizure disorders | | | | | | |
|    Strokes | | | | | | |
|    Brain damage/head injuries | | | | | | |
|    Other (specify on back) | | | | | | |
| G. Autoimmune and other diseases | | | | | | |
|    Cancer | | | | | | |
|    Asthma | | | | | | |
|    Crohn's disease—colitis | | | | | | |
|    Migraine headaches | | | | | | |
|    Thyroid disease | | | | | | |
|    Diabetes | | | | | | |
|    Other (specify on back) | | | | | | |
| H. Died | | | | | | |

<u>MATERNAL GENOGRAM</u> (to be completed with interviewer)

Please include only the child's maternal grandparents, mother, maternal aunts and uncles (mother's sisters and brothers), and their children—first cousins (*i.e.* children of aunts and uncles only). Please mark the first initial of each family member in the box representing him/her so that individuals with important abnormalities can be identified in later questions about the family. Do not forget to include deceased family members in the genogram and in all subsequent questions; mark them with an oblique line across the box. Do not forget to mark the child (propositus) with an arrow.

<u>Maternal Family History</u>

Please indicate the number of individuals having the characteristic in each box. Place a zero (0) in all boxes containing no family member so that there are no empty boxes. Please include deceased family members in the count.

|  | Handedness | | | |
|---|---|---|---|---|
| Child's: | Right | Left | Both | Don't know |
| Grandfather |  |  |  |  |
| Grandmother |  |  |  |  |
| Aunts |  |  |  |  |
| Uncles |  |  |  |  |
| Female first cousins |  |  |  |  |
| Male first cousins |  |  |  |  |

263

<u>Maternal Family History</u>

Please indicate the number of affected individuals in each box. Place a zero (0) in all boxes containing no family members with that condition so that there are no empty boxes. Please use the first initials on the genogram to identify members and write details about them on the back of the page.

| | Grandpa | Grandma | Aunts | Uncles | First cousins | |
| --- | --- | --- | --- | --- | --- | --- |
| | | | Child's | | | |
| | | | | | Male | Female |
| A. Stuttering | | | | | | |
| B. Speech/language delay/disorder | | | | | | |
| C. Motor difficulties | | | | | | |
| D. Learning/behavioral/developmental problems | | | | | | |
|    Reading | | | | | | |
|    Spelling | | | | | | |
|    Writing | | | | | | |
|    Mathematics | | | | | | |
|    Autism | | | | | | |
|    Mental retardation | | | | | | |
|    Hyperactivity | | | | | | |
|    Attention deficit | | | | | | |
|    Conduct disorder | | | | | | |
|    Eating disorder | | | | | | |
|    Other (specify on back) | | | | | | |
| E. Psychiatric disorders | | | | | | |
|    Schizophrenia | | | | | | |
|    Major depression | | | | | | |
|    Manic depression | | | | | | |
|    Anxiety disorders | | | | | | |
|    Psychiatric hospitalizations | | | | | | |
|    Other (specify on back) | | | | | | |
| F. Neurological disorders | | | | | | |
|    Tourette syndrome/tics | | | | | | |
|    Seizure disorders | | | | | | |
|    Strokes | | | | | | |
|    Brain damage/head injuries | | | | | | |
|    Other (specify on back) | | | | | | |
| G. Autoimmune and other diseases | | | | | | |
|    Cancer | | | | | | |
|    Asthma | | | | | | |
|    Crohn's disease—colitis | | | | | | |
|    Migraine headaches | | | | | | |
|    Thyroid disease | | | | | | |
|    Diabetes | | | | | | |
|    Other (specify on back) | | | | | | |
| H. Died | | | | | | |

# APPENDIX 4

## NEUROLOGICAL EVALUATION

**Comments**

This appendix lists the items included in the neurological evaluation of the 556 children entered into the study. Each item was scored on a three-point scale: normal/near-normal; mildly/moderately abnormal; very abnormal/unable to do, no data. We prepared a manual to instruct the neurologists in giving the examination and a coding scheme to provide summary scores so as to give even weights to the different parts of the examination represented by uneven numbers of items. The manual and coding scheme, together with a revised neurological examination form for preschool children and integral scoring sheet are obtainable from the authors. We provide here some critical comments to enable readers intending to employ such an evaluation to profit from our experience.

• Ideally, design a form that can be read optically into a computer, to bypass the transcribing of scores onto a screen, which is time-consuming and adds another layer of potential errors.

• It is desirable but may not always be possible to separate reasons for lack of data. A classification of 'No data' if you didn't make observations or didn't examine is clear, but deciding whether a child refused (negativistic) or couldn't perform an item (for reasons of mental retardation, attention disorder or other non-sensorimotor cause) is not always obvious. We advise providing discrete codes for these.

• We strongly advise having items that can be scored by observation, without the need for active participation, to minimize this problem, *e.g.* gait, posture, abnormal movements, etc.

• The section on stereotypies and self-injurious behaviors should be expanded, inasmuch as these are strong markers for autism and are purely observational items.

• The sensory examination is unreliable in preschool children and should be omitted.

• The oromotor examination can be shortened. The rapid syllable repetition is sensitive but unreliable in that age group and can be omitted because too many children do not cooperate.

• The mental status and language parts need change; as it stands, some items are unsatisfactory because they encompass both decreased and increased behaviors, or have to do with quantity as well as quality under a single item.

• Play with representational toys is critically important: it provides the core of the mental status examination and strongly discriminates autistic from non-autistic children, even though it is confounded by age and IQ. It provides the best sample of language because the neurologist is less liable to fire a barrage of questions to the child, which will result in mostly single word answers, than during the rest of the examination.

**Neurological evaluation items**

A. IDENTIFYING DATA
• Sex
• Date of birth
• Date of examination
• Age (in months) on day of examination

B. GENERAL FINDINGS
• General state (of health)
• General state (physical)
• Appearance (including shape of head, if unusual, dysmorphic features, malformations)
• Ears—otoscopic examination

- Visual acuity
- Head circumference

## C. GROSS MOTOR
- Gait—walking
- Gait—running
- Gait—on toes
- Gait—on heels
- Jump on 2 feet
- Hop (age ≥5y)
- Tandem gait [have child walk 2m (6ft) along tape or stripe on floor] (age ≥5y)
- Standing on one foot for 5 seconds (age ≥5y)

## D. FINE MOTOR (disregard mirror movements)
- Finger to nose (intention tremor and past-pointing)
- Patting (on hard surface)
- Apposing index finger to thumb (5 or more times)
- Appose 4 fingers to thumb sequentially
- Pile 2.5cm (1″) blocks
- Build with 2.5cm blocks (age ≥3y, 3-block bridge; ≥4y, 6-block pyramid; ≥5y, 5-block gate)
- Draw (age ≥3y, line, circle; ≥4y, also square; ≥5y, also square and triangle)

## E. TYPE OF MOTOR DEFICIT
- Apraxia
- Spasticity (supine) (arms, legs)
- Spasticity (gait)
- Rigidity (lead pipe to passive movement) (arms, legs)
- Hypotonia (resistance to passive movement, joint laxity) (arms, legs)
- Weakness (arms, legs)

## F. ABNORMAL POSTURE OR INVOLUNTARY MOVEMENTS
- Tremor—intention and/or postural
- Choreoathetosis
- Dystonia
- Tics

## G. SENSORY EXAMINATION
- Tactile localization (single stimulus)
- Tactile localization (double simultaneous)

## H. CRANIAL NERVES
- Visual fields to confrontation (gaze preference?)
- Ocular motility
- Strabismus
- Nystagmus
- Facial movements—upper motor neuron (lower face)
- Facial movements—lower motor neuron (upper + lower face)

## I. OROMOTOR FUNCTION
- Drooling
- Jaw movements: up and down
- Jaw movements: side to side
- Tongue movements: side to side (to corner of lips)
- Tongue movements: in and out
- Tongue movements: curl up and down

266

- Click and/or tsk tongue
- Put tongue in R and L cheek
- Palate
- Purse lips (whistling position)
- 'Kiss'
- Pa-pa-pa-pa-pa-pa-pa (at least 5 times)
- Ta-ta-ta-ta-ta-ta-ta (at least 5 times)
- Kae-kae-kae-kae-kae-kae-kae (like 'kept'—at least 5 times)
- Syllable repetition
  —Children aged 3 and 4:  Pa-ta-pa-ta (5 times or more)
  —Children aged 5 and above:  Pa-ta-ka-pa-ta-ka (5 times or more)

## J. BEHAVIOR
- Alertness—state of arousal
- Interpersonal interaction
- Cooperation
- Attention
- Activity level
- Affect
- Appropriateness of behavior
- Stereotypies, self-mutilation, etc.
- Play (Use doll house or other toy suitable for child's age. Play with the child so as to elicit conversation.)

## K. LANGUAGE AND COMMUNICATION
- Communicative use of speech
- Communicative use of gestures (including facial expression)
- Amount of language (too much or too little)
- Intelligibility
- Prosody (melody and rhythm of speech)
- Sentence structure
- Fluency
- Pointing on command
- Naming to confrontation  ("What's that?')
- Echolalia
- Comprehension of commands
- Comprehension of questions
- Seizures (observed only)

## L. TYPE OF DISABILITY (summary of impression)
- Sensorimotor
- Oromotor
- Language deficit—production
- Language deficit—comprehension
- Cognitive deficit
- Autistic behaviors

## M. PRESUMED LOCALIZATION OF PATHOLOGY (based on sensorimotor data only)

# APPENDIX 5

## WING SCHEDULE OF HANDICAPS, BEHAVIOUR AND SKILLS (HBS) *

*Lorna Wing*

This schedule was compiled for use with children and adults who are moderately, severely or profoundly retarded (as defined in the International Classification of Diseases, 9th Revision), and also for those who are severely retarded in some but not all aspects of their development (*e.g.* due to autism or developmental speech disorders).

It is intended as a measure of achievements and problems as they are shown in everyday activities and not in formal intelligence tests. Each item contains questions which discriminate very low levels of performance. The schedule is therefore not appropriate for those who are not retarded in any respect.

### INSTRUCTIONS
*System of coding*
This schedule is designed to describe the person's level of functioning and present behaviour. It can be adapted for history taking by asking for the age at which each step in the developmental sequences was attained and the age range during which each item of behaviour was shown.

Two kinds of items are included:
(1) Those indicating the stage of development reached (*e.g.* use of language, ability to walk, dress and feed). The sub-items under each heading are arranged in order according to the usual sequence of development. The higher the stage reached, the higher the score. The subject (S) should be rated on his latest achievement. The usual level of current performance should be rated—not the occasional 'high point' which is not characteristic. The ages noted on the left of the developmental sub-items give an approximate indication of when the relevant skill is likely to have emerged during the course of normal development.**
(2) Those concerning abnormal or difficult behaviour (*e.g.* disturbance of sleep, echolalia, stereotypic movements, physical aggression). The sub-items under each heading are arranged in order of severity, and the least abnormal behaviour receives the highest 'score'. The subject should be rated on his behaviour over the past month, or whatever period of time has been chosen for the study concerned.

Each sub-item is numbered. The number for the sub-item which best describes the level of skill or behaviour of the child concerned is entered on the schedule page or into the appropriate space on the coding sheet.

For each item, 9 = not known or not applicable (use 99 for items with 2-digit codes). If 9 is used when the evidence is equivocal, note examples of the behaviour and the reasons why a decision could not be made.

---

*The HBS was originally designed as a research tool in 1970, before the advent of current 'politically correct' terminology. The term 'handicap' was then in common usage for what is now referred to as 'disability'. The pronoun 'he/his' was adopted throughout because the majority of children with communication disorders are boys.

The HBS has provided the basis for a more detailed schedule, the Diagnostic Interview for Social and Communication Disorders (known as the DISCD) which is now being developed as a clinical instrument.

**For certain items, sub-items are included that represent deviations from the normal course of development. Developmental age-equivalents do not apply to these items.

For each developmental item, instructions are given for when 0 (= skill absent) should be used and when 9 is appropriate.

*Administration of the schedule*

The schedule is not intended as a questionnaire which always has to be administered in the same way and using the same words. The informant should be questioned, using phrases that he or she can understand, in order to establish how the subject functions or behaves. The questions should be rephrased until it is quite clear that an accurate rating has been obtained.

Suggestions for introductory questions are made for each section—the replies determine how the questioning should proceed. The questioning in each individual case must be adapted to the knowledge of the subject's level of functioning which is gained as the interview proceeds. In some cases, as, for example, that of someone with severe physical disabilities, it is unnecessary to ask the questions concerning activities of which he is incapable, and the items should be coded as 0 or 9 as appropriate. However, such subjects should be given a rating for their behaviour whenever it is reasonable to do so. For example, a person who cannot walk cannot jump up and down, but may be able to flap his arms (see Section 26, Abnormal bodily movements).

Leading questions which suggest a specific answer should be avoided as far as possible when introducing each item, but, eventually, specific questions, using examples as illustrations, are necessary to make sure that the correct rating is made. If you feel the informant cannot grasp the idea behind the questions, and cannot give useful examples of the subject's behaviour, rate 9.

When dealing with items which rate level of development, it is best to begin the questioning at approximately the level at which you expect the subject to perform, based on information from previous items, or from acquaintance with the subject.

When dealing with items which rate abnormal behaviour, it is best to phrase the initial question in a fairly neutral manner, to avoid any tendency for the informant to deny abnormality.

Some items are rated on the frequency of abnormal behaviour. Others are rated on severity rather than frequency, because this is more appropriate in certain cases. If a subject shows variable behaviour on such items (*e.g.* insistence on routines, clinging to objects—Section 27), then rate the problem as present if it has occurred within a specified time period (defined according to the purposes of the study) and has lasted long enough to present difficulties of management.

For each item, concrete examples of the subject's behaviour should be noted.

Sometimes a person can be given a high rating on one item, but does not show the behaviour necessary for one or more of the lower levels of achievement. In this case, note the rating which occurs below the 'gap' in achievement, as well as that for the highest level reached. The decision as to which one is entered in the list of codes depends on the purpose of the study.

The ratings should be based on each person's actual behaviour and not on what the informant thinks the child could do if he tried.

When the schedule has been completed, the items should be considered again in case changes in earlier ratings are necessary in the light of information obtained later in the interview.

1. MOBILITY
   Throughout this section, if a subject is unable to walk for any reason, use 0.

   a. Walking on level surfaces
      How much can S move around? How much help does he need to sit up/walk?

|       | 00 | Cannot lift head |
|-------|----|------------------|
| 4 mo  | 01 | Can lift head |
| 6 mo  | 02 | Turns onto back when lying prone, and vice versa |
|       | 03 | Sits up with support (*e.g.* cushion, special chair) |
| 7 mo  | 04 | Sits up without support |
| 9 mo  | 05 | Crawls or shuffles along at least a few yards |
|       | 06 | Pulls himself upright by holding on to furniture, etc. |
|       | 07 | Can stand unsupported, not holding on, for a minute or more |
|       | 08 | Walks with support |
| 1 y 2 mo | 09 | Walks without support indoors, but needs pram, or pushchair, or wheelchair when taken out for longer distances |
| 1 y 5 mo | 10 | Walks without support, no need for pram or pushchair |
| 2 y   | 11 | Runs more than 50 yards (45 metres). |

   b. Walking up and down stairs
      How does S manage stairs?

|       | 0 | Cannot walk upstairs |
|-------|---|----------------------|
| 1 y 6 mo | 1 | Walks upstairs with help (not crawling) |
| 2 y 6 mo | 2 | Walks upstairs without help, bringing feet together on each step |
| 3 y   | 3 | Walks upstairs without help, alternating feet on stairs, but walks downstairs bringing feet together on each step |
| 4 y   | 4 | Walks up and down stairs, alternating feet |
|       | 5 | Climbs up and down wall bars without help |
| 5 y   | 6 | Climbs with marked agility |

2. SKILLED MOVEMENTS
   Throughout this section, if the subject cannot perform these actions for any reason, use 0.

   a. Riding a tricycle or bicycle
      Can S sit on a tricycle? Can he ride it by himself?

|       | 0 | Cannot ride a tricycle |
|-------|---|------------------------|
| 2 y 6 mo | 1 | Sits on tricycle but pushes it along with feet on floor |
| 2 y 9 mo | 2 | Rides a tricycle a few yards, pedalling |
| 4 y   | 3 | Rides tricycle well |
|       | 4 | Rides bicycle a few yards, pedalling |
| 7 y   | 5 | Rides bicycle well |

   b. Manual dexterity
      How much can S do with his hands and fingers?

|       | 0 | Does not use hands at all |
|-------|---|---------------------------|
|       | 1 | Grasps but cannot let go |
| 3 mo  | 2 | Grasps with whole hand - can let go |
| 9 mo  | 3 | Grasps with finger and thumb |
| 9 mo  | 4 | Uses both hands in tasks needing two hands to complete |
| 1 y 1 mo | 5 | Uses both hands but shows definite preference for right or left |
| 1 y 10 mo | 6 | Can unwrap sweet—clumsily |
| 2 y+  | 7 | Can unwrap sweet—neatly |

c. <u>Hand–eye coordination</u>
Does S play with a ball? Can he throw a ball? Can he catch?

| | | |
|---|---|---|
| | 0 | Cannot throw a ball at all |
| 9 mo– | 1 | Throws ball indiscriminately |
| 1 y 6 mo | | |
| 2 y | 2 | Throws ball fairly accurately |
| 3 y | 3 | Holds out arms to catch a ball but does not coordinate hand and eye |
| | 4 | Catches a ball clumsily |
| 4 y | 5 | Catches a ball neatly |

3. <u>FEEDING</u>
For items *a*, *b* and *c*, if subject is unable to feed himself, chew, etc., for any reason, use 0.

a. <u>Feeding</u>
(Those who cannot sit up)—How do you manage with feeding?
(Those who can sit up)—Can S feed himself, or do you have to feed him? Can he use a spoon or a fork (even if he prefers fingers)?

| | | |
|---|---|---|
| | 00 | Always has to be fed |
| 9 mo | 01 | Feeds himself with fingers |
| 1 y | 02 | Feeds himself with spoon—messy, may need help |
| 1 y 6 mo | 03 | Feeds himself with spoon, no help, little or no mess |
| 3 y | 04 | Feeds himself with spoon and fork |
| Between | (05 | Feeds with spoon and fork but uses knife for spreading butter, etc. |
| 5 y and 8 y | (06 | Feeds himself with knife and fork but needs help with cutting difficult foods |
| | (07 | Feeds himself with knife and fork without help |
| | (08 | Can manage all foods for himself (boiled eggs, fish with bones) |
| 9 y | 09 | Can manage all foods for himself and helps himself at table |

b. <u>Ability to chew</u>
Can S chew his food?

| | | |
|---|---|---|
| | 0 | Needs a liquid diet |
| | 1 | Chews minced or mashed food |
| 1 y | 2 | Chews some solid food |
| 2 y | 3 | Chews meat and other hard food |

c. <u>Drinking</u>
Does S need a special cup or bottle, or can he drink from an ordinary cup?

| | | |
|---|---|---|
| | 0 | Needs a special drinking container (*e.g.* bottle or feeding cup) |
| 8 mo | 1 | Drinks from a cup with help (helps to hold cup) |
| 1 y 6 mo | 2 | Holds own cup—but some spilling |
| 2 y | 3 | Holds own cup without spilling |
| 2 y 6 mo–3 y | 4 | Can get himself a drink from a jug or a tap |

d. <u>Dribbling</u>
Does S dribble a lot? Does he often have a runny nose? Do you have to wipe his mouth and chin or nose often to keep him dry?

| | | |
|---|---|---|
| | 0 | Dribbles and has a runny nose frequently |
| | 1 | Dribbles frequently, but no problem with runny nose |
| 1 y | 2 | No problem with dribbling, but frequently has a runny nose |
| | 3 | No problems |

N.B. If 0, 1 or 2 is rated, then a rating should also be made under Section 28j, <u>Difficult or objectionable personal habits</u>, depending on the degree to which the problem makes S socially unacceptable.

4. WASHING

Throughout this section, if S is unable to wash himself for any reason, use 0.

a. Washing

Can S wash himself at all or does he need help?

|  |  |  |
|---|---|---|
|  | 0 | Always needs to be washed |
|  | 1 | Beginning to try to wash and dry hands |
| 2y 7mo | 2 | Dries own hands without help |
| 3y 7mo | 3 | Gets hands acceptably clean and dry without help |
| 4y–5y | 4 | Washes and dries hands and face, without help |
|  | 5 | Baths himself with help |
| 6y 3mo | 6 | Baths himself without help but needs supervision |
| 8y 10mo | 7 | Baths and dries himself without help (can be left alone in the bathroom and will complete the task himself, except for washing and drying hair) |
| 12y 5mo | 8 | Can bath, dress, shave, cut nails, wash and dry hair, without help, or with help on rare occasions only |

5. DRESSING

Throughout this section, if S is unable to dress and undress himself, etc., for any reason, use 0.

a. Dressing

How much help does S need with dressing? If you dress him, does he do anything to help, or is it like dressing a doll?

|  |  |  |
|---|---|---|
|  | 00 | Has to be dressed and gives no help at all |
| 1y | (01 | Holds out arms or legs |
|  | (02 | Helps by putting arms in sleeves or head through neck if garment is held for him |
| 2y | 03 | Puts on shoes (may not fasten) |
|  | 04 | Puts on coat (may not fasten) |
| 2y 6mo | 05 | Pulls up pants and then arranges other clothing properly |
| 3y | 06 | Can pull clothes over head unaided |
| 4y | 07 | Dresses himself completely but may not do up fastenings (zips, laces, buttons) —but needs clothes arranged in sequence and right way round (otherwise puts items on in wrong order, back to front, etc.) |
| 5y | 08 | Dresses himself completely and gets clothes right way round (may need some help with difficult garments) |
| 12y 5mo | 09 | Can be left to choose own clothes from wardrobe without help, makes appropriate choice to suit weather, type of occasion, etc. |

b. Buttons

Can S do up buttons?

|  |  |  |
|---|---|---|
|  | 0 | Cannot do up buttons |
| 3y 6mo | 1 | Does up large and easy buttons (*e.g.* on coat) |
| 4y | 2 | Can do up most buttons—needs help with buttons on cuffs |
| 5y | 3 | Can do up all buttons |

c. Undressing

(Adapt questions to reply for dressing)

|  |  |  |
|---|---|---|
|  | 00 | Has to be undressed and gives no help at all |
| 1y | 01 | Holds out arms or legs |
| 1y 6mo | 02 | Pulls off socks and shoes (if unfastened for him) |
| 2y | 03 | Takes arms out of sleeves (can take coat off) |
| 2y–3y | 04 | Pulls off pants |
| 3y | 05 | Pulls off clothes over head |

| 3y–4y | 06 | Undresses himself with some help |
| 4y | 07 | Undresses himself except for laces, or laces and buttons |
| 5y | 08 | Undresses himself without help |
| 6y 9mo | 09 | Undresses and goes to bed, turns out light, etc., without assistance or supervision |

d. Hair brushing and combing

Do you have to brush and comb his hair or can S do this for himself?

| | 0 | Does not brush and comb own hair |
| 2y | 1 | Brushes and combs hair with help |
| 5y | 2 | Brushes and combs hair without help, and hair looks acceptably tidy |

(N.B. Age may be lower or higher depending on hair style)

6. CONTINENCE

If subject is incontinent for any reason, or cannot perform the skills in c and d, use 0.

a. Incontinence during day

Is S wet or dirty during the day? What do you do about toilet training?

| | 0 | Doubly incontinent during day |
| | 1 | Incontinent of urine during the day |
| 2y | 2 | Usually clean and dry if taken to toilet or pot - occasional accident |
| 3y | 3 | Reliably clean and dry if taken to toilet or pot |
| | 4 | Takes himself to toilet or pot if told |
| | 5 | Takes himself to toilet or pot without being told—occasional accident |
| 3y–4y | 6 | Takes himself to toilet or pot without being told—completely reliable |

b. Incontinence during the night

Is S wet or dirty at night? Can you avoid this by lifting him during the night?

| | 0 | Doubly incontinent, or encopretic at night—weekly or more often |
| | 1 | Doubly incontinent, or encopretic at night—less than weekly |
| | 2 | Enuretic—weekly or more often |
| | 3 | Enuretic—less than weekly |
| | 4 | Dry at night if lifted during night |
| 3y | 5 | Dry at night—no problem |

c. Indication of toilet needs

How do you know when S wants to go to the toilet?

| | 0 | Never indicates need to use toilet |
| | 1 | Involuntary indication (goes red in the face, restless movements, etc.) |
| 1y 6mo | 2 | Sometimes indicates by speech or gesture that he needs to use toilet (occasionally indicates when it is too late) |
| 2y | 3 | Asks to go to toilet, by speech or gesture, in good time, whenever this is necessary, (e.g. can ask or indicate if he is in an unfamiliar place and does not know where to find the toilet) |

d. Cleaning and dressing after toilet

Can S look after himself when he goes to the toilet? Does he need help with cleaning himself and with his clothes?

| | 0 | Needs cleaning and help with clothes after using toilet |
| | 1 | Some supervision necessary |
| 3y 10mo | 2 | No supervision necessary |

7. COMPREHENSION OF SPEECH

Throughout this section if S is known to be too deaf to hear speech, use 9. Otherwise use the appropriate rating.

a. General level of comprehension of speech

How much does S understand when you speak to him? Can he obey some simple instructions? Can he understand something a little more complicated?

0 No response when spoken to

1 Responds to name only

1 y–1 y 3 mo   2 Understands simple phrases in context, because of a learned sequence of events, *e.g.* 'Give Mummy a kiss', 'Come and get your dinner', 'Time for bed'. The cues come from actions and gestures with the words. The individual words are not recognized on their own (*e.g.* would kiss mother if his *actions* were appropriate even if mother *said* 'Give Mummy an apple')

1 y 3 mo–2 y   3 Knows the meaning of some words, even if not linked to a special learned phrase (*e.g.* understands and responds appropriately to a phrase that is not said regularly every day, *e.g.* 'Where is your teddy bear?' Also can respond to, *e.g.*, 'Give me your cup'. Use examples based on the phrases the informant says S understands)

2 y–2 y 6 mo   4 Can follow instructions involving two named objects, *e.g.* 'Put the doll on the chair', 'Put the brush in the drawer'. (N.B. These must not be familiar phrases learnt in context)

2 y 6 mo+   5 Can be sent out of the room to fetch two or more objects reliably (*e.g.* 'Go upstairs and fetch Mummy's handbag and gloves')

3 y   6 Understands a sequence of commands (*e.g.* 'First put your paints in the cupboard, then wash your hands and then lay the table')

4 y   7 Understands instructions involving decisions (*e.g.* 'See if your coat is in the hall, and, if not, then look for it in your bedroom')

b. Understanding of prepositions

Does S know what you mean if you use words like 'in', 'on', 'under', 'behind', or 'before', 'after'?

0 Does not understand these words

2 y   1 Understands some but not all

3 y   2 Fully understands all these words

(Use example of 'under the cupboard' as opposed to 'in the cupboard')

8. ABILITY TO USE SPEECH

For items *a* and *b*, if S is known to be too deaf to hear speech, use 9 or 99. Otherwise use the appropriate ratings. If S is mute in some situations but speaks in others, rate him on his performance in the environment where he does speak.

a. Development of grammar

How much can S talk? What can he say? Can he make sounds that have any meaning? (Rate on level that S has attained and not just on his willingness to speak. Do not give credit for meaningless echolalia.)

00 No speech or sounds at all, or makes noises (not normal baby sounds) without meaning

3 mo   01 Babbles, gurgles, coos, laughs without meaning

9 mo   02 Babbles or makes noises with meaning

1 y 4 mo   03 Gives the names of some people or things when asked

1 y 8 mo   04 Spontaneously says names of several familiar objects for some purpose

2 y   05 Says phrases of two words (*e.g.* 'Want dinner', 'Have sweet')

| 2y–3y | 06 | Says some longer phrases with nouns and verbs, missing out the small linking words (*e.g.* 'When time go on holiday?') |
| | 07 | Talks in spontaneous sentences using small linking words—present tense only |
| | 08 | Can form sentences using 'but', 'because', etc. |
| 4y | 09 | Uses past, present and future tenses, and complex grammatical constructions (*e.g.* 'Perhaps I will go out tomorrow if it has stopped raining') |

b. Asking questions
Does S ever try to ask you questions? What sorts of questions? How does he ask this—what does he say?

|  | 0 | Does not ask questions |
| | 1 | Asks for objects using a simple, learnt phrase |
| 3y | 2 | Asks a limited range of questions only (*e.g.* 'Where are we going?', 'Who is that?', 'When are we going home?') |
| 4y | 3 | Asks more complex 'why' and 'how' questions (*e.g.* 'Why does the sun go down at night?, 'How does it work?', 'Why is X unhappy?') |

c. Intelligibility—execution of speech
How easy is it to understand what S says? (Rate item only if S has phrases of 2 words or more, otherwise use 9. If speech is only meaningless echolalia, use 9.)

|  | 0 | All, or almost all speech unintelligible |
| | 1 | Most speech unintelligible but a few words can be understood |
| | 2 | Speech can be understood by people who know S well—but with difficulty |
| | 3 | Speech can be understood by people who know subject well—fairly easily |
| 3y | 4 | Speech can be understood by strangers—but with difficulty |
| 4y | 5 | Speech easily understood by strangers—but pronounces some letters incorrectly |
| 5y | 6 | No problems |

(N.B. The lower ratings should be used if problems are caused by poor pronunciation or articulation *or* by rapidity, jerkiness, inaudibility or other abnormalities of delivery of speech.)

d. Intelligibility—content of speech
Does what S says make sense to people who know him well? Rate item only if S has sufficient speech to make it possible to rate the content, otherwise use 9. If speech is entirely echolalia, use 9.

|  | 0 | Speech is garbled, nonsensical, vague, inconsequential even to those who know him well—marked problem |
| | 1 | Sometimes a problem, or minor problem |
| | 2 | Content of speech may seem odd to strangers, but people who know S well recognize its relevance |
| | 3 | No problem |

9. COMPREHENSION OF SIGN LANGUAGE
(relevant for those who cannot understand speech)
Throughout this section if S is known to be too visually impaired to see signs, use 9 or 99. Otherwise use the appropriate ratings.

a. General level of comprehension of sign language
Has anyone tried to teach S a sign language? How much does he understand when you sign to him? Can he obey some simple instructions? Can he understand something a little more complicated?

|  | 00 | No response when signed to, though attempts made to teach signs |
| | 01 | Responds to name only |

275

| 1 y–<br>1 y 3 mo | 02 | Understands simple signs in context because of a learned sequence of events, *e.g.* 'Give Mummy a kiss', 'Come and get your dinner', 'Time for bed'. The cues come from actions and gestures with the words. The individual signs are not recognized on their own (*e.g.* would kiss mother if his *actions* were appropriate even if mother *signs* 'give Mummy an apple') |
|---|---|---|
| 1 y 3 mo–<br>2 y | 03 | Knows the meaning of some signs, even if *not* linked to a special learned phrase, *e.g.* understands and responds appropriately to a phrase that is not signed regularly every day (*e.g.* 'Where is your teddy bear?' Also can respond to, *e.g.* 'Give me your cup.' (Use examples based on the signs the informant says S understands) |
| 2 y–<br>2 y 6 mo | 04 | Can follow instructions involving two named objects, *e.g.* 'Put the doll on the chair', 'Put the brush in the drawer.' (N.B. These must not be the familiar phrases learnt in context) |
| 2 y 6 mo+ | 05 | Can be sent out of the room to fetch two or more objects reliably (*e.g.* 'Go upstairs and fetch Mummy's handbag and gloves') |
| 3 y | 06 | Understands a sequence of commands (*e.g.* 'First put your paints in the cupboard, then wash your hands and then lay the table') |
| 4 y | 07 | Understands instructions involving decisions (*e.g.* 'See if your coat is in the hall and, if not, then look for it in your bedroom') |
| | 08 | Cannot comprehend speech, but no attempt made to teach signs |
| | 09 | Comprehends speech |

b. Understanding of prepositions

Does S know what you mean if you use signs to indicate 'in', 'on', 'under', 'behind', or 'before', 'after'?

| | 0 | Does not understand these signs |
|---|---|---|
| 2 y | 1 | Understands some but not all |
| 3 y | 2 | Fully understands all such signs<br>(Use example of 'under the cupboard' as opposed to 'in the cupboard') |
| | 3 | Cannot comprehend speech, but no attempt made to teach signs |
| | 4 | Comprehends speech |

*(Specify on coding sheet type of sign language used)*

10. ABILITY TO USE SIGN LANGUAGE

(Relevant for those who cannot use speech.)

For items *a* and *b*, if S is known to be too visually impaired to see signs, use 9 or 99. Otherwise use the appropriate ratings. If S uses no signs in some situations but signs in others, rate him on his performance in the environment where he does use signs.

a. Development of grammar

Can S make signs that have any meaning? (Rate on level that S has attained and not just on his willingness to use signs. Do not give credit for meaningless echopraxia.)

| | 00 | No use of signs, though attempts have been made to teach some signing |
|---|---|---|
| 3 mo | 01 | Makes a few 'signs' but these have no meaning |
| 9 mo | 02 | Copies signs only when prompted |
| 1 y 4 mo | 03 | Signs the names of some people or things when asked (not a direct copy) |
| 1 y 8 mo | 04 | Spontaneously uses signs for several familiar objects for some purpose |
| 2 y | 05 | Signs phrases of two words (*e.g.* 'Want dinner', 'Have sweet') |
| 2 y–3 y | 06 | Signs some longer phrases with nouns and verbs |
| | 07 | Signs in simple spontaneous sentences |
| | 08 | Can form sentences using 'but', 'because', etc. |
| 4 y | 09 | Uses past, present and future tenses, and complex constructions |

10 Cannot speak, but no attempt made to teach signs
11 Uses speech

b. <u>Asking questions</u>
Does S ever try to ask you questions, using signs? What sorts of questions? How does he do this—what does he try to ask with his signs?

0 Does not ask questions
1 Signs for objects using a simple, learnt phrase
2 Signs a limited range of questions only (*e.g.* 'Where are we going?')
3 Asks more complex questions (*e.g.* 'How does it work?')
4 Cannot speak, but no attempt made to teach signs
5 Uses speech

3y
4y

11. <u>ABNORMALITIES OF SPEECH OR SIGN LANGUAGE</u>
Throughout this section if no speech or formal sign language at all, use 9.

a. <u>Immediate echolalia (or echopraxia)</u>
Have you ever heard S copying words that other people have just spoken, rather like a parrot? (Does he copy signs in an empty way?)

0 Marked
1 Minor
2 No problem

b. <u>Delayed echolalia or repetitive use of words or phrases (or signs)</u>
Does S tend to have certain words or phrases that he uses over and over again? Some or all of these may be words or phrases used in the past by other people, but the source may be unknown

0 Marked
1 Minor
2 No problem

c. <u>Reversal of pronouns</u>
Does S use words like 'you' and 'I'? Does he use them correctly? Does he always or usually call himself 'you', 'he' or his own name, because he is using phrases copied from other people without modification (*e.g.* 'Do you want a biscuit?' = 'I want a biscuit'; 'John had better put on his coat' = 'I must put on my coat')? (If S uses no personal pronouns, rate 9.)

0 Marked
1 Minor
2 No problem

d. <u>Idiosyncratic use of words or phrases (or signs)</u>
Does S use words or phrases whlch have a special meaning peculiar to himself, *e.g.* 'Tram-bus' meaning a single deck bus, 'Go on green riding' meaning he wants to play on the swings in the park? (The origins may or may not be known.)

0 Marked
1 Minor
2 No problem

e. <u>Repetitive speech</u>
(To be distinguished from pure echolalia which is not part of a conversation.) Does S tend to talk to you about the same things over and over again? [Rate item only if S has enough speech (or signs) to hold a 'conversation', otherwise use 9.]

0 Repetitive speech very marked (*e.g.* repeats some questions over and over again and does not seem to take in answer. Always reverts to same topic of conversation regardless of context. Frequently makes irrelevant remarks which recur in conversations. May talk incessantly about abstruse subjects. The above occurs in a conversational context)
1 Conversation partly repetitive, partly varied and appropriate
2 Minimal or no problems

f. Muddling of sequence of words and phrases
Does S ever get words in the wrong order (*e.g.* 'put salt it on', 'shake-milk', 'take park to doggy')? (Rate only if S has phrases or sentences, otherwise use 9.)

0 Marked
1 Minor
2 No problem

g. Tone of voice
Does his voice have normal changes in tone and pitch or does it always sound the same? (Voice is flat or monotonous, or all phrases have exactly the same intonation as each other. The voice may sound 'mechanical'.) (Rate only if S has spoken phrases of two words or more; otherwise use 9.)

0 Marked
1 Minor
2 No problem

12. COMPREHENSION OF NONVERBAL COMMUNICATION
This section refers to understanding of spontaneous gestures common to people sharing the same culture. The understanding of formal sign language is rated under Section 9. Throughout this section, if S is too visually impaired to see gestures, use 9.

a. Understanding of gesture and miming
How much does S understand gestures?

0 No understanding of gesture
3 mo    1 Understands concrete demonstration (*e.g.* holding up coat to show it is time for a walk or touching a chair to ask him to sit down). (Normal child at 3 mo knows when it is bathtime, etc.)
1 y     2 Understands pointing, beckoning
By 2 y  3 Clearly understands nodding and shaking of the head to mean yes and no
        4 Understands more complex social gestures (*e.g.* shaking fist to mean anger or 'thumbs-up' sign to mean things are going well)

b. Understanding of facial expressions
How much can you control his behaviour by your facial expression without saying anything?

0 No understanding of facial expression
By 2 y  1 Behaviour can be controlled by exaggerated expressions
By 3 y  2 Behaviour can be controlled by small changes of facial expression (including a slight frown or lift of an eyebrow)

13. ABILITY TO USE NONVERBAL COMMUNICATION
Throughout this section, if S is too visually impaired to see gestures, or too physically handicapped to make movements, use 9.

a. Copying gesture
Can S copy any movements or actions that you show him?

278

| 9 mo | 0 | Cannot copy other people's movements (*e.g.* clapping, waving, a dance step, a miming game). Does not learn even if limbs are moved for him |
|---|---|---|
| | 1 | Cannot copy movements but can learn if limbs are moved for him |
| | 2 | Can copy simple movements (*e.g.* clapping, waving bye-bye) but not complicated ones |
| | 3 | Copies many different movements (*e.g.* in miming games) but tends to be stiff, awkward or inaccurate |
| 1 y 6 mo–2 y | 4 | Can copy many movements well (singing games with hand movements, dance steps) |
| 3 y 9 mo | 5 | Can act in plays or do a little song and dance with appropriate movements and facial expression, etc. Does actions convincingly (memory of actions is needed for this) |

b. Use of symbolic gesture (with or without speech)
Does S use any gestures like pointing or nodding his head to mean 'Yes'? and other body language with specific meaning?

0 Never nods to mean 'Yes' or shakes head to mean 'No' or uses 'thumbs up' sign, pretends to shake fist, etc.

(Shakes head by 10 mo; nodding by 2 y)

1 Sometimes uses such gestures and/or uses only a limited number, and/or makes markedly limited movements when gesturing

2 Uses the normal range and frequency of these gestures clearly, and knows their meaning

c. Use of facial expression
Can you tell how S is feeling from the expression on his face?

0 Face almost expressionless

1 Has some facial expressions

2 Clear and frequent changes in facial expression (compare with normal people of same age, *e.g.* can look surprised, puzzled, scorn-ful as well as happy and miserable)

d. Gesture as a substitute for speech
How well can S communicate in gesture? [This can be rated (a) for subjects who *cannot* express themselves in speech and (b) for subjects who *can* speak. For the latter, ask about behaviour when trying to converse with someone who cannot understand, or for communicating at a distance, etc. Vary the question depending on the subject's level of speech.]

0 No gesture at all

1 Shows needs by concrete demonstration (*e.g.* takes food from cupboard, leads people by hand)

9 mo 2 Points by touching the object concerned

1 y 3 Points to objects from a distance

2 y–3 y (4 Shows needs by simple gestures (*e.g.* points to teapot and then cup, or points to ( mother's handbag, then to ice-cream van)

(5 Shows need by miming (*e.g.* pretends to drink if thirsty)

N.B. This question refers to *spontaneous* gestures common to people sharing the same culture. The use of formal sign language is rated under Section 10.

14. INTEREST IN COMMUNICATION (Verbal and non-verbal)
Throughout this section, if S does not communicate for any reason, use 0.

a. Usual method of obtaining needs
If S wants something, such as a drink, how does he let you know? (Rate on S's preference, not his capability.)

279

|     | 0 | Never communicates or seems to want anything |
| --- | --- | --- |
|     | 1 | Screams or makes noises without specifically indicating his needs |
|     | 2 | Mostly gets what he wants for himself |
|     | 3 | Takes you by the hand and leads you to the object |
| 1 y | 4 | Points to the object |
|     | 5 | Gestures or mimes (not a formal sign language) |
|     | 6 | Tries to say the words, and gestures at the same time |
|     | 7 | Makes requests in words |
|     | 8 | Makes requests in formal sign language |

b. Initiation of communication

Does S talk to or communlcate in any way with other people (even if this is in a one-sided, egocentric manner)?

0 Never communicates in speech, or babbling, gurgling, facial expression, gesture, mime, eye contact, etc.
1 Communicates needs only
2 Minimal response if others initiate
3 Willing response if others initiate communication
4 Sometimes initiates communication
5 Frequently initiates communication with parents/staff, but not peers
6 Shy in a group with strangers, etc., but initiates communication when at ease with peer group. (N.B. differentiate from 4)
7 Easily initiates communication with peer group

c. Sharing of interests

Does S like to point things out to you so that you can share the interesting experience? The emphasis here is on *sharing* interests.

|     | 0 | No attempt to communicate with others |
| --- | --- | --- |
| 7 mo–8 mo | 1 | Will look when attention is drawn to things in immediate environment |
| 9 mo–1 y | 2 | Spontaneously shares interest with other people in-a simple way (*e.g.* shows he wants to be talked to, points things out to others for interest, brings toys, etc. to show) |
| 3 y 2 mo | 3 | Gives narrative accounts of his experiences spontaneously, reasonably coherently and with detail (speech or gesture or mime or signs) |

15. EDUCATIONAL ACHIEVEMENTS

Throughout this section, if S cannot perform skills for any reason, use 0.

a. Visuospatial skills

Does S play with rattles, bricks, etc.? Can he make jigsaw puzzles? Can he do fitting and assembly tasks?

|     | 00 | Does not hold objects in hands |
| --- | --- | --- |
| 3 mo | 01 | Holds objects in hands—no exploration of them |
| 5 mo | 02 | Examines objects for simple sensations (tastes, smells, strokes, etc.) |
| 9 mo–10 mo | 03 | Handles and rattles and bangs objects on floor, etc. |
| 1 y | 04 | Rolls appropriate baby toys along the floor |
| 1 y 6 mo | 05 | Builds tower of 2–5 bricks if shown how to do this |
| 2 y | 06 | Builds towers of 6 bricks or more |
| 2 y–2 y 9 mo | 07 | Can arrange objects in order of size, *e.g.* nest of cubes |
| 3 y 6 mo | 08 | Can make a simple jigsaw puzzle of 10 or more pieces, or simple constructional toy, or perform a simple assembly task |
| 5 y+ | 09 | Can make complicated constructional toys or can assemble a complex object |

b. Use of scissors
Can S use scissors?

0 Cannot cut with scissors
2 y   1 Can with help
3 y   2 Can without help

c. Three-dimensional modelling
Does S play with plasticine, or with any toys meant for making models, such as Meccano, or make objects in pottery?

0 None
1 Plays with clay, Lego, etc., but makes no shapes
2 y 6 mo–3 y   2 Tries to make shapes—results unrecognizable
4 y   3 Makes recognizable shapes

d. Drawing—executive skill
Can S use a pencil? Does he try to draw pictures?

0 Does not use pencil at all
1 Makes a few marks on paper
1 y 3 mo–   2 Scribbles all over the paper, does not break point or tear paper
1 y 8 mo
3 y   3 Makes simple patterns—circle or square
3 y   4 Tries to draw objects—unrecognizable
4 y   5 Draws recognizable objects, but proportions are peculiar
5 y+   6 Draws recognizable objects with fairly good proportions

e. Drawing—content
What kinds of things does S draw?

0 No content
2 y+   1 Individual objects
6 y+   2 Individual objects against background
8 y+   3 Action scene, involving movement or interaction between objects or people

f. Painting
Does S use brushes and paints?

0 None
1 y   1 Finger paints
1 y 3 mo   2 Marks with brush, one colour
3 Uses more than one colour
3 y   4 Attempts picture, inappropriate colours
5 y   5 Attempts picture, appropriate colours

g. Colouring inside lines
Can S colour inside guide lines?

0 Does not use pencil or paints
1 y   1 Scribbles over paper
3 y–4 y   2 Tries to keep inside lines but fails
5 y   3 Can keep inside lines

h. Interest in picture books
Does S like pictures or picture books?

0 Never looks at picture books
1 y 3 mo   1 Looks at picture books but turns pages over very fast—soon loses interest (or will look at one picture but will not turn pages in a book)
2 Looks at picture books, turning pages slowly for a minute or two
1 y 6 mo–2 y   3 Looks at picture books, turning pages slowly, for longer than two minutes

i. Understanding of pictures
Does S point out things he sees in pictures?

0 Does not point out objects or scenes
1y 6mo 1 Picks out individual elements (*e.g.* horse, cow, pig, etc.)
2y–2y 6mo 2 Recognizes nature of whole scene (e.g. farmyard)

j. Interest in mirror-images
Does S look in a mirror? Does he know himself?

0 Does not recognize himself in a mirror
1 Some brief interest in his own mirror-image
2y 2 Obviously recognizes himself in a mirror
2y+ 3 Spontaneously uses a mirror to check on his own appearance

k. Response to photographs
Does S recognize anyone in a photograph?

0 Does not recognize himself or others in photographs
1y 6mo–2y 1 Recognizes himself and/or others in photographs

l. Reading
Can S read any words?

0 Has no understanding of written words
3y 6mo–4y 1 Can recognize own name
2 Can match words to pictures
4y–5y 3 Can recognize up to 10 familiar words
5y–6y 4 Can read simple first reading books and comprehend them (possibly made up by teacher)
7y+ 5 Can read books for children aged 7+ and comprehend them
8y 7mo 6 Reads on own initiative

m. Writing
Can S write any letters or words?

0 Cannot write any letters of the alphabet
4y 1 Can write some letters by copying
4y 6mo 2 Can write simple words by copying
5y 3 Can write some letters without copying
5y 3mo 4 Can write a few simple words without copying
6y 5 Can write 12 or more words without copying—correct spelling
9y 8mo 6 Can write a short letter on own initiative

n. Numbers
Can S count? Does he understand what numbers mean?

0 Has no understanding of numbers
3y 1 Can count to 2 (knows meaning)
4y 2 Has one-to-one correspondence (*e.g.* can give 2 cups, 3 pencils, etc.)
5y 6mo 3 Can classify objects using a single numerical attribute (*e.g.* can match 3 cats with 3 dogs, 4 cups with 4 mice, etc.)
5y–7y (4 Has concept of numbers up to 10 (*e.g.* can say how many pencils there are when
( shown pencils all bunched together—does not reply 'one')
(5 Can do simple addition
(6 Has the concept of numbers up to 30
(7 Can do simple addition and subtraction

o. Money
Does S know money is needed to buy things?

|          | 0 | Has no idea of the value of money |
| 3 y 6 mo | 1 | Has some idea that money is needed to buy things |
| 6 y–7 y  | 2 | Can identify coinage |

p. Days, months, years
   Does S know the names of any of the days of the week?

|      | 0 | Has no idea of days, months, years |
| 6 y  | 1 | Can name days of week with some understanding |
| 7 y  | 2 | Can name months of the year with some understanding or can give dates correctly |

q. Telling the time by the clock
   Can S tell the hours on the clock?

|      | 0 | Has no idea of time of day |
| 5 y  | 1 | Can tell hours and half hours on the clock |
| 7 y  | 2 | Can tell time by clock fairly well (quarter hours at least) |

r. Understanding of time
   Does S have any idea about time?

|         | 0 | Understands nothing outside his own immediate experience (if that) |
| 2 y     | 1 | Understands if told in simple terms year of events occurring on same day (*e.g.* 'We are going to the park after dinner'). (If S has no understanding of the future he may think he is going for a ride in a car at once if told he is going out tomorrow) |
| 3 y–4 y | 2 | Understands if told of familiar events occurring next day or later (*e.g.* 'We will visit Granny next week') |

16. ENTERTAINMENTS

a. Television, films, plays, etc.
   Does S enjoy watching TV? (If S is too visually impaired to see TV, use 9.)

|         | 0 | No interest in TV |
|         | 1 | Likes simple items such as a car chase, sport, a moving train, picture of water, etc.—is interested in the movement, not the meaning |
| 3 y–4 y | 2 | Enjoys cartoons, musicals, simple shows for children |
|         | 3 | Can follow a very simple story for children on TV |
| 5 y     | 4 | Can follow a fairly complicated story on TV |

b. Stories read out loud
   Does S enjoy listening to stories? (Include stories or plays heard on the radio.)

|          | 0 | No interest in stories |
|          | 1 | Listens but does not really understand the story |
| 1 y 6 mo | 2 | Understands simple narration of his own recent experiences |
| 2 y      | 3 | Can follow a simple story adapted to his level |
| 4 y–5 y  | 4 | Can follow a new story read from a book or a radio play |

17. IMAGINATIVE ACTIVITIES

a. Level of play and imaginative activities
   Does S have any pretend play or other imaginative activities? (If S has no play or other imaginative activities for any reason, use 0. If he is too old for pretend play, ask about past behaviour. Also, ask about more adult imaginative activities such as the ability to make up stories, to join in with fantasies such as 'What would happen if creatures from outer space landed on earth', etc. Adapt ratings appropriately.)

|          | 0 | No play with model toys (no interest in the function of trains, cars and dolls, although he may handle them in the same way as any other objects) |
| 1y–<br>1y 6mo | 1 | Plays with real household equipment using it for its real purpose—no interest in miniatures (*e.g.* sweeps with real broom, digs with real spade) |
| 1y 3mo–<br>1y 6mo | 2 | Holds doll, toy animals as if real, at least some of the time (hugs and kisses) |
| 1y 9mo | 3 | Goes through simple sequences of actions with toys (*e.g.* pushes toy trains and cars along floor as if real, and makes appropriate noises, or tucks doll in bed) |
|          | 4 | Will pour out and give pretend cup of tea to other person *spontaneously*. (If S only drinks from cup himself, rate 3) |
| 2y 6mo | 5 | Goes through longer sequences of actions with toys, *e.g.* has a doll's tea party, sets up a garage, road and road bridges for play with toy cars |
| 3y | 6 | Plays simple make-believe games with other children |
| 4y | 7 | Pretends to be, *e.g.*, a cowboy or nurse, using special dressing-up clothes, with other children and with awareness of the dramatic role, not just putting on clothes, not just copying |
| 8y 3mo | 8 | Has imaginative play. Has been through stage of believing in Father Christmas, but now knows he doesn't exist |

b. Spontaneity of play or other imaginative activities
Does S invent pretend play or other imaginative activities for himself or does he just copy other people's activities with no ideas of his own? (If S has no pretend play or other imaginative activities, use 9. Refer to answer already given to item *a* above.)

0 All imaginative activities are copied
1 Some copying, some inventive
2 Most are spontaneous and inventive (apart from normal willingness to join in with suggestions from others at appropriate times)

(N.B. From 12 months to 18 months a normal child copies play, but elaboration soon occurs.)

18. ABNORMAL IMAGINATIVE ACTIVITIES
Throughout this section, if S has no imaginative activities, use 9. (Refer to previous section, 17*a*.)

a. Stereotypic play or other symbolic activities
If S does have some relevant activities, does he play in many different ways (or draw, invent stories, etc.) or does he have just a few very special interests only, such as loading and unloading a toy truck, continually ironing, playing at Batman, talking about science fiction, etc. For adults, adapt questions to suit age and level of function.

0 Imaginative activities confined to making models or drawings of same object(s). Does not play with models. No action in, or stories told about drawings (*e.g.* draws series of identical dolls, cars, etc.)
1 Has imaginative activities but limited to one or two themes which recur over and over again (*e.g.* putting a doll to bed, loading and unloading a truck, acting Batman, drawing, modelling and acting out symbolic but repetitive themes such as lively scenes of aeroplanes crashing with much action and detail). These activities are not modified by suggestions from others. They do not develop in complexity nor incorporate new themes—though one theme may be replaced by another after a time (*e.g.* from Batman to Bionic Man)
2 Minor problems—a bit repetitive but some flexibility
3 Has imaginative activities appropriate for mental age

b. Fantasies

Does S talk about daydreams and fantasies? (Ask only if S has enough speech and symbolic activity.)

0 Constant preoccupation with fantasy interfering with activities
1 Present, but not interfering with activities
2 Minor or absent—normal for age

19. EYE CONTACT

Throughout this section if S is too visually impaired to make eye contact, use 9. If S does not look at people in authority but has good eye contact with his companions, rate on the latter. If he has been taught to look at certain specific people, but has poor eye contact with others, especially his age peers, rate on the latter.

a. Amount of eye contact

How easy is it to get S to look at you? Does he make eye contact with his everyday companions, or people he meets occasionally? Does he make or break eye contact in a way that seems easy and normal?

0 Actively avoids eye contact—turns whole body, head or eyes away if others try to make contact
1 Usually avoids, or looks past or through others, but occasionally makes contact in a brief glance
2 Has a blank, unfocused stare, but no active avoidance of eye contact
3 Makes eye contact, but inappropriately. May stare hard and long, hold another person's head to fix their gaze, but also may not make eye contact at socially appropriate times, *e.g.* on first meeting
4 Eye contact appropriate

b. Social use of eye contact

Does S try to give you messages with his eyes?

0 Does not use eye contact to help social interaction, convey information, etc. Does not look when strangers enter a room. (This should be differentiated from the person with normal eye contact who *sometimes* does not look up because of total absorption in activities)
1 Looks at familiar people, for reassurance that actions are correct, or to check if being observed prior to some forbidden act. Does not usually look at strangers entering a room
2 Uses eye contact to ask for help or invite play, cuddling, etc.
3 Uses eye contact to share a joke or convey subtle social meanings—use this code only if there is a real sharing of understanding on a symbolic, abstract level

20. SOCIAL RESPONSIVENESS

Throughout this section if S is socially unresponsive for any reason, use 0.

a. Spontaneous show of affection

Is S affectionate? Does he show he wants to be held or cuddled? (Do not rate physical contact without social recognition.)

0 Never shows affection to others spontaneously
1 Sometimes shows affection spontaneously
2 Frequently shows affection spontaneously (even if only to parents/staff).

(N.B. Rate in relation to mental age, *e.g.* an older child or adult may no longer show physical affection, but may show feelings in other ways.)

b. Response to age peers—ability to make friendships

How does S react to other companions of his own age? Does he like having them around?

285

| | | |
|---|---|---|
| –6 mo | 0 | No interest in age peers (include those who actively withdraw from contact, or show, in any way, dislike or fear of others, which is not just due to shyness) |
| 6 mo | 1 | Accepts or enjoys presence of age peers but does not join in activities (not just due to shyness) |
| 2 y | 2 | Accepts or enjoys presence of age peers and plays or carries out other activities in parallel, though does not interact with the group |
| 3 y | 3 | Interacts (actively or passively), at least in a small group, but has no special friend |
| 4 y | 4 | Seems to prefer some people to others, but has no special friend |
| 5 y+ | 5 | Makes friendships, even if soon broken |

(N.B. Rate on enjoyment of company of age peers, not simply willingness to join in activities.)

21. SOCIAL PLAY

Throughout this section, if S does not play for any reason, use 0. Physically handicapped people should be rated on the level of their actual performance.

a. Level of social play

What sort of games will S play—even if he has to be pushed to join in?

| | | |
|---|---|---|
| | 0 | No play at all |
| | 1 | Likes tickling, romping games |
| 9 mo | 2 | Plays 'peep-bo' and similar baby games |
| 2 y+ | 3 | Plays very simple games of chasing, etc. |
| 3 y 3 mo | 4 | Joins in simple group games ('Nuts in May', etc.) |
| 5 y 2 mo | 5 | Plays simple competitive games (*e.g.* racing, simple football, etc.) |
| 5 y 8 mo | 6 | Plays simple table games with others and understands rules and aims (ludo, dominoes, etc.) |
| 8 y 3 mo | 7 | Cooperative play in a group (*e.g.* organized football, complex dramatic play, etc.) |

b. Willingness to join in leisure activities of age peers

Is S happy to join in games or other leisure activities with his age peers? Does he have to be pushed into them?

| | | |
|---|---|---|
| | 0 | Does not join in with age peers |
| | 1 | Will join in if parent/staff insists and supervises |
| | 2 | Will join in, and continue to engage, if others initiate. Takes passive role |
| 3 y | 3 | Shy about joining in, but joins in actively with companions he knows well |
| | 4 | Joins in actively, appropriately for mental age |

(N.B. Subject's own activities should not be considered in above rating, *e.g.* if he initiates a game of chasing but will not join with others in different games, rate 0 and make note.)

22. SOCIAL INTERACTION

All subjects can be rated.

a. Quality of social interaction

The following rating is made on the basis of the information obtained from the interview so far, plus any further questioning that may be needed, and *direct observation* of the subject. Rate on behaviour within own social group, not with staff or parents or well-known caregivers. This section is not strictly a hierarchy of development. Give S the rating which most nearly describes him, taking into account all aspects of his social behaviour. Rate on the usual, not on the 'best' behaviour.

0 Does not interact—aloof and indifferent

1 Interacts to obtain needs, otherwise indifferent

2 Responds to (and may initiate) *physical* contact only—including 'rough and tumble' games, chasing, cuddling, etc.

3 Generally does not initiate, but responds to *social* (not just physical) contact, if others, including age peers, make approaches. Joins in passively, *e.g.* as baby in game of mothers and fathers, or, for adults, in adult social situations. Tries to copy, but with little understanding. Shows some pleasure in passive role (unlike Groups 0, 1, 2, who move away once physical needs are satisfied)

4 Makes *social* approaches actively, but these are usually inappropriate, naive, peculiar, or bizarre—'one sided'. The behaviour is not modified according to needs, interests and responses of person approached

5 Shy, but social contacts appropriate for mental age with well-known people, including age peers. Also use for children who refuse to talk to adults, but interact with other children. For older children and adults, this rating can be used for those who are not gregarious, but who can interact appropriately with people they like. Also use for those who have periods of social withdrawal due to psychiatric illness or moodiness, but who interact normally between

6 Social contacts appropriate for mental age with children and adults. Looks up with interest and smiles when approached. Responds to the ideas and interests of people of similar mental age and contributes to the interaction. Non-mobile people without speech can show social interest by means of eye contact and 'eye pointing'

23. ABNORMAL RESPONSE TO SOUNDS

Throughout this section, if S is totally deaf, use 9.

a. Distress caused by sounds

Do any sounds upset S (*e.g.* vacuum cleaner, aeroplane, fire engines, road drills, etc.)? Is he distressed by sounds that don't affect others?

0 Marked

1 Minor

2 No problem

b. Fascination with sounds

Does S have an unusual interest in some sounds? (not music) (*e.g.* friction drive cars, bells, water hissing in pipes, etc.)? Does he spend much time listening to these sounds?

0 Marked

1 Minor

2 No problem

c. Other

Does S show any other unusual responses to sounds (*e.g.* totally ignores loud sounds but reacts to some that are almost inaudible to other people)? *(Specify on coding sheet)*

0 Marked

1 Minor

2 No problem

24. ABNORMAL RESPONSE TO VISUAL STIMULI

For items *a* and *b*, if S is too visually impaired to see anything, use 9, but partially sighted subjects may have these problems to a marked degree.)

a. Bright lights and shiny objects
Is S unusually interested in shiny things (*e.g.* silver paper, tinsel, patches of sunlight, or street lights at night)?

0 Marked
1 Minor
2 No problem

b. Interest in watching things spin
Does S get unusually excited if he sees things spinning (*e.g.* a spinning top, wheels of toy cars, spin drier, record, etc.)?

0 Marked
1 Minor
2 No problem

For items *c* and *d*, if S is too visually impaired to see anything, use 9, but partially sighted people may have these problems to a marked degree. If S is too physically handicapped to use his hands, use 9.

c. Twisting or turning hands or objects near eyes
Does S twist or flick his hands or objects near his eyes?

0 Marked
1 Minor
2 No problem

d. Interest in studying angles or objects
Does S like to look at objects from many different angles for no obvious reason? (Demonstrate, for example, with a small cube.)

0 Marked
1 Minor
2 No problem

e. Other
Does S have any other unusual responses to visual stimuli (*e.g.* frequently makes holes in pieces of paper and looks through them; makes tears come into his eyes to obtain unusual visual effect)? (*Specify on coding sheet*)

0 Marked
1 Minor
2 No problem

25. ABNORMAL PROXIMAL SENSORY STIMULATION
Throughout this section if S is too physically handicapped to carry out these activities, use 9, but make a rating if possible.

a Mouthing of objects
Does S tend to put everything into his mouth?

0 Marked
1 Minor
1 y 6 mo    2 No problem

b. Smelling objects or people
Does S tend to explore objects or people by smelling them?

0 Marked
1 Minor
2 No problem

c. Touching objects

Does S have an unusual interest in the feel of surfaces (*e.g.* fur coats, nylon stockings, hair, smooth plastic)?

0 Marked
1 Minor
2 No problem

d. Scratching and tapping surfaces

Does S scratch or tap on different surfaces, apparently in order to *feel* the sensation?

0 Marked
1 Minor
2 No problem

e. Repetitive destructive activities

Does S tear or break things in an aimless repetitive way (*e.g.* tears all paper into small pieces, picks at wallpaper, removes all loose parts from toys, etc.)?

0 Marked
1 Minor
2 No problem

f. Repetitive, aimless manipulation of objects (not near eyes)

Does S flick things like pieces of string, sticks, etc.? Does he tap two objects together, roll pieces of cotton in his fingers, push toy cars to and fro without any real pretend play, etc.? (If S makes more elaborate, but still repetitive use of objects, code under 27*b*.)

0 Marked
1 Minor
2 No problem

g. Self-injury

Does S bite or scratch or cut himself or push objects into his nose or ears producing injury if not prevented?

0 Marked
1 Minor
2 No problem

h. Self-stimulation without injury

Does S have any habits like prodding his eye, regurgitating food to rechew it, self-induced vomiting, tapping his chin, grinding his teeth, etc.?

0 Marked
1 Minor
2 No problem

i. Other

Does S have any other activities which appear to provide repetitive sensory stimulation, not classified elsewhere (*e.g.* making repetitive noises)? *(Specify on coding sheet)*

0 Marked
1 Minor
2 No problem

26. ABNORMAL BODILY MOVEMENTS

Throughout this section, if S is too physically handicapped to carry out these activities, use 9, but make a rating if possible.

289

a. Jumping with excitement
   Does S jump up and down with excitement, more than his normal age peers?

0 Marked
1 Minor
2 No problem

b. Unusual movements of hands or arms
   Does S flap his hands or arms when he gets excited?

0 Marked
1 Minor
2 No problem

c. Spinning
   Does S like spinning himself round or running round in circles, more than his normal age peers?

0 Marked
1 Minor
2 No problem

d. Rocking (sitting)
   Does S rock himself when sitting down?

0 Marked
1 Minor
2 No problem

e. Rocking (standing up)
   Does S rock himself when standing up?

0 Marked
1 Minor
2 No problem

f. Tip-toe walking
   Does S walk on tip-toe?

0 Marked
1 Minor
2 No problem

g. Aimless movement
   Does S move around aimlessly, wandering about without any real purpose?

0 Marked
1 Minor
2 No problem

h. Other
   Does S have any other abnormal bodily movement not classified in this section?
   *(Specify on coding sheet)*

0 Marked
1 Minor
2 No problem

27. ROUTINES AND RESISTANCE TO CHANGE
    Throughout this section, if S is too physically handicapped to carry out any of these activities, use 9, but make a rating if possible.

a. Dislike of change in the normal routine
Is S abnormally distressed if everyday routines are changed (*e.g.* sequence of dressing, sitting on same chair at table, route taken to familiar places, arrangement of ornaments or furniture)?

0 Marked
1 Minor
2 No problem

b. Routines invented by the child (involving sequences of actions)
Does S have some special routines of his own (*e.g.* makes lines of all kinds of objects, tapping on chair before sitting down, standing up and turning round several times during each meal, etc.)?

0 Marked
1 Minor
2 No problem

c. Food fads
Does S have very unusual food fads (*e.g.* will eat only Marmite sandwiches)?

0 Marked S
1 Minor
2 No problem

d. Clinging to objects
Does S have any special objects he likes to carry around with him? Does he get very upset if he loses them?

0 Marked
1 Minor
2 No problem

e. Interest in special objects or parts of objects
Is S fascinated by one type of object, *e.g.* light switches, church steeples, people's teeth, etc?

0 Marked
1 Minor
2 No problem

f. Special fears
Is S frightened of anything? Does he mind the dark, big dogs, trains, etc? Do these fears interfere with everyday activities?

0 Marked
1 Minor
2 No problem

(N.B. Rate as marked only if the fear is unusually intense, persistent, and S cannot be comforted or reassured, and it interferes with everyday activities.)

28. BEHAVIOUR PROBLEMS WITH LIMITED OR NO SOCIAL AWARENESS
Throughout this section all subjects can be rated.

a. Wandering
Does S run away or wander, unless constantly supervised?

0 Marked
1 Minor
2 No problem

b. Destructiveness
Does S tear books, wallpaper, spoil furniture, own clothing, etc., unless constantly supervised?

0 Marked
1 Minor
2 No problem

c. Noisiness
Does S frequently scream or shout or make other loud noises (not crying or moaning)?

0 Marked
1 Minor
2 No problem

d. Temper tantrums
Does S frequently have temper tantrums?

0 Marked
1 Minor
2 No problem

e. Aggressive behaviour
Is S frequently aggressive toward others (including spitting at them)?

0 Marked
1 Minor
2 No problem

[N.B. If S is aware of the social implications of his actions (*e.g.* tries to justify himself if scolded) do not rate here, but rate under Section 29a, Difficulties with other people.]

f. Hyperactivity
Does S never sit still (even when interested in food, TV, etc.)?

0 Marked
1 Minor
2 No problem

g. Behaviour in public places
Is S too difficult to take out because of marked problems in public places (*e.g.* grabs things in shops, speaks loudly and tactlessly, screams, takes off clothes, etc.)?

0 Marked
1 Minor
2 No problem

h. Lack of cooperation
Does S strongly resist attempts to make him join in, learn new things, or to change his behaviour—screams, temper tantrums, scratches, bites, kicks if these are tried, or else passively resists?

0 Marked
1 Minor
2 No problem

i. Crying and moaning
Does S cry or moan a great deal, appearing miserable most of the time, with no known cause?

0 Marked
1 Minor
2 No problem

j. <u>Difficult or objectionable personal habits</u>
Does S spit, smear, make himself vomit, hoard rubbish, eat rubbish,
continuously eat or drink, have inappropriate swearing, inappropriate sexual
behaviour without social awareness, etc?

0 Marked
1 Minor
2 No problem

k. <u>Scatters or throws objects around</u>
Does S create chaos aimlessly?

0 Marked
1 Minor
2 No problem

l. <u>Other behaviour problems</u>
Does S have any other behaviour problems with limited or no social awareness?
*(Specify on coding sheet)*

0 Marked
1 Minor
2 No problem

(N.B. If any of the problems in this section are due to repetitive behaviour, rate
here and also rate under the appropriate item in Section 23, 24, 25, 26 or 27.)

29. <u>BEHAVIOUR PROBLEMS WITH SOCIAL AWARENESS</u>
Throughout this section all subjects can be rated.

a. <u>Difficulties with other people</u>
Does S frequently tease, bully, refuse to take turns, make trouble, etc.? (This can
include physical aggression with full social awareness.)

0 Marked
1 Minor
2 No problem

b. <u>Rebellious behaviour</u>
Is S frequently rebellious, awkward or cheeky?

0 Marked
1 Minor
2 No problem

c. <u>Pestering for attention</u>
Does S frequently pester for attention?

0 Marked
1 Minor
2 No problem

d. <u>Lying, cheating, stealing</u>
Does S lie, cheat or steal, or show other delinquent behaviour, at any
opportunity?

0 Marked
1 Minor
2 No problem

e. Other behaviour problems
Does S show any other behaviour problems with social awareness that cannot be classified under items a, b, c or d? *(Specify on coding sheet)*
0  Marked
1  Minor
2  No problem

30. SLEEPING PROBLEMS
This question should be asked only if informant is with S at night or a night report is written. All subjects can be rated if information is available.

a. Night sedation
Does S have any tablets or other medicine at night? Is this to help him sleep?
0  On sedation every night
1  Occasional
2  None

b. Disturbance of sleep
Does S cause disturbance to others because of waking in night, restlessness, noisiness, or because late in going to sleep or waking very early in the morning? (If S is on night sedation, rate on his behaviour when the medication has been given.)
0  Marked
1  Minor
2  No problem

31. PRACTICAL SKILLS
Throughout this section, if S cannot perform for any reason, use 0.

a. Tidying, cleaning, etc.
Can S give you any help with cleaning and tidying?

|  |  |  |
|---|---|---|
| | 0 | Does not take part in any domestic task |
| 1 y 9 mo | 1 | Helps a little but with no skill (*e.g.* may carry cup to kitchen with close super-vision) |
| 2 y | 2 | Does simple, immediate tasks (*e.g.* carrying things, holding things on request, putting something on shelf) |
| 3 y | 3 | Fetches or carries to and from another room, or takes a simple message to someone in another room |
| 3 y 7 mo | 4 | Gives some help with tasks involving a sequence of actions (*e.g.* clearing or laying table, dusting, tidying up) |
| 8 y 6 mo | 5 | Helps regularly in completing tasks (as in 4) without need for supervision |
| 10 y 11 mo | 6 | Does some tasks on own initiative for payment |
| 14 y 8 mo | 7 | Is responsible for some routine domestic task (*e.g.* cleaning car, weeding garden) |

b. Cookery, woodwork, etc.
Can S help with cooking, do any sewing, woodwork, etc.?

|  |  |  |
|---|---|---|
| | 0 | Does not take part in any creative work |
| 1 y 6 mo | 1 | Gives minimal help with cooking, woodwork, etc., under close supervision (*e.g.* stirs cake mix, breaks up jelly cubes, hammers nail in wood) |
| 3 y 6 mo–4 y | 2 | Can complete a small task under close supervision (*e.g.* make a jelly, mix pastry, sew a hem, sandpaper wood) |
| 8 y 6 mo | 3 | Can complete such small tasks with minimal or no supervision |
| 11 y 3 mo | 4 | Can perform and complete more complex creative tasks (*e.g.* cook bacon and eggs, sew a kettle holder, simple woodwork) |

c. <u>Any special skill(s)</u>
Is there anything S is especially good at? (Rate this on all the information obtained throughout the interview. There is no need to ask this question if S is clearly profoundly handicapped in all areas, *or* if it is already clear that he does have some outstanding skill.) *(Specify on coding sheet)*

0 No unusual skill
1 Has some special skill which is well above general level of functioning

32. <u>INITIATIVE AND PERSEVERANCE</u>

a. <u>Acquisition of objects</u>
How does S try to get things for himself? (If S cannot perform for any reason, use 0.)

|         |   |                                                                                                                          |
|---------|---|--------------------------------------------------------------------------------------------------------------------------|
|         | 0 | Does not try to pick up objects                                                                                          |
| 3 mo+   | 1 | Grasps objects within arm's length                                                                                       |
| 4 mo+   | 2 | Reaches for objects nearby but beyond arm's length                                                                       |
| 1 y     | 3 | Looks for objects that are out of sight, covered or hidden                                                               |
| 1 y 9 mo| 4 | Some ability to overcome obstacles in order to acquire objects opens doors, stands on chair to reach up high, uses stick to bring objects nearer) |
| 3 y–4 y | 5 | Good ability to overcome obstacles. Can acquire most objects that he wants (unbolts doors, uses keys, etc.)              |

b. <u>Spontaneous initiation of activities</u>
If S is left on his own, will he find something to do for himself? If S cannot perform for any reason use 0.

0 No spontaneous activities
1 Occasionally initiates activities
2 Frequently initiates activities (even if these are repetitive in nature)

c. <u>Nature of chosen activity</u>
If S does find something to do, is his activity varied and constructive or does he just repeat the same thing over and over? (If S does not find any activity, use 9.)

0 Mostly or always repetitive
1 Sometimes repetitive, sometimes varied
2 Mostly or always varied.

d. <u>Attention span</u> (for activities chosen or known to be enjoyed by S)
If S does find or readily accept something to do to occupy himself, how long will he remain occupied without needing your attention? (Rate activity involving objects even if repetitive, but do not count body rocking, hand-twisting or similar self-directed activities. If, for any reason, S has no self-chosen or readily accepted activity, use 0.)

|       |   |                                                                              |
|-------|---|------------------------------------------------------------------------------|
|       | 0 | No self-chosen activities with objects                                       |
|       | 1 | Engages in such activities for less than 15 minutes and then needs attention |
| 5 mo  | 2 | Engages in such activities for 15 minutes or more                            |

e. <u>Attention span</u> (for tasks given by others)
If you give S something to do will he persevere with it by himself or do you have to help him and supervise him? (If, for any reason, S makes no attempt to carry out any task, use 0.)

0 No attempt to carry out task
1 Task attempted with adult supervision (one to one)
2 Task completed with minimal supervision
3 Task completed with no supervision

33. LEVEL OF INDEPENDENCE
Throughout this section, all subjects can be rated.

a. Understanding of danger
   Does S have any understanding of danger?

            0  No understanding of danger
            1  Avoids hot stoves, sharp things
2y         2  Understands danger of falling from heights, ledges, etc.
5y         3  Understands danger from traffic
10y–11y   4  Full understanding of danger

b. Need for supervision
   How far can you let S go by himself?

           00  Needs constant supervision
1y         01  Can move around room unattended
1y 8mo    02  Can walk about house unattended
           03  Can walk around garden unattended (depending on size of garden)
4y 8mo    04  Can walk around local street or estate unattended
5y 1mo    05  Can go around local street, estate or park on a tricycle, bicycle, scooter or skates (if streets are traffic-free)
5y 10mo   06  Can go to school or workshop or other centre alone
           ( Items 4, 5 and 6 above—ages vary depending upon safety of streets)
9y 5mo    07  Can go around home town or local area alone, beyond own street or estate
15y 10mo  08  Can go to nearby towns or areas alone, makes own arrangements
18y 1mo   09  Can go alone to distant places that are relatively remote and strange

c. Staying at home alone
   Could you ever leave S alone at home, while you cross the road to post a letter, or go to a nearby shop?

           0  Could never be left at home alone
           1  Could be left alone for a minute or two
10y        2  Could be left alone for an hour or so
11y–12y   3  Could be left alone for half a day
14y–15y   4  Could be left alone all day

d. Shopping
   Does S go shopping with you? Does he show you things he wants?

           0  Does not do shopping, or is taken to shops but does not ask for things by speech or gesture
1y 6mo–2y  1  Goes to shops with mother or other supervisor and asks him for things he wants
3y 6mo–4y  2  Goes to shops with mother or other supervisor and makes small purchases with her supervision
5y 10mo   3  Goes to local shops alone with written list and exact money
7y         4  Has pocket money which he spends for himself
9y 5mo    5  Buys one or two things for himself with money given for this purpose. Makes his own decisions. Is responsible for the change

e. Telephone calls
   Could S answer the telephone? Could he make a telephone call?

           0  No ability to use telephone
3y–4y     1  Can answer telephone and fetch another person if required
7y–8y     2  Can make local telephone calls, look up a number, and hold a conversation

# INDEX